INTERPERSONAL PSYCHOTHERAPY FOR DEPRESSED ADOLESCENTS

Interpersonal Psychotherapy for Depressed Adolescents

Second Edition

LAURA MUFSON
KRISTEN POLLACK DORTA
DONNA MOREAU
MYRNA M. WEISSMAN

THE GUILFORD PRESS
New York   London

© 2004 The Guilford Press
A Division of Guilford Publications, Inc.
72 Spring Street, New York, NY 10012
www.guilford.com

Paperback edition 2011

Printed in the United States of America

This book is printed on acid-free paper.

Last digit is print number: 9 8 7 6

Library of Congress Cataloging-in-Publication Data

Interpersonal psychotherapy for depressed adolescents / Laura Mufson.— 2nd ed.
    p. cm.
  Includes bibliographical references and index.
  ISBN 978-1-60918-226-7 (paperback : alk. paper)
  ISBN 978-1-59385-042-5 (hardcover : alk. paper)
  1. Depression in adolescence—Treatment. 2. Interpersonal psychotherapy. 3.
Adolescent psychotherapy. I. Mufson, Laura.
  RJ506.D4I58 2004
  616.85′27′00835—dc22

                                                          2004002941

About the Authors

Laura Mufson, PhD, is Director of the Department of Clinical Psychology at the New York State Psychiatric Institute and Associate Professor of Clinical Psychology in Psychiatry at Columbia University College of Physicians and Surgeons. Dr. Mufson was the first to adapt interpersonal psychotherapy (IPT) for adolescents and has been conducting research on interpersonal psychotherapy for depressed adolescents for over a decade. She travels extensively, training clinicians in treatment techniques for IPT.

Kristen Pollack Dorta, PhD, is a clinical psychologist currently in private practice. Dr. Dorta has been instrumental in the implementation of interpersonal psychotherapy for depressed adolescents in school-based mental health clinics and the training of school-based clinicians.

Donna Moreau, MD, is Clinical Associate Professor of Psychiatry at Columbia University College of Physicians and Surgeons and Director of the Children's Anxiety and Depression Clinic at Children's Hospital of New York–Presbyterian Hospital.

Myrna M. Weissman, PhD, one of the originators of interpersonal psychotherapy, is Professor of Psychiatry and Epidemiology at Columbia University College of Physicians and Surgeons and the Joseph L. Mailman School of Public Health. She is also Director of the Division of Clinical and Genetic Epidemiology at the New York State Psychiatric Institute and has published extensively on interpersonal psychotherapy, including coauthoring (with John C. Markowitz and Gerald L. Klerman) *A Comprehensive Guide to Interpersonal Psychotherapy.*

Preface

This book has three aims: (1) to provide a general overview of the nature and current treatment practices of adolescent depression; (2) to introduce the experienced adolescent therapist to the theoretical formulation and practical application of interpersonal psychotherapy for depressed adolescents (IPT-A); and (3) to update our original IPT-A treatment manual published in 1993 to include over a decade of experience using the manual to treat myriad adolescents suffering from depression. IPT-A is a 12-week-long psychotherapy with weekly face-to-face sessions interspersed with telephone contacts. Treatment focuses primarily on the depressed adolescent but frequently also involves the parents. The four problem areas originally developed in IPT for adults are applied to adolescents and include grief, interpersonal role disputes, role transitions, and interpersonal deficits.

Part I of this volume provides a brief overview of adolescent depression, including diagnosis, assessment, clinical course, and other treatments for adolescent depression. The rationale for the adaptation of IPT to treat adolescent depression is presented in this section. Part II of the book is the actual treatment manual written for the clinician who is trained to conduct psychotherapy for adolescent disorders. It is organized as a step-by-step description of the therapeutic tasks for the three phases of the psychotherapy. Part III addresses the special issues that arise when working with adolescents and how they can be addressed while staying within the IPT-A treatment framework. Part III also includes a discussion of the current and future research in IPT-A that is currently under way.

The results of our efficacy study of IPT-A, as well as the study conducted by the IPT research group in Puerto Rico, demonstrated that IPT-A is an efficacious treatment for depression in adolescents. The recently completed effectiveness study of IPT-A in comparison to treatment as usual for depressed adolescents in school-based health clinics also demonstrates the effectiveness of IPT-A in a community setting and in treating adolescents with a spectrum of depression disorders. As a result of this most recent study, we have gained experience and insight into training therapists from diverse backgrounds to work in a range of settings with varied constraints on training and supervision. This book includes many of the insights we gained from training these clinicians to conduct IPT-A. More studies on the effectiveness of IPT-A that include larger, more heterogeneous samples conducted in a variety of community settings are needed.

Currently there are few formal training programs in IPT-A independent of the research setting. We hope to develop more training sites to offer a variety of levels of training in IPT-A. We believe that, even without attending one of these formal training programs or conference-sponsored workshops, clinicians with experience in the treatment of adolescents will be able to adopt elements of the IPT-A approach by reviewing the manual presented here. Similarly, for those less experienced practitioners, we hope that exposure to IPT-A through this book will encourage them to seek further training in IPT-A and its use in clinical practice. Our ultimate goal is for more clinicians to have exposure to IPT-A and to utilize the elements of IPT-A both in research and in clinical practice because we believe it to be an effective treatment model that is acceptable to adolescents.

This second edition provides new and more extensive scripts and clinical vignettes to help guide the reader in the implementation of IPT-A and updates the efficacy data from clinical trials conducted using IPT-A. The most significant modification of the manual in this edition is the elimination of the single-parent-families problem area and inclusion of these issues in a subgroup category under role transitions. This modification is an outgrowth of our continued experience using the manual, which suggested that the majority of the adolescents who experienced the problem area of single-parent families did so largely in the context of a role transition. While we were aware of this from the inception of IPT-A, at that time we felt that the special issues for adolescents dealing with family structural change needed to be separated into a distinct problem area. Continued experience has changed our perception and has led us to conclude that the issues once addressed under single-parent families are best understood as a special circumstance in the context of role transition.

Nonetheless, we still believe that the circumstances are often unique and require some separation from the larger transitional issues. The transitions associated with changes in family structure are typically outside of the control of the adolescent and are generally not normative or expected. The problems that arise from the structural change are often a result of the parents' difficulty in negotiating the change or transition, and their difficulties lead to stress and depression in their adolescent. In addition, the adolescent, in trying to deal with these stresses, often finds himself in the middle of many disputes with both the custodial and noncustodial parents in addition to having difficulties in making the transition to the new family structure. By incorporating these problems into the role transitions problem area, we also are able to acknowledge that these family structural changes not only occur in single-parent families but also can characterize the challenges adolescents face in adapting to stepfamilies and foster families. We therefore are returning to the four-problem-area model for IPT-A, with a special subproblem area of family structural change under the problem area of role transitions.

Our continued clinical work with depressed adolescents and the challenges we faced when disseminating the treatment in the community provided the impetus for revising the book at this time. We have gained significant experience over the past decade treating depressed adolescents and training a multitude of clinicians, so that we strongly felt we could enhance the original manual and make the treatment more accessible to clinicians and researchers alike. We are acutely aware of the potentially crippling effects of depression on adolescents, and we have been motivated to improve the dissemination of effective treatments to more clinicians. Many depressed adolescents will improve within the first few weeks of nonspecific psychotherapeutic interventions and will leave treatment despite concerted efforts on the therapist's part to maintain the therapy. Many of these adolescents will return with future depressive episodes, but many others will not return to receive necessary treatment. Instead, the latter group will suffer the impairing social and interpersonal consequences of their depressive episode until many years later when they may again seek treatment as adults. We hope that IPT-A, specifically tailored to the adolescent's developmental tasks, will address the need for effective treatments for adolescent depression. We also hope that the enhanced explication of techniques, strategies, and guidelines for the structuring of the therapy sessions will facilitate clinicians' use of the principles and techniques of IPT-A in new research endeavors as well as in general clinical practice.

UPDATE 2011

Since the initial publication of this edition in 2004, we have undertaken new projects to adapt IPT-A for prepubertal depression, as a prevention program for adolescents at risk for depression, for adolescents suffering from bipolar disorder, and as a prevention program for adolescent girls at risk for weight gain. We also are exploring an adaptation of IPT-A with increased parental involvement for adolescents with significant parent–child conflict. Many of these adaptations are still in the preliminary stages of evaluation, but we are hopeful that they too will prove to be beneficial for these other populations. We have ongoing projects training community-based clinicians to conduct IPT-A in community mental health centers and school-based mental health programs utilizing the revised manual. Since publication in 2004, IPT as a treatment model for adolescents has been deemed to have "well-established efficacy" by the APA Task Force on the Promotion and Dissemination of Psychological Procedures guidelines (David-Ferdon & Kaslow, 2008). We are confident that the empirical support for the treatment model and the availability of the manual will promote clinicians' use of IPT-A both in general clinical practice as well as in new research endeavors.

REFERENCE

David-Ferdon, C., & Kaslow, N. J. (2008). Evidence-based psychosocial treatments for child and adolescent depression. *Journal of Clinical Child and Adolescent Psychology, 37*, 62–104.

Acknowledgments

We would like to thank the many foundations and government agencies that have helped to support the work in interpersonal psychotherapy for depressed adolescents (IPT-A) over the past decade. Specifically, we would like to thank the NARSAD Foundation for providing funds to new investigators, the National Institute of Mental Health (NIMH) in awarding Laura Mufson an NIMH First Award that enabled her to conduct the first controlled clinical trial of IPT-A, and the Substance Abuse and Mental Health Services Administration for funding Laura Mufson to conduct the first effectiveness study of IPT-A in school-based health clinics. In addition, we are very grateful to the NIMH Research Intervention Center in Child Psychiatry under the leadership of Dr. David Shaffer for providing invaluable help in carrying out the IPT-A research program over the past decade.

Developing a strong research program is not a solo endeavor. Many people have contributed their support of IPT-A research—most particularly, the Outpatient Pediatric Psychiatry Department at Children's Hospital, New York Presbyterian Medical Center, the New York City Board of Education, and the New York school-based health clinics that allowed us to enter their world and who shared with us their challenges in treating depressed adolescents. We are excited that the work in IPT-A is continuing to grow and expand to areas of group treatment, prevention, and treating the medically ill. Many individuals have provided their support and insight to the production of this book, including Jami F. Young, PhD, Helena Verdeli, PhD, Kathleen Clougherty, MSW, Trish Gallagher, PhD, Agnés Tabah, and Tanya Stockhammer, PhD. We would like to thank Marilyn Camacho, BA, and Rina Kawano for their help in the researching, editing, and production of the manuscript. We would also like to thank Linda Pilgrim for her tireless and generous work in putting the manuscript into its final form.

Laura Mufson would like to thank her husband, Bennett Leifer, for his constant support and encouragement of her work, his sharing of ideas, and his partnership in raising their children that enabled her to write this book. She also wants to thank her children, Josh and Nina, for understanding the importance of this work, for their sacrifice of some "Mommy time" to allow this book to be completed, and for their boundless love and constant reminder of the true joys of life.

Kristen Pollack Dorta would like to thank Dr. Mufson for her mentorship and guidance. She also would like to thank her family and her husband's family for their support and endless "babysitting time" that made her contributions to this book possible. Finally, she would like to thank her husband, Nelson Dorta, and her children, Ana and Lukas, for their love and constant reminder of all that really matters.

This interpersonal psychotherapy (IPT) adaptation for adolescents is based on the work of the late Gerald L. Klerman, MD, husband of Myrna M. Weissman. Dr. Klerman was the originator of IPT, enthusiastically trained Dr. Mufson, and encouraged the adaptation of IPT for depressed adolescents. His early papers on the Youthful Age of Melancholia in the 1970s foresaw the epidemic of depression in young people documented in the epidemiological studies of the 1980s. This book derives directly from the first manual for IPT, titled *Interpersonal Psychotherapy for Depression* (Klerman, Weissman, Rounsaville, & Chevron, 1984), and its revision, *A Comprehensive Guide to Interpersonal Psychotherapy* (Weissman, Markowitz, & Klerman, 2000). The initial phase of treatment, including the diagnostic procedures and medical model as well as the problem areas, all derive from IPT as it was originally conceived and tested by Dr. Klerman and described in these books. This adaptation takes into account the developmental adaptations of the treatment for adolescents. Dr. Klerman's interest in and energy dedicated to developing effective treatments and his high standards for clinical and research practice continue to serve as the foundation upon which we build an ever growing IPT-A program. Most important, we would like to thank the many adolescents who have agreed to participate in the development and study of IPT-A. Without them, this work would not have been possible. We hope that IPT-A will provide relief from the symptoms and relationship difficulties that accompany adolescent depression and that dissemination of IPT-A and other efficacious therapies will enable more adolescents to receive effective treatment.

LAURA MUFSON
KRISTEN POLLACK DORTA
DONNA MOREAU
MYRNA M. WEISSMAN

Contents

PART I

Overview

CHAPTER 1

The Nature of Depression in Adolescents

This chapter provides an overview of the epidemiology, nature, and course of child and adolescent depression, as well as associated outcomes of the disorder. While the book's main topic is adolescents, it is important to review data on both children and adolescents to gain a developmental perspective on adolescent depression. The influence of comorbidity also is discussed in regard to the diagnostic complexities and treatment of adolescent depression.

NOT ALL ADOLESCENTS ARE DEPRESSED

Traditional psychoanalytic and psychological theory proposed that all adolescents have periods of depression because they experience conflicts within themselves commonly referred to as "adolescent turmoil." This was thought to be a normal stage of development. G. Stanley Hall (1904) was the first to give this concept the name "Sturm und Drang," or "storm and stress." He believed that normal adolescents experience wide mood swings and variable functioning, but that this did not signify psychopathology. Eissler (1958) described the adolescent as a slave to his impulses and prone to antisocial behavior, anxiety, and depression. The notion of adolescent turmoil as a normal state received wide clinical support (Blos, 1961; Freud, 1958).

More recently, however, longitudinal and epidemiological studies have refuted the view that adolescent turmoil is normative (Offer, 1969; Offer, Ostrov, & Howard, 1982; Rutter, Graham, Chadwick, & Yule, 1976). Adolescents have periods of feeling lonely and isolated from peers and experience conflicts with family and teachers, but for most adolescents these periods do not persist for any significant length of time or severely impair functioning. Studies of community-based samples of adolescents find significantly less adolescent turmoil present (Offer, 1969). Rutter et al. (1976) in the Isle of Wight study found that although some turmoil is a fact of adolescence, parent–child alienation and evidence of an impaired significant interpersonal relationship are more common features of adolescents showing psychiatric problems.

An important research and clinical task is to differentiate between "normal" adolescents and those with psychiatric disturbances in need of attention. Studies by Offer (1969) and Rutter et al. (1976) suggest that socially withdrawn adolescents with dramatic mood swings, cognitive distortions, and increasing conflicts with parents and peers are those adolescents more likely to be psychiatrically ill. Initially, there was disbelief that these disorders could occur prior to late adolescence. This view was replaced by the belief that these symptoms did exist but appeared in children and adolescents as a behavioral disturbance. The disorder known as "masked depressive reaction" was coined to refer to the presentation of these emotional and behavioral disturbances (Cytryn & McKnew, 1972). DSM-III unmasked the illness and formalized the existence of depression in children and adolescents, paving the way for research on the etiology and treatment of youth depression (Waslick, Kandel, & Kakouros, 2002).

DEFINING ADOLESCENT DEPRESSION

Clinical Presentation

Children and adolescents are referred for an evaluation for depression based on a number of behavioral and mood symptoms that may be manifest to peers, family members, or school personnel. Sometimes, adolescents report feeling intolerable sadness and hopelessness and take it upon themselves to alert an adult to their need for help. The illness of depression has varying components, as described in DSM-IV. Children and adolescents may present as feeling sad a significant portion of the day and for the majority of the week. The sadness may appear as extreme moodiness, irritability, and even a pervasive feeling of boredom or lack of interest in most facets of life. Sometimes these feelings are overtly obvious to those people surrounding the adolescent, but at other times they may only become apparent upon direct questioning of the child or adolescent.

These feelings of sadness may be accompanied by disturbances in sleep, such as difficulty in falling asleep, in staying asleep during the night, or waking up too early in the morning and not being able to fall back to sleep. Similarly, there may be disturbances of appetite, either loss of appetite or overeating. Other symptoms of depression experienced by children and adolescents include the following: feelings of hopelessness about the future; difficulty concentrating on school work and a frequent drop in grades; frequent tearfulness or crying; feelings of low self-esteem; lack of energy and/or motivation; feelings of guilt about having done something wrong in the past or currently that might be the cause of the depression illness; and for some adolescents, thoughts about wanting to be dead or actually about how to hurt oneself. Not all adolescents experience all symptoms, and they experience their own symptoms to varying degrees of severity and impairment.

A common consequence or precursor to depression is school difficulties, which can take the form of academic underachievement, poor school attendance, or actual school failure (Hammen, Rudolph, Weisz, Rao, & Burge, 1999). Depression can cause problems in concentration and motivation that make it difficult for the youth to keep up with his schoolwork, both at home and in class, and to perform consistent with his premorbid level of functioning. In extreme cases, it may result in significant school refusal (King & Bernstein, 2001) or school dropout. In turn, undiagnosed learning problems can engender low self-esteem and feelings of frustration, hopelessness, and helplessness that can presage the development of depressed mood.

Diagnostic Criteria

There is more than one type of mood disorder that may be experienced by adolescents. Adolescents also may experience a subsyndromal depression in which they experience dysphoric mood and several other symptoms, but not to the level of severity that leads to significant impairment, or prolonged duration of symptoms, or to meeting criteria for a specific depression disorder. The various disorders are elaborated on in DSM-IV and include the following: major depressive disorder, dysthymic disorder, depressive disorder not otherwise specified, as well as adjustment disorder with depressed mood. The disorders are distinguished from one another other by level of symptom severity, acute or chronic course, and whether or not the symptoms are a response to a specific stressor.

An ongoing discussion in the field focuses on whether or not the use of adult diagnostic criteria is appropriate for children and adolescents.

DSM-IV does not have a separate diagnostic category for depression in children and adolescents. To be diagnosed with major depressive disorder, an adolescent must report sad mood, anhedonia, or irritability in addition to four other co-occurring symptoms such as sleep disturbance, appetite disturbance, low self-esteem, psychomotor retardation, or suicidal ideation every day for most of the day for at least 2 weeks (American Psychiatric Association, 2000a). For diagnosing children and adolescents with major depressive disorder, the only modification is a substitution of irritability for depressed mood as the primary mood state and the reconceptualization of the weight loss criteria to include failure to maintain a normal expected growth and weight gain, accounting for normal expectations of growth and weight gain for children and adolescents. To be diagnosed with dysthymic disorder, the adolescent may report depressed mood and two or more symptoms of depression; however, the presence of the symptoms is for a longer duration. The criteria for dysthymic disorder have been adapted for children and adolescents in regard to the duration of symptoms, being adjusted from a 2-year to 1-year duration. Otherwise, all other criteria for major depressive disorder and dysthymia are identical for children, adolescents, and adults.

There are questions as to whether some child and adolescent depressions are missed by not using developmentally adjusted criteria. The effects of developmental changes in cognition and emotional expression on the presentation of depression over time have yet to be fully delineated. From childhood to adolescence, there appears to be a transition from predominantly vegetative symptoms to more inner psychological or cognitive ones. The ability to assess guilt and inner emotional experiences is often complicated by children's more limited cognitive and verbal skills. Adolescents, in comparison to children, are thought to begin to resemble adults in their depth of despair, negative self-cognitions, sense of hopelessness, sleep and appetite disturbance, propensity for suicide, and accompanying anxiety and agitation (Bemporad & Lee, 1988; Birmaher, Ryan, Williamson, Brent, & Kaufman, 1996b; Kashani, Rosenberg, & Reigh, 1989; Ryan et al., 1987). Differences include lack of pervasive anhedonia in the adolescents; more reactivity to external situations or stressors; irritability at times, rather than depressed mood; and lack of similar drug response to tricyclic antidepressants (Carlson & Strober, 1979; Mitchell, McCauley, Burke, & Moss, 1988). Researchers (Birmaher et al., 1996b; Kovacs, 1996; Ryan et al., 1987) conclude that developmental changes across childhood and adolescence have only mild to moderate effects on the expression of a limited number of affective symptoms in children with major depression, and that, for the most part, depression presentation is not significantly different between youths and adults to require different diagnostic criteria.

THE COURSE OF ADOLESCENT DEPRESSION

Longitudinal studies of clinical samples find that episodes of major depression in children and adolescents have a median duration of 7–9 months from onset to recovery (Kovacs, Feinberg, Crouse-Novak, Paulauskas, & Finkelstein, 1984; Kovacs, Devlin, Pollack, Richards, & Mukerji, 1997a; McCauley et al., 1993). Another 20% of these adolescents have episodes lasting 15 months or longer. The course of the episode varies based on whether it is an acute or chronic illness and the severity of the symptomatology. Clinically it often appears that adolescents have episodically intense periods of depression interspersed with periods of improved functioning in comparison to the adult model of a more pervasive and long-lasting period of depression (Angst, Merikangas, Scheidegger, & Wicki, 1990). Adolescents with dysthymic disorder have a median episode length of approximately 4 years (Kovacs, Akiskal, Gatsonis, & Parrone, 1994). Keller, Beardslee, Lavori, and Wunder (1988) reported that the probability of persistent depression after 1 year was 21% and after 2 years it was 10%. Approximately 70–80% of adolescents recover from major depression after 1 year, increasing to 86–98% after 2 years (Kovacs, 1996; Kovacs et al., 1997a; Kovaks, Obrosky, Gatsonis, & Richard, 1997b; McCauley et al., 1993). These rates parallel rates of chronicity and recovery that occur in adult depression (Keller et al., 1988).

Childhood depression places one at significant risk for recurrence in adolescence (Garber, Kriss, Koch, & Windholm, 1988; Kovacs et al., 1984; Pine, Cohen, Gurley, Brook, & Ma, 1998). Impairment in psychosocial functioning at school, with friends, and with family is associated with having major depression and can persist after the depression episode resolves, placing the adolescent at risk for future adverse events and recurrent episodes (Puig-Antich et al., 1985a, 1985b; Rao et al., 1995; Williamson et al., 1998). Few studies have thoroughly examined the course of adolescent depression, but early onset of mood disorder has been shown to predict recurrent mood episodes, with 70% of youth experiencing a recurrence within 5 years of the initial onset of the major depressive disorder (Kovacs et al., 1994; Rao et al., 1995). In addition, depressed adolescents appear to be at high risk for developing mania or hypomania in the ensuing years (Geller, Zimmerman, Williams, Bolhofner, & Craney, 2001; Kovacs et al., 1994). Similarly, studies following adolescents into adulthood (Angst et al., 1990; Lewinsohn, Rohde, Klein, & Seeley, 1999; Rao, Hammen, & Daley, 1999; Warner, Weissman, Fendrich, Wickramaratne, & Moreau, 1992), as well as studies following children into adulthood (Harrington, Fudge, Rutter, Pickles, & Hill, 1990; Weissman et al., 1999b), find 30–50% rates of recurrence into adulthood as well as chronic psychosocial problems (Garber et al., 1988; Kandel & Davies, 1986; Keller et al., 1988; Kovacs et al., 1984; Puig-Antich et al., 1993).

RISK FACTORS

Risk factors are conditions or characteristics that increase the onset or recurrence of the disorder rather than specifically cause depression (Costello et al., 2002). Risk factors associated with depression include age of onset, female gender, low socioeconomic status, family history, and family relationships. The importance of age and gender in the changing prevalence rates of depression has already been discussed. Low socioeconomic status has been associated with adult depressive symptoms (Cytryn, McKnew, Zahn-Waxler, & Gershon, 1986) and more recently with psychiatric disorders in children and adolescents, including depression (Costello et al., 1996). In general, poverty and low socioeconomic status are seen as risk factors for a variety of mental health problems, with little evidence of a specific and unique association with depression disorder in children and adolescents. Studies consistently find that those children and adolescents with major depression have mother–child relationships that are marked by low warmth and low family cohesion as well as parents characterized by high irritability, anger, and punitiveness (Fendrich, Warner, & Weissman, 1990; Kashani, Burbach, & Rosenberg, 1988; Puig-Antich et al., 1985a; Reinherz et al., 1989, 1993). There is increasingly strong evidence from high-risk family studies that major depression runs in families and that being the child of a depressed parent places one at increased risk for the development of major depression (Angold et al., 1987; Beardslee et al., 1983; Hammen, Burge, Burney, & Adrian, 1990; Klein, Lewinsohn, Seeley, & Rohde, 2001; Kovacs et al., 1997a; Orvaschel, 1990; Puig-Antich et al., 1989; Weissman, Leckman, Merikangas, Gammon, & Prusoff, 1984a; Weissman et al., 1987a). Comorbidity associated with adolescent depression is important to consider in the development of psychotherapeutic and psychopharmacological interventions. For a complete review of risk factors, see Costello et al. (2002).

Comorbidity

Comorbidity is the occurrence of more than one psychiatric disorder at the same time. It commonly occurs in children and adolescents who are depressed. Depression in children and adolescents is likely to be preceded, accompanied, or followed by other disorders (Pine et al., 1998).

Disorders that have been found to be associated with major depression in adolescence include attention-deficit/hyperactivity disorder (ADHD) (Biederman et al., 1987), anxiety disorders (Alessi, Robbins, & Dilsaver, 1987; Bernstein & Garfinkel, 1986; Kovacs, Gatsonis, Paulauskas, & Richards, 1989), behavior and conduct disorders (Alessi & Robbins, 1984; Marriage, Fine, Moretti, & Haley, 1986), and eating disorders (Swift, Andrews, & Barklage, 1986). A number of studies examined the order of onset of disorders and concluded that unipolar depression follows the onset of other disorders except for substance abuse and panic disorder, which usually co-occur in mid- to late adolescence (Costello, Erkanli, Federman, & Angold, 1999; Kessler & Walters, 1998; Rohde, Lewinsohn, & Seeley, 1991). Among children and adolescents with a major affective disorder, about one-third also have a comorbid diagnosis of conduct disorder or a similar behavior problem (Carlson & Cantwell, 1980; Kashani et al., 1987; Kovacs et al., 1989; Puig-Antich, 1982). Ryan et al. (1987) found that mild conduct problems were present in 25% of adolescents but were disruptive in only 11% of the adolescents. Depression comorbid with conduct disorder is associated with greater impairment in functioning (Kovacs et al., 1989). Angold, Costello, and Erkanli (1999) conducted a meta-analysis of studies on prevalence rates and found that anxiety disorders were 8.3 times as common in depressed versus nondepressed children and adolescents. They also reported oppositional defiant disorder and conduct disorder as, respectively, 6.6 times as common and 5.5 times as common in depressed versus nondepressed children and adolescents.

The interactive effects of comorbid disorders on impairment in functioning and the long-term course of the disorders are still not clear; however, comorbidity does complicate treatment outcome perhaps by making it more difficult to achieve recovery in the shorter treatment durations. More clinical trials involving depressed youth with comorbidities are needed and are currently under way to begin to answer the question of which interventions best address the complexity of problems presented by the comorbidities.

ASSOCIATED OUTCOME OF DEPRESSION

It may often be a suicide attempt or expression of suicidal ideation that engenders an adolescent's first foray into the mental health system. It is not uncommon for depressed adolescents either to have attempted suicide or more frequently to have expressed to someone the desire to kill oneself or the thought that life isn't worth living and that they would be better off dead. Depression has been identified as a leading risk factor for suicide ideation, attempts (Gould et al., 1998), and completed suicides (Shaffer et al., 1996b), but not all suicidal behavior is associated with a mood disorder. Still, among adolescents, 5–10% will commit suicide within 15 years of the initial episode of major depression (Rao, Weissman, Martin, & Hammond, 1993; Weissman et al., 1999a). Levy & Deykin (1989) found that when major depression was present in adolescents, the rate of suicidal ideation or behavior was markedly higher for both males and females, even in an untreated sample. Half the students who admitted to having made a suicide attempt did not meet diagnostic criteria for major depression at any time. Weissman et al. (1999a), in a longitudinal follow-up study of depressed children and adolescents, found an almost 8% completed suicide rate, significantly higher than the rate for the general population as well as for the nondepressed comparison group. Evaluation for suicidality is an absolutely necessary component of an evaluation for a mood disorder, just as it is imperative to assess for a mood disorder in youth presenting with a suicidal crisis.

CONCLUSION

Major depression, as well as other depressive disorders, occurs in children and adolescents. Depression is associated with significant impairment and morbidity. Most importantly, it is demonstrated to be a recurrent disorder reemerging in adulthood for many children and adolescents. There are significant psychosocial impairments that occur in the acute stages, continue after recovery, and persist into adulthood. These psychosocial impairments are either of an interpersonal type or lead to interpersonal difficulties. Adolescents who are members of families with a history of affective disorders and whose families experience interpersonal problems are at significant risk for depression themselves.

There is a significant pattern of underrecognition and undertreatment of adolescent depression both in clinically referred and nonreferred populations (Keller, Lavori, Beardslee, Wunder, & Ryan, 1991). The impairment and recurrence rates highlight the importance of having in one's armamentarium a psychosocial intervention to treat adolescent depression and its interpersonal impairments, no matter what the biological substrate and genetics of depression may be. Adolescents with more acute onset of depression have an illness that tends to resolve more rapidly and may lend itself better to a treatment that is brief and deals with the current problem. These adolescents may prefer to return for treatment when needed rather than being in treatment and in the patient role for a prolonged period of time. IPT-A is a brief, focused treatment that seems to appeal to many adolescents for these reasons. More chronic forms of the disorder may require a longer duration of treatment (Goodman, Schwab-Stone, Lahey, Shaffer, & Jensen, 2000; Kovacs et al., 1994); however, this still bears investigation. The next chapter provides an overview of types of treatment for depressed children that may target these different forms of the disorder.

CHAPTER 2

Current Psychosocial Treatments for Adolescent Depression

In clinical practice, depressed adolescents frequently receive psychotherapies that have been shown to be efficacious in the treatment of adults (Hersen & Van Hasselt, 1987). In contrast to the small number of treatments that have been tested empirically in depressed adolescents, numerous ones are used clinically. The literature describing psychosocial interventions for depressed youth has included many case studies and small single-subject designs. Until recently, scientifically rigorous randomized, controlled clinical outcome studies were lacking. The majority of the recent clinical trials investigated the efficacy of cognitive-behavioral treatments, with a smaller number examining interpersonal psychotherapy. Clinical trials generally include children with depression symptoms and adolescents with major depression and/or dysthymia. Many of these studies need replication due to a number of methodological limitations that include (1) small sample sizes, (2) inclusion of nonreferred versus referred children, (3) treatment of mild to moderate versus severe symptoms, (4) treatment of depressive symptomatology versus criterion-based diagnosis, and (5) lack of comparison with another already established treatment (Kovacs, 1997).

WHAT IS AN EMPIRICALLY BASED TREATMENT?

Guidelines set forth by the Task Force on Promotion and Dissemination of Psychological Procedures (1996) specify several conditions that must be met for a treatment to be considered efficacious: (1) The treatment must be manual-based; (2) sample characteristics must be detailed; (3) treatment must be tested in a randomized clinical trial; and (4) at least two different investigatory teams must demonstrate intervention effects (Kaslow & Thompson, 1998). Only one treatment, The Coping with Depression Course for Adolescents (Lewinsohn, Antonuccio, Steinmetz, & Teri, 1984), is close to meeting well-established criteria (Lewinsohn, Clarke, Rohde, Hops, & Seeley, 1996). These intervention studies are limited in another way by the fact that the majority of treatment approaches in use are downward extensions of adult treatment modalities (Mueller & Orvaschel, 1997) and may lack appropriate developmental adaptations for this age group.

There is evidence suggesting that depressed adolescents are a largely underserved population (Burns, 1991; Hoberman, 1992; Keller et al., 1991; Wu et al., 1999), in part because they often are not identified and partially due to economic, social, personal, familial, and cultural obstacles to their access to treatment. Myriad psychotherapies are used to treat adolescent depression; however, only a handful of them have been demonstrated to be efficacious in clinical trials (Mufson & Velting, 2002). With the advance of managed care and the establishment of standards of care for treatment, increased emphasis has been placed on the use of "evidence-based" therapies for both research purposes as well as general clinical practice. Given the substantial rates of depressive disorders in adolescents and the concomitant negative developmental trajectory, it is critical to develop new treatments and further establish the efficacy of these and other treatments for adolescent depression.

There are treatments for which there is evidence, although they do not always meet full criteria as well-established treatments using the task force guidelines. These treatments include specific adaptations of cognitive-behavioral therapy (CBT) and interpersonal psychotherapy (IPT). Various versions of CBT are the most widely studied of the psychotherapies. Other commonly used treatments include the following: psychodynamic psychotherapy, psychoanalysis, behavior therapy, family therapy, and group therapy. The goal of each of these treatments is to alleviate the psychological symptoms and improve functioning using various techniques to alter the behavior, thoughts, or attitudes of the patient that are felt to be contributing to the problems. Specifically, the more immediate goal is to relieve suffering from dysphoric symptoms. The longer-term goal of treatment is to limit the functional impairment from the symp-

toms (e.g., poor interpersonal relationships, family conflict, school refusal), and to prevent chronicity and recurrence of the depressive episodes. The specific causes of mood disorders are unknown; therefore, it
is very likely that there will be no single cause of depression and that no
one treatment will apply to all depressed persons. This chapter provides
a brief introduction to treatments other than IPT-A for adolescent depression.

COGNITIVE THERAPY

The defining characteristics of cognitive treatment are that it is directive,
structured, often time-limited, and emphasizes changing cognitions that
are associated with behavioral events and problem-solving skills (Kovacs,
1979; Matson, 1989). The underlying construct is that a person's
cognitions determine how a person feels (Emery, Bedrosian, & Garber,
1983). There are several modifications of the general cognitive tenets
originally developed by Aaron Beck (Beck, 1967).
    The goals of cognitive therapy are (1) to obtain symptom relief and
(2) to uncover beliefs that lead to depression and subject them to reality
testing (Emery et al., 1983). The techniques used to accomplish these
goals include monitoring the negative cognitions; helping the patient to
make the connections between cognition, affect, and behavior; and
learning to identify and alter dysfunctional beliefs (Beck, Rush, Shaw &
Emery, 1979). The goal has been to decrease the reinforcement of the adolescent's dysfunctional cognitions.
    Cognitive therapy differs from psychodynamic treatment in that the
therapist does not make interpretations of unconscious factors. It differs
from interpersonal psychotherapy for depressed adolescents (IPT-A) in
its focus on dysfunctional belief systems, whereas IPT-A would focus on
dysfunctional interpersonal communication processes. Several different
CBT manuals have been developed, but they all share the same basic theoretical foundation. There is reasonably good evidence for the efficacy
of CBT in the treatment of depression in adolescents (Harrington,
Whittaker, & Shoebridge, 1998; Lewinsohn & Clarke, 1999; Reinecke,
Ryan, & DuBois, 1998); however, some room for improvement remains.
For a review of the studies, see Mufson and Velting (2002).

BEHAVIORAL APPROACHES

The behavioral component of CBT has its roots in reinforcement theory.
One of the major behavioral models of depression focuses on the loss of

positive reinforcement. Lewinsohn, Weinstein, and Shaw (1969) found that depressed individuals appeared to lack access to sufficient schedules of positive reinforcement due to either the complete absence of reinforcement or the individual's inability to access them due to a lack of appropriate skills. The low rate of positive reinforcement for one's behavior can lead to depression. In turn, the depressive affect being displayed further decreases the individual's chances of receiving positive reinforcement for his behavior, thereby exacerbating or increasing the depression. The goal is to increase positive reinforcement from the pleasurable activities directly and from improved interpersonal relationships that may be a secondary outcome of the activities. Lewinsohn's treatment for depression has focused on teaching adolescents the skills necessary to obtain the needed positive reinforcement to break the depressive feedback cycle, such as increasing pleasurable activities, problem solving, social skills, assertiveness training, and emotion regulation (Lewinsohn, Clarke, Hops, & Andrews, 1990).

PSYCHODYNAMIC PSYCHOTHERAPY

Psychodynamic psychotherapy is commonly used to treat depressed adolescents. A number of thoughtful papers by leading clinicians have described their clinical experience and theoretical perspectives on psychotherapy for the depressed adolescent (Bemporad, 1988; Cytryn & McKnew, 1985; Kestenbaum & Kron, 1987; Liebowitz & Kernberg, 1988; Nissen, 1986). The principles derive from psychoanalytic theories. In the simplest terms, they are based on the premise that symptoms of distress are a result of unconscious conflicts. These symptoms can be addressed and decreased through such interventions as confrontation, clarification, and interpretation (Liebowitz & Kernberg, 1988). Within the psychodynamic psychotherapy framework, there are several types of psychodynamic psychotherapy: child psychoanalysis, expressive or exploratory child psychotherapy, supportive psychotherapy, and expressive supportive child psychotherapy. The specific application and goals of each of these therapies is described in Liebowitz and Kernberg's (1988) excellent review of psychodynamic psychotherapies for children.

IPT-A differs from psychodynamic psychotherapy with adolescents in its time-limited framework, its focus on current interpersonal issues rather than intrapsychic ones, and the more directive stance of the therapist in the actual therapy sessions. To date, there have been no controlled clinical trials of psychodynamic psychotherapy with depressed adolescents.

FAMILY THERAPY

Family therapists conceptualize depression as occurring within the family system. The family therapy model is based on the belief that people are a product of their social context or family system, and that the individual cannot be understood in isolation without some understanding of the larger context (Nichols, 1984). Disequilibrium among the family members, improper alliances, or communication difficulties can result in the creation of an identified patient who manifests the family's problems in his or her depression. Therefore, the therapist addresses the adolescent's depression by addressing the pathology in the family system. Within the family therapy modality, there are several different types of treatment, ranging from systems family therapy (Haley, 1976), structural family therapy (Minuchin, 1974), to contextual family therapy (Boszormenyi-Nagy & Krasner, 1986). There is no one specific model of a dysfunctional family that has been linked to depression in children and adolescents.

In reviewing the empirical studies, the term "family-based therapy," instead of "family therapy," has been applied to the body of work. This shift in terminology reflects the increasing integration of three family-oriented treatment orientations: behavioral, psychoeducational, and systems therapy (Diamond, Serrano, Dickey, & Sonis, 1996). Despite the empirical and theoretical support for the role of family factors in the development, maintenance, and relapse of child and adolescent depression, there are few studies of family-based treatments for depressed adolescents. Fristad, Gavazzi, and Soldano (1998) have developed a family-based psychoeducational program to be used in conjunction with other treatments. However, no efficacy data have yet been published on this approach. Diamond and Siqueland (1995) developed an attachment-based family therapy (ABFT) that is based on the assumption that attachment failures and concomitant negative family environments prevent children from developing the necessary coping skills to handle the familial and environmental stressors that can lead to or exacerbate depression. The treatment aims to find solutions to the attachment failures, to work with parents to become better caregivers, and to improve communication between adolescents and their parents, which will result in a reduction in depression (Diamond, Reis, Diamond, Siqueland, & Isaacs, 2002). These models are currently undergoing further investigation of their efficacy for adolescent depression.

GROUP PSYCHOTHERAPY

One of the main goals of group therapy for almost any psychiatric problem is to put the adolescent in contact with peers who have similar difficulties, who can provide support for one another, and provide one another with opportunities to practice new skills for interpersonal relationships. The specific goals of group therapy can include (1) enabling the individual to perceive the similarity of one's needs to others', (2) generating alternative solutions to particular conflicts, (3) learning more effective social skills, and (4) increasing awareness of others' needs and feelings (Corey, 1981). Many groups are time-limited with set goals and programs to accomplish within that time, such as social skills groups, while others are more open-ended. The social skills groups differ from IPT-A because the group format precludes more intensive focus on the individual adolescent's specific interpersonal problems and provides fewer opportunities to follow each adolescent's particular interpersonal issues to successful resolution. As discussed above, there have been clinical trials of a structured type of cognitive-behavioral group for depressed adolescents (Clarke, Hops, Lewinsohn, & Andrews, 1992; Clarke, Hawkins, Murphy, & Sheeber, 1995; Clarke, Rohde, Lewinsohn, Hops, & Seeley, 1999; Lewinsohn et al., 1990; Reynolds & Coats, 1986) in addition to social skills groups, which have demonstrated some efficacy (Fine et al., 1989; Fine, Forth, Gilbert, & Haley, 1991). The efficacy of a group adaptation of interpersonal psychotherapy for depressed adolescents (IPT-AG; Mufson, Gallagher, Dorta, & Young, 2004b) is currently under investigation.

PHARMACOTHERAPY

The effects of a depressive episode for an adolescent are so far-reaching that therapeutic intervention needs to include both pharmacological and psychosocial strategies as options. Clinicians should be able to generally address parents' and the adolescent's questions regarding the biochemical basis of depression and to emphasize the necessity of a treatment intervention that deals with the accompanying psychosocial and interpersonal impairment. Initial studies of pharmacotherapy for adolescent depression were conducted with tricyclic antidepressants, which were generally not found to be as effective with adolescents as they were with depressed adults (Birmaher & Brent, 2002). More recent research has focused on the selective serotonin reuptake inhibitors (SSRIs). Several clinical trials have demonstrated the efficacy of paroxetine (Keller et al., 2001), fluoxetine (Emslie et al., 1997, 2002) and sertraline (Wagner et al., 2003) for the treatment of adolescent depression. Nonetheless, response rates in these studies are typically between 60 and 70%, which still leaves room for improvement or the need to provide adjunctive treatment to improve the response rates. Recently, amid concerns of a relationship between paroxetine and an increase in suicidal events in depressed children and adolescents, paroxetine is no longer indicated as a first-line treatment for depression in this population. In clinical practice, medication use for depressed children and adolescents has increased dramatically in the past decade and is a common first-line treatment for adolescent depression. For a complete review of pharmacotherapy for adolescent depression, see Birmaher and Brent (2002). The use of medication in conjunction with IPT-A is discussed in Chapter 18.

CONCLUSION

Given the involvement of environmental influences in the course of adolescent depression, psychosocial treatments are likely to have a place as effective treatments either alone or in combination with pharmacological treatment. Despite the focus of controlled clinical trials on evidence-based manualized treatments for adolescent depression, numerous therapeutic orientations are widely used in clinical practice. These other treatments need to be carefully assessed regarding their efficacy with adolescents. Whether IPT-A will be effective in reducing the long-term psychosocial impairments associated with depression first presenting in adolescence remains to be seen. Further clarification of the course of illness, recurrence and recovery rates, and associated impairment and comorbidity are needed to implement treatment strategies that will be effective over the long term. IPT-A has been found to be effective in several clinical trials of acute treatment, and other trials are under way (Mufson et al., in press-a; Mufson, Weissman, Moreau, & Garfinkel, 1999; Rosselló & Bernal, 1999). Chapter 3 delineates the major principles and theoretical foundation for IPT-A, formulated to address those interpersonal issues believed to play a significant role in the maintenance of depression and identified as important targets for intervention. In addition, the chapter provides an overview of the initial studies using IPT as well as the IPT-A clinical trials. A full description of a treatment case and discussion about how a CBT therapist in comparison to an IPT-A therapist would approach the treatment of the depressed adolescent is included in Chapter 20.

CHAPTER 3

The Origins and Development of Interpersonal Psychotherapy for Depression

Interpersonal psychotherapy (IPT) is a brief, time-limited psychotherapy that was initially developed in the late 1960s for the treatment of nonbipolar, nonpsychotic, depressed adult outpatients. The treatment is based on the premise that, regardless of the underlying cause of depression, the depression is inextricably intertwined with the patient's interpersonal relationships. IPT's goals are (1) to decrease depressive symptomatology and (2) to improve interpersonal functioning by enhancing communication skills in significant relationships (Klerman, Weissman, Rounsaville, & Chevron, 1984). IPT is a unique departure from other types of psychotherapeutic interventions because its focus is on current interpersonal conflicts, and it is one of the first therapeutic modalities to be operationalized in a treatment manual. IPT can be administered after appropriate training by experienced psychiatrists, psychologists, and social workers. It can be used alone or with medication. IPT for depressed adolescents (IPT-A) is an innovative adaptation of a psychotherapeutic treatment that already has been shown to be effective in clinical trials. This chapter describes the development, concepts, and evidence for the efficacy of IPT as well as IPT-A. By reviewing IPT's history and development, the reader will gain a greater understanding of the conceptual framework that serves as the foundation for this adaptation.

BACKGROUND

Theoretical and Empirical Sources

IPT does not make any assumptions about the etiology of depression. However, IPT does assume that the development of clinical depression occurs in a social and interpersonal context and that the onset, response to treatment, and outcomes are influenced by the interpersonal relations between the depressed patient and significant others. This assumption is supported by the writings of Adolf Meyer and Harry Stack Sullivan as well as by more recent empirical investigation of the interpersonal model of depression.

The ideas of Adolf Meyer, whose psychobiological approach to understanding psychiatric disorders places great emphasis on the patient's relation to his or her environment (Meyer, 1957), form the theoretical foundation for IPT. Meyer views psychiatric disorders as an expression of the patient's attempt to adapt to his environment. An individual's response to environmental change is determined by prior experiences, particularly early experiences in the family and the individual's affiliation with various social groups. Harry Stack Sullivan, a colleague of Meyer, has written extensively about his own theories on interpersonal relationships (Sullivan, 1953).

According to Sullivan (1953), *psychiatry* is the study of interpersonal relationships under any and all circumstances in which these relationships exist. Sullivan states in his interpersonal theory of emotions that interpersonal behavior of other individuals forms the most significant class of events and objects that trigger emotions in people. He states that a large part of mental disorders results from and is perpetuated by inadequate communication. He emphasizes that a person's actions need to be understood and derive meaning from their historical or present interpersonal context. An appropriate treatment therefore would offer ways to identify interpersonal problems, clarify the conflict, and help the person to experiment with alternative behaviors (Horowitz, 1996).

Kiesler expands on the theory and develops an elaborate model of interpersonal communication and relationships focusing on issues of complementarity in communication and the patient's "evoking messages" (Kiesler, 1979). According to Kiesler, the therapist's job is to identify specific problematic interpersonal issues and how they manifest themselves in the patient's style of interpersonal communication. Then, through metacommunication about his interpersonal style, the therapist helps to correct his problematic communications both with the therapist and others in the patient's life (Kiesler, 1979). While Klerman and Weissman's original model of IPT does not use the same specific language as Kiesler and Leary, nor the specific techniques of the interpersonal circumplex and impact messages (Kiesler, 1983), the techniques are very consistent and target the same goals of (1) changing communication and (2) solving interpersonal problems in order to change the level of satisfaction to be achieved from interpersonal relationships and thereby improve one's emotional well-being. The interactional perspective of depression addresses the reciprocal influences of a depressed person's communications occurring between the person and his significant others. This is consistent with IPT's goals of helping the patient understand how changing certain communications will change the responses that he elicits in his relationship and thereby change the emotional valence of that relationship, which will, in turn, reduce his feelings of depression.

The interpersonal theory of emotions has roots in early attachment theory, as does interpersonal psychotherapy (Klerman et al., 1984). Bowlby states that people have a propensity and need to make strong affectional bonds to particular others and experiences (e.g., separation or loss of these relationships) and give rise to emotional distress, including depression (Bowlby, 1978). Adolescence is a time when early attachments may lessen and become supplemented by new ones. These attachment transitions can be difficult to traverse and can result in depression. Many conflicts between parents and adolescents may be due to the effects of the adolescent's exploration and extension of relationships with peers on perceived attachment to his parents. IPT recognizes the importance and role of attachment in depression. It focuses on conflicts or transitions as well as grief in relationships that may affect the adolescent's feelings and perceptions of attachment and contribute to depression. IPT is a natural outgrowth of the attachment theorists' emphasis on exploring patterns of interaction with significant others and how these patterns may be repeated in other relationships or be causing difficulties in these relationships, manifested in the patient's response to particular life events. This leads to the same treatment goals of teaching the patient different ways to communicate and interact, changing the affective experience of the relationship.

The Social Context of Depression

IPT is based not only on theory but also on empirical research, including studies associating stress, life events, and social impairment with the onset and clinical course of depression. Longitudinal studies demonstrating the social impairment of depressed women during the acute phase of their depressive episode, as well as during their recovery, highlight the need for a treatment intervention that would directly address the persistent social problems of depressed adults (Klerman et al., 1984). Brown,

Harris, and Copeland (1977) have demonstrated the role of intimacy and social supports as protection against depression in the face of adverse life stress and have supported the perceived importance of good social relations for emotional well-being.

Brown and Harris (1978), in *The Social Origins of Depression*, focus on the role of social factors in depression. They show that interpersonal factors are crucial in the creation of vulnerability to life stress. The most potent of these factors is the lack of an intimate and confiding relationship. The interactional theorists have sought to extend these findings by demonstrating that depressed persons engage the environment in ways that lose support from significant others and actually elicit depression-supporting feedback (Coyne, 1976), making the person vulnerable to increased depression. Studies demonstrate that experiences such as early parental loss (Brown & Harris, 1978), having a depressed parent (Weissman, Warner, Wickramaratne, Moreau, & Olfson, 1997), and poor parenting (Parker, 1979) contribute to the development of depression in adolescence and later in life, supporting the orientation of both the adult manual as well as the adolescent adaptation. Interestingly, another group of researchers has focused on the role of adaptive interpersonal functioning in protecting against depression. They have demonstrated that coping strategies, such as approach instead of avoidance, direct problem solving, and seeking out information from others rather than making assumptions, can buffer people against the depressogenic effects of negative life events (Holahan, Moos, & Bonin, 1999). These protective techniques are the very focus of the middle phase of IPT and are significant strategies used to facilitate recovery from depression as well as to prevent relapse or recurrence.

ORIGINS IN ADULT WORK

IPT itself has evolved over nearly 25 years of treatment and research experience with ambulatory depressed adult patients. The development began in 1968 as part of a clinical trial for depressed outpatients intended to test approaches to preventing relapse following reduction of acute symptoms of depression with pharmacotherapy (Klerman et al., 1984). By the mid-1960s it was clear that the new antidepressants were effective in reducing acute depressive symptoms. Sleep, appetite, and mood usually improved in 2–4 weeks. However, the relapse rate was high, and it was unclear how long medication should be continued and whether there was any advantage to adding psychotherapy. The intent of standardizing the psychotherapy in a manual for the first clinical trial was to ensure a consistent approach among therapists. The intent, however, was not to develop a new psychotherapy but to describe what we believed was a treatment that included the best and most important components of good clinical practice with depressed patients.

Clinical Depression as Conceptualized in IPT

Clinical depression, within the IPT framework, is conceptualized as having three component processes (Klerman et al., 1984; Weissman, Markowitz, & Klerman, 2000):

1. *Symptom formation,* involving the development of the depressive affect, signs, and symptoms that may derive from psychobiological or psychodynamic mechanisms, or both.
2. *Social functioning,* involving social interactions with other persons, which derives from learning based on childhood experiences, concurrent social reinforcement, and current personal efforts at mastery and competence as a result of the depression; and
3. *Personality,* involving more enduring traits and behaviors; the handling of anger and guilt and overall self-esteem that constitute the person's unique reactions and patterns of functioning and that may contribute to a predisposition to symptom development.

IPT, as it was originally developed, intervenes in the first two processes. Due to the brevity of the treatment, low level of psychotherapeutic intensity, and focus on the current depressive episode, IPT does not purport to have an impact on the enduring aspects of personality.

In fact, in IPT, there is the intentional avoidance, during the treatment of the acute symptomatic episode, of issues related to personality functioning and character pathology. The reluctance to focus on personality traits is most pronounced in work with adolescents. Our clinical experience has shown us that very often behaviors demonstrated by the adolescents during the acute illness that appear to be personality traits (e.g., dependency, splitting and viewing people as all bad or all good, instability of relationships) tend to resolve with the alleviation of symptoms. This suggests that these characteristics are more secondary as symptoms of the Axis I depression and its effect on relationships at this stage of life rather than any enduring personality pathology.

We define IPT at three levels: (1) strategies for approaching specific tasks, (2) techniques used to accomplish these tasks, and (3) therapeutic stance. IPT resembles other therapies in techniques and stance, but not in strategies as they are applied to specific tasks. The therapeutic strategies of IPT are to help the patient master the interpersonal context of the depression. Strategies include (1) education; (2) clarification of feelings and expectations; (3) clarification of roles in family, peer group, and community; and (4) facilitation of social competence. Techniques can include communication analysis, interpersonal problem solving, and modeling as well as role playing.

IPT has been evaluated in a number of studies for depression both as an acute and a maintenance treatment. These controlled clinical trials provide the foundation for clinical practice utilizing IPT and for efforts to modify IPT for application to other clinical conditions. IPT has been tested alone, in comparison, and in combination with tricyclics in six clinical trials with depressed patients, three of acute treatment (Elkin et al., 1989; Sloane, Stapes, & Schneider, 1985; Weissman et al., 1979) and three of maintenance treatment (Frank et al., 1990; Klerman, DiMascio, Weissman, Prusoff, & Paykel, 1974; Reynolds & Imber, 1988; Weissman et al., 1974). Five completed studies have included a drug comparison group (Elkin et al., 1989; Frank et al., 1990; Klerman et al., 1974; Reynolds & Imber, 1988; Sloane et al., 1985; Weissman et al., 1979), and four have included a combination of IPT and drugs (Klerman et al., 1974; Kupfer, Frank, & Perel, 1989; Reynolds & Imber, 1988; Weissman et al., 1979). For a comprehensive review of the past studies and current adaptations of IPT, see *A Comprehensive Guide to Interpersonal Psychotherapy* (Weissman et al., 2000).

There are similarities and differences between IPT and the other major psychosocial treatments along several dimensions, including duration of treatment; whether the patient's problem is defined as lying in the distant past, the immediate past, or the present; explicit attention to the interpersonal context; and the use of specific therapeutic techniques. In brief, IPT deals with current, not past, interpersonal relationships, focusing on the patient's immediate social context just before and following the onset of the current depressive episode. Past depressive episodes, early family relationships, previous significant relationships, and friendship patterns are assessed in order to understand overall patterns in the patient's interpersonal relations. The psychotherapist does not frame the patient's current situation as a manifestation of internal conflict or as a recurrence of prior intrafamilial maladaptive patterns but rather explores the patient's current disorder in terms of interpersonal relations. In contrast to CBT, the IPT-A therapist focuses on changing relationship patterns rather than distorted cognitions, and there is less focus on systematic homework assignments targeting the cognitive distortions. They are similar in their goals of improving interpersonal problem-solving skills and assisting the adolescent in gaining a sense of social and emotional competence.

Rationale for Use with Adolescents

The rationale for the adaptation of IPT for adolescents lies in research evidence, the developmental relevance of the treatment, and the clinical need in the community. As stated above, clinical research conducted in the 1970s and 1980s had clearly established the efficacy of IPT for the treatment of depression in adults (DiMascio et al., 1979; Elkin et al., 1989; Weissman et al., 1979). At the same time, other research has demonstrated the similarities between adolescent and adult depressive symptoms (Ryan et al., 1987). Chronic and significant psychosocial impairment and interpersonal difficulties are associated with adolescent depression (Hammen, 1999; Marx & Schulze, 1991; Puig-Antich et al., 1993; Stader & Hokason, 1998). They occur in acute stages, continue after recovery, and persist into adulthood. There is little question that major depression has an adverse effect on a child's academic performance, family and peer relationships, and overall functioning. Depression may increase alcohol and drug use and may lead to suicide attempts. In a study of prepubertal depressives, Garber and colleagues (1988) find that depressed adolescents have significant adjustment difficulties in social activities, family relationships, and significant partner relationships, while another study states that depressed children view themselves as less socially competent (Altmann & Gotlib, 1988). In a study of prepubertal children, after they had sustained recovery from their index episode, Puig-Antich and colleagues (1985a, 1985b) show that, while the children's school functioning improves, they still suffer impairment in familial and peer relationships. Thus, while their depression has resolved, they are left with interpersonal deficits.

IPT-A is an intervention that is specifically aimed at treating the interpersonal problems that are associated with adolescent depression. IPT-A focuses largely on current interpersonal issues that are likely to be areas of the greatest concern and importance to adolescents. Discussing interpersonal events is something adolescents can relate to and are accustomed to doing in their daily lives. The current adaptation, IPT-A, has modified the treatment goals and strategies of the specified problem areas to address the developmental tasks and abilities of adolescents. IPT-A focuses on damaged interpersonal relationships, particularly those occurring within the family. Parents and siblings are encouraged to become involved in the treatment either for support of the adolescent, for direct intervention to change patterns in familial relations, or to affect intrafamilial communications. Thus, it effectively addresses the psychological context associated with depression: familial conflict, social competence, affective expression, and effective communication. Familial relationships are models for extrafamilial intimate relationships. Strategies for changing the adolescent's interpersonal relationships with family members can be extrapolated by the adolescent to relationships outside of the family system. IPT-A attempts to address these associated symptoms and impairments and to provide the adolescent with skills that will be helpful in the future as well as present interpersonal context.

OVERVIEW OF BASIC PRINCIPLES OF IPT-A

IPT-A is designed as a once-a-week, 12-week-long treatment. The goals of the treatment are to reduce depressive symptoms and to address the interpersonal problems associated with the onset of the depression. The two main approaches for achieving these goals are to identify one or two problem areas as the focus of treatment and to emphasize the interpersonal nature of the problem as it occurs in current relationships. The treatment is divided into three phases: (1) the initial phase, (2) the middle phase, and (3) the termination phase. The initial phase focuses on confirmation of depression diagnosis, psychoeducation about the illness, exploration of the patient's significant interpersonal relationships, and identification of the problem area that will be the focus of the remainder of the treatment. Symptom relief begins with helping the patient understand that the vague and uncomfortable symptoms are part of a known syndrome that responds to various treatments and has a good prognosis. The major problem associated with the onset of the depression is identified, and an explicit treatment contract to work on this problem area is made with the patient. The topical content of the sessions is, therefore, not open-ended. The identified problem areas of IPT-A include grief reactions, parent–child disputes, peer conflicts, difficulty making transitions between stages in life, coping with stresses associated with changes in family structure, and communication problems.

During the middle phase of treatment, the therapist focuses on identifying specific strategies that can help the adolescents negotiate their interpersonal difficulties, within one or two problem areas, more successfully. For example, adolescents are taught communication skills to express their feelings regarding conflicts or disappointments in their relationships and life circumstances such as an absent father, an inconsistent father, or conflict about dating rules. Techniques include expression of affect, clarification of expectations for relationships, communication analysis, interpersonal problem solving, and role playing new methods of interaction.

The goal of the termination phase is to clarify warning symptoms of future depressive episodes, identify successful strategies used in the middle phase, foster generalization of skills to future situations, emphasize mastery of new interpersonal skills, and to discuss the need for further treatment.

MODIFICATIONS MADE FOR ADOLESCENTS

IPT has been selected for use with adolescents due to its developmental relevance to the adolescent population. However, several alterations have been made to the IPT manual to increase the model's appropriateness for the treatment of adolescent depression. Although the overall goals and problem areas of IPT are employed in IPT-A, the latter also includes a discussion, within the problem area of role transitions, of a specific type of role transition for adolescents that is due to family structural change. This separate discussion of a specific transition is included given the frequency with which it occurs for adolescents, its empirically demonstrated connection to depressive symptoms, and the interpersonal challenges and difficulties that are associated with this situation. A second adaptation is the addition of a parent component to the treatment protocol. Although IPT-A is an individual treatment, for many adolescents some degree of involvement on the part of the parent or guardian is often advisable and critical in promoting the well-being of the adolescent and in encouraging the success of the treatment. Parent involvement in IPT-A is flexible and can range from no involvement to attendance at several sessions. Recommendations typically include, in the least, involvement at the initial phase in order to be educated about the disorder and the treatment. The role of the parent or guardian in treatment is presented for each phase of the treatment, as described later in this volume.

The objectives of treatment have been altered slightly to take into account developmental tasks, including individuation, establishment of autonomy, development of interpersonal relations with members of the opposite sex and with potential romantic partners, coping with initial experiences amid death and loss, and managing peer pressure. Second, the techniques employed in the treatment for working toward the goals of decreasing depressive symptoms and improving interpersonal functioning have been geared toward adolescents. Techniques employed specifically with adolescents include giving them a rating scale of 1–10 to rate their mood, which is concrete and makes it easier for them to monitor improvement; doing more basic social skills work; conducting explicit work on perspective-taking skills to counteract adolescent black-and-white thinking about solutions to problems; and learning how to specifically with adolescents include giving them a rating scale of 1–10 to rate their mood, which is concrete and makes it easier for them to monitor improvement; doing more basic social skills work; conducting explicit work on perspective-taking skills to counteract adolescent black-and-white thinking about solutions to problems; and learning how to negotiate, specifically, parent–child tensions. Strategies have been developed to include family members in various phases of the treatment as needed and to address special issues that arise in the treatment of adolescents, such as school refusal, physical or sexual abuse, suicidality, aggression, and involvement of a child protective service agency. These strategies are more fully discussed in the chapter on special issues in working with adolescents.

OVERVIEW OF EFFICACY

The efficacy of IPT-A has been demonstrated in three randomized controlled clinical trials (Mufson et al., 1999, 2004a; Rosselló & Bernal, 1999). In the clinical trial conducted by Mufson and colleagues, IPT-A is superior to clinical monitoring with respect to decreasing depressive symptoms and increasing rates of recovery from depression and rates of retention in treatment. In addition, adolescents who received IPT-A demonstrate significant improvement in certain areas of social functioning and interpersonal problem-solving skills as compared to adolescents who received clinical monitoring. These findings, together with the results of Rosselló and Bernal (1999), demonstrate the effectiveness of IPT with depressed adolescents.

Current empirical investigations of IPT-A aim to reach a broader range of depressed adolescents by providing treatment in community-based practice settings. Adaptations are being made to make treatment delivery accessible to more teens. In the third clinical trial, Mufson and colleagues conducted an effectiveness trial comparing IPT-A to treatment as it is usually delivered in school-based health clinics located in impoverished urban communities. The study demonstrates the ability to train community clinicians to conduct IPT-A effectively as well as shows that IPT-A is significantly more effective compared to treatment as usual (TAU) in decreasing depression symptoms and improving global and social functioning in depressed adolescents (Mufson et al., 2004a). Mufson and colleagues also have a small-scale, randomized trial of the group version of IPT-A under way. If effective, the group version of IPT-A (Mufson et al., 2004b) possibly could be a more cost-effective treatment. A more complete discussion of IPT-A research can be found in Chapter 19 on current and future research. Preliminary feedback suggests that the group model is at least acceptable and feasible. Findings from these studies will hopefully be part of the solution to the public health need to provide more empirically based, efficacious treatments for depressed adolescents.

CONCLUSION

IPT has arisen out of the tradition of the interpersonal theorists and their emphasis on the importance of good interpersonal relationships for mental health. The significant evidence for the efficacy of IPT with depressed adults both as an acute and maintenance treatment served as the impetus for the adaptation of IPT for depressed adolescents. Importantly, there is increasing evidence for the efficacy of IPT-A. The development of psychotherapies specifically designed for depression that are time-limited and of brief duration is a significant advance in psychotherapy research.

The chapters that follow present the detailed treatment manual for IPT-A. This edition of the manual has been modified based on over a decade of experience treating adolescents both in hospital-based clinics as well as in the community, specifically in school-based health clinics. We hope to share the knowledge that we have gained from training diverse types of clinicians and participating in their experiences in applying IPT-A to a variety of adolescents suffering from depression. These experiences have culminated in this revised and expanded version of the IPT-A treatment manual, characterized by a more detailed delineation of our treatment principles, techniques, and therapeutic processes.

PART II

Application of Interpersonal Therapy for Depressed Adolescents

CHAPTER 4

Diagnosis of Depression and Suitability of Interpersonal Psychotherapy for the Adolescent

Prior to the initiation of IPT-A, a thorough diagnostic evaluation of the adolescent should be undertaken to gather information on current symptoms as well as previous psychiatric, family, developmental, medical, social, and academic history. The goals of the diagnostic assessment are:

1. To make a current clinical diagnosis using DSM-IV diagnostic criteria.
2. To ascertain the adolescent's level of psychosocial functioning and pinpoint areas of interpersonal problems.
3. To assess which treatment would be most appropriate for the adolescent.

To these ends, all available sources of information should be accessed, including the adolescent, parents and other family members, teachers and other school personnel, and other caretakers such as pediatricians and clergy. The importance of obtaining as much information as possible from people who see the patient in various roles and circumstances should be explained to the adolescent and the parents, who will hopefully provide consent to speak to the other important people in the adolescent's life. Without this permission, the therapist is not at liberty to speak to anyone other than the patient and the parents.

DIAGNOSING THE DEPRESSION

Diagnostic procedures include clinical interviews with the adolescent and the parents about the adolescent, as well as interviews with other key figures in the adolescent's life. Self-report instruments to be completed by the adolescent also can be useful. While these instruments have been designed for research purposes, they can be helpful to the general clinician. The instruments provide guidelines for a systematic review of disorders, for obtaining information systematically from a variety of sources so the clinician can compare the quality and/or nature of the information obtained from the sources, and closely monitor changes in the adolescent's psychological state. They are not a substitute, however, for clinical acumen and are most effective in a clinical situation when skillfully woven into the assessment and therapeutic process.

Psychological testing also can be a useful addition to the clinical diagnostic interview, particularly if there is a possibility of a learning disability complicating a depression. A recent comprehensive physical examination should be required for all patients in order to rule out organic causes of the depression, such as hypothyroidism, and side effects of medications, such as steroid treatment or birth control pills. Prior to initiating IPT-A, it is important to confirm that there is no medical condition causing the current symptoms.

Adolescent and Parent Reports of Depression Symptomatology

One of the primary steps in diagnosing children and adolescents and assessing their functioning is to obtain information about the presence and severity of specific symptoms (Kazdin, French, Unis, & Esveldt-Dawson, 1983). The IPT-A therapist is interested in obtaining information about current and past depressive symptoms; history of current depression, including possible precipitant, type, and course of previous psychiatric illness; psychosocial history and current psychosocial functioning; and family and medical history. Most typically, this information is obtained from the adolescent as well as the parent(s). When evaluating the information that is obtained, it is important to consider the quality of the adolescent's relationship to the informant.

There are considerable discrepancies between parents' and children's reports about the degree and nature of children's psychopathology (Angold, 1988; Edelbrock, Costello, Dulcan, Kalas, & Conover, 1985; Kashani, Orvaschel, Burke, & Reid, 1985; Kazdin et al., 1983; Leon, Kendall, & Garber, 1980; Lobovits & Handal, 1985; Moretti, Fine, Haley, & Marriage, 1985). Parents and children may use different criteria of severity for determining when a behavior is worth mentioning, and as observers parents may be unable to perceive what is problematic for their child. In addition, parents may have different areas of concern that are reflected in their responses (Kashani et al., 1985). Angold et al. (1987) concluded that parents are relatively unlikely to report symptoms that their children do not report, but children often report symptoms that their parents do not report. This is particularly true in the area of reports on suicidality, ideation, or attempts (Velez & Cohen, 1988; Walker, Moreau, & Weissman, 1989).

Depressive symptoms can often be silent or misinterpreted. Some parents or teachers might consider the adolescent's silence and isolation as a "phase." Irritability or anger may be the first symptom manifested by the adolescent. If the roots of the adolescent's behavior are not assessed, the adolescent can be labeled simply as a problem that needs to be dealt with in a disciplinary manner. For a complete picture of the child's psychopathology, it is prudent to obtain information from as many sources as possible, including parents and teachers; however, the more accurate information is likely to be obtained from the adolescent. It is important to interview adolescents directly for an accurate and complete picture of their internal emotional state (Angold, 1988).

The clinician's ability to obtain and synthesize information is key to making an accurate assessment and diagnosis. The astute clinician will often re-interview someone with new information obtained from another informant. Discrepancies should be addressed directly with each informant in an attempt to clarify the point in question. The clinician needs to keep an open mind at all points of treatment, to be able to integrate new information and reformulate diagnostic assessments accordingly.

How to Conduct the Pretreatment Evaluation

Step 1

During the pretreatment evaluation, the therapist will meet with both the adolescent as well as the participating family members. It is often helpful to first meet with the adolescent and his family together to explain the strategy for conducting the initial evaluation, such as when the therapist will meet with the adolescent alone, parents alone, and then the family together, in addition to the topics the therapist hopes to cover in the evaluation. We recommend that the therapist, following this brief joint meeting, begin the next stage of the evaluation with the adolescent alone.

Step 2

While alone with the adolescent, the therapist explains the limits of confidentiality, specifically that the session content will not be shared with the parents unless the therapist is concerned about the adolescent being a danger to himself or others. The therapist also explains that there may be times when it would be helpful for the treatment to share other information with the parent. In such cases, the therapist will discuss the issue of confidentiality, and the patient and therapist will jointly decide whether or not to share the information to facilitate the treatment.

The therapist then asks the patient his reasons for seeking treatment, the recent history of the depression, specific symptoms of depression, and associated psychosocial functioning, such as suicidality, drug abuse, and antisocial behavior. The therapist should review past depressive episodes, the presence of any past manic or hypomanic episodes, environmental or interpersonal precipitants, and previous treatments or methods of resolution. Social, academic, and/or family consequences of the depression should also be explored. Suicidal intent must be carefully assessed because it may be a contraindication to outpatient treatment (see Chapter 16). All of this information should be obtained so that the therapist can begin to make a determination about treatment recommendations and whether IPT-A is a suitable treatment modality. While evaluating these symptoms, the therapist should keep in mind whether or not the symptoms indicate a possible need for medication due to severity and impairment.

Step 3

After obtaining the adolescent's view of his current difficulties, it is important to meet with the family, especially parents, to seek their perspective on their adolescent's difficulties. A comprehensive history of the adolescent's symptoms, including type, duration, and social functioning, should be obtained from the parent(s). Often the parents add a valuable perspective on the current struggles of the adolescent. It is also the first opportunity that the therapist has to begin to educate the family about what it means to have a psychiatric illness like depression. It is similarly important at this time to obtain permission from the parents to contact the school for information regarding academic performance as well as social behavior with peers.

Depression in adolescents can be complicated by such comorbid disorders as conduct disorder, anxiety disorders (including panic disorder), or substance use disorder. The reader is referred to DSM-IV for a symptom review of such comorbid disorders as conduct disorder, anxiety disorders, substance abuse/dependence, and learning disabilities (American Psychiatric Association, 2000a). The adolescent should be assessed for the presence of these disorders before initiating treatment. Comorbidity with any of these disorders can result in multiple missed appointments, failure to focus on the tasks of therapy, or various life crises including legal complications.

DETERMINING AN ADOLESCENT'S SUITABILITY FOR IPT-A

An integral part of the assessment process is determining an adolescent's suitability for IPT-A based upon diagnosis, severity of illness and impairment, as well as an assessment of the family environment and willingness to engage in treatment. Based on our clinical experience, the following characteristics of an adolescent make IPT-A a good treatment choice:

1. The adolescent's ability to establish a therapeutic relationship with the therapist and willingness to work in a one-to-one therapeutic relationship in a time-limited therapy.
2. An agreement between the adolescent and therapist that there seem to be difficulties of an interpersonal nature that may be causing problems at this time.
3. A family who supports the therapy or at least will not prematurely terminate the adolescent's treatment.

The therapist can gauge the adolescent's ability to relate to the therapist during the assessment process by the adolescent's willingness to come to sessions and to be honest and open with the therapist about his feelings. An adolescent who is eager to discuss feelings and problems and is willing to explore connections among feelings, events, and relationships is a particularly good candidate for IPT-A. IPT-A is probably most effective with adolescents who have had an acute onset of depressive symptoms and historically have not had severe interpersonal problems with friends or family. In such cases, there is often an identifiable precipitant to the depression, and the depression has resulted in interpersonal problems. IPT-A also can be helpful to adolescents with long-standing interpersonal problems, but the goals for improvement may need to be more circumscribed.

IPT-A is designed for use with adolescents, ages 12–18 years, who have an acute onset major depression or other milder forms of depression such as dysthymia, an adjustment disorder with depressed mood or depression not otherwise specified. Adolescents are suitable for the treatment if they are of normal intelligence and are not actively suicidal. Depressed adolescents with psychotic symptoms or primary diagnoses of manic depression, substance abuse, anxiety disorders, or conduct disorders have not been treated with IPT-A. Depressed adolescents with comorbid anxiety disorders, attention deficit disorder, and oppositional defiant disorder have been treated with IPT-A.

CONCLUDING THE PRETREATMENT EVALUATION

At the end of the evaluation, if the adolescent appears suitable for IPT-A, the therapist should inform the adolescent and family of the adolescent's diagnosis of depression and educate them about the depressive condition. The education process includes a review of symptoms and types of treatment as well as reassurance and guidance in managing symptoms. The goal of the initial guidance is to foster a feeling that the adolescent has already begun working on the problem. This feeling may facilitate his commitment to the treatment and engagement in the therapeutic relationship.

The therapist should stress the importance of conducting such a thorough evaluation for making an accurate assessment of the adolescent's problems and deciding upon an appropriate treatment. At the same time, the therapist should praise the adolescent for working hard in these sessions to give the therapist a picture of his experience of depression and for recognizing the need for treatment. At this point, a discussion of psychotherapy should ensue, reviewing the different types of therapy available, the possibility of treating the depression with medication, and the therapist's desire to initiate a treatment of interpersonal psychotherapy. A brief explanation of the therapy rationale can be given to both the adolescent and parents. They are then instructed to return the next week to actually begin the therapy program. At that time, education about depression will continue, as will education about the focus and course of psychotherapy. The therapist should provide an opportunity for the adolescent and parent to ask any questions they may have about the evaluation process before concluding the meeting.

SUMMARY

The goal of the pretreatment evaluation is to gather as much information as possible about the patient's symptoms and interpersonal functioning to determine whether or not he, in fact, does have a depression and whether or not IPT-A would be an appropriate treatment for him. To make these decisions, the therapist needs information on the family's history, the patient's medical history, developmental and academic history, as well as an assessment of possible comorbid disorders that might preclude IPT-A from being the treatment of choice. The pretreatment evaluation enables the therapist to get a sense of the parents' perspective on their adolescent's mental health and their level of support for the treatment. The therapist should contact the school for additional information that may inform the treatment choices for the adolescent. A thorough evaluation enables the therapist to quickly focus on the depression and its interpersonal consequences once interpersonal psychotherapy has actually begun.

CHAPTER 5

Conducting Session 1 in IPT-A

The two main goals of IPT-A are (1) to decrease the depressive symptoms and (2) to improve the interpersonal problems associated with the onset of the depressive episode. The initial visits (sessions 1–4), along with the pretreatment session, are devoted to diagnosing the depression, obtaining an interpersonal inventory, identifying one or more problem areas, and negotiating the therapeutic contract. During the initial phase of IPT-A the therapist has seven objectives:

1. Confirm the depression diagnosis according to current diagnostic systems.
2. Complete psychoeducation about depression and the therapy process.
3. Conduct an interpersonal inventory (i.e., review of significant relationships) and relate the depression to the interpersonal context.
4. Identify the interpersonal difficulties in one or more principal problem areas.
5. Explain the theory and goals of interpersonal therapy.
6. Explain the patient's and parents' expected roles in the treatment.
7. Set the stage for the work of the middle phase.

This chapter focuses on the confirmation of diagnosis and the completion of the initial psychoeducation process (objectives 1 and 2). The interpersonal inventory (objective 3) is detailed in Chapter 6. Identifying the problem area, explaining the theory of IPT-A, assigning roles in treatment, and establishing the therapeutic contract (objectives 4–7) are taken up in Chapter 7.

TASKS OF SESSION 1

To achieve objectives 1 and 2, there are several tasks the therapist needs to complete by the conclusion of the first session. To achieve the first objective of confirming the diagnosis, the therapist's first task is to conduct another brief but thorough review of depression symptoms. To achieve the second objective of psychoeducation, the therapist must perform the following additional tasks:

1. Confirm the suitability of the patient for IPT-A.
2. Explain the nature of depression in adolescents.
3. Explain treatment options.
4. Explain the limited "sick role" as assumed by the patient during therapy.
5. Introduce the basic principles of IPT-A.
6. Obtain a commitment to treatment and explain the goals for session 2.

The therapist must use her clinical knowledge and acumen to assess if, when, and how to involve the adolescent's parents in conducting tasks 1–6 involved in the second objective. It is preferable to involve the parents in the first session by breaking up the initial IPT-A session into a combination of meetings with the adolescent and parent together, adolescent alone, and parent alone, as was done in the pretreatment evaluation. When this is possible, it is ideal if the therapist can extend the therapy session to 75–90 minutes as needed to cover the material. If it is not possible, the therapist should try to meet with the parent alone at another time to accomplish tasks 1–6 with the parent prior to session 2 with the adolescent.

Task 1: Review of Depression Symptoms

The detailed review of the patient's symptoms has four purposes:

1. To assist the therapist in confirming the depression diagnosis.
2. To show the patient that his symptoms are part of a known syndrome that is understood and that can be effectively treated.
3. To help place the symptoms in their interpersonal context.

TABLE 5.1. Criteria for Major Depressive Episode

A. Five (or more) of the following symptoms have been present during the same 2-week period and represent a change from previous functioning; at least one of the five symptoms must be either (1) depressed or irritable mood or (2) loss of interest or pleasure.

> Note: Do not include symptoms that are clearly due to a general medical condition, or mood-incongruent delusions or hallucinations.

(1) depressed mood most of the day, nearly every day, as indicated by either subjective account or observation by others (e.g., appears tearful). **Note:** In children and adolescents, can be irritable mood.
(2) markedly diminished interest or pleasure in all, or almost all, activities most of the day, nearly every day (as indicated by either subjective account or observation made by others)
(3) significant weight loss when not dieting or weight gain (e.g., a change of more than 5% of body weight in a month), or decrease or increase in appetite nearly every day. **Note:** In children, consider failure to make expected weight gains.
(4) insomnia or hypersomnia nearly every day
(5) psychomotor agitation or retardation nearly every day (observable by others, not merely subjective feelings of restlessness or being slowed down).
(6) fatigue or loss of energy nearly every day
(7) feelings of worthlessness or excessive or inappropriate guilt (which may be delusional) nearly every day (not merely self-reproach or guilt about being sick)
(8) diminished ability to think or concentrate, or indecisiveness, nearly every day (either by subjective account or as observed by others)
(9) recurrent thoughts of death (not just fear of dying), recurrent suicidal ideation without a specific plan, or a suicide attempt or a specific plan for committing suicide

B. The symptoms do not meet criteria for a Mixed Episode.

C. The symptoms cause clinically significant distress or impairment in social, occupational, or other important areas of functioning.

D. The symptoms are not due to the direct physiological effects of a substance (e.g., a drug of abuse, a medication) or a general medical condition (e.g., hypothyroidism).

E. The symptoms are not better accounted for by Bereavement, i.e., after the loss of a loved one, the symptoms persist for longer than 2 months or are characterized by marked functional impairment, morbid preoccupation with worthlessness, suicidal ideation, psychotic symptoms, or psychomotor retardation.

Note. From American Psychiatric Association (2000a, p. 356). Copyright 2000 by the American Psychiatric Association. Reprinted by permission. See DSM-IV-TR for other depression diagnoses.

4. To illustrate for the patient the active nature of his role and the therapist's role in the treatment.

At the conclusion of the review, the patient should know that the depression symptoms are (1) time-limited, (2) reflective of a disorder that can be treated successfully, and (3) that he will likely be able to function better with treatment.

The review of symptoms should enable the therapist to confirm a DSM-IV diagnosis of major depression (see Table 5.1) and confirm the comorbid diagnoses identified in the pretreatment evaluation. To this end, the following symptoms should be probed:

Depressed Mood

Has there ever been a time when you felt sad, down, empty, moody, like crying, unhappy, or when you had a bad or unhappy feeling inside most of the time? How long during the day did it last? A long time or short time? The whole morning? All afternoon? From waking up in the morning until lunch? Less? More? Is it worse in the morning or later in the day?

Anhedonia

Has there ever been a time when you just could not have as much fun as usual? Or were having much less fun than your friends? How long did it last? Did you enjoy anything at that time? Has there been a time when you felt bored most of the time? When was that? Do you know why you were feeling that way? Could you have changed it? Could you have found anything to do that was fun? Was there anything you enjoyed or you felt like doing at that time?

Separation Issues

Do these sad feelings happen only when you are away from your [major attachment figure] or your family? What was going on in your life when you felt that way or before you felt that way? Had anything happened that upset you? Was something bothering you?

Grief Reaction

Has someone you were very close to died recently, or have you recently had a pet die? Is the way you feel now different from when someone close to you (or a pet) has died?

Lack of Reactivity

When you are sad, do you feel better when something good happens?

Appetite and Weight

Have you lost your appetite or lost weight? How much? Are you hungrier than usual, or have you gained weight? How much?

Initial Insomnia

Do you have trouble sleeping? What is your usual bedtime and awakening time? Do you have trouble falling asleep? How long does it take? What keeps you awake? What thoughts do you have when you get into bed?

Middle Insomnia

Do you wake up during the night and then cannot go back to sleep right away?

Terminal Insomnia

Do you wake up before you have to? Do you feel rested upon awakening? How much earlier do you wake up?

Hypersomnia

Have you been sleeping more than usual? How much more? Do you take naps during the day?

Agitation

Do you have trouble sitting still, or do you walk back and forth?

Retardation

Do you talk or move more slowly than usual?

Fatigue

Are you very tired? Do you have less energy than usual?

Diurnal Variation

Do you feel worse in the morning or afternoon? Is it significantly worse or just a little bit worse?

Depersonalization

Do you ever feel like you are outside of yourself, watching yourself do things or say things but not feel like you are part of it? Like you are watching yourself in a movie?

Paranoid Symptoms

Have you felt as though people are talking about you? That strangers are talking about you? Do you worry that someone or a group is trying to hurt you? Who? What are they trying to do? Why would they want to hurt you?

Obsessive and Compulsive Symptoms

Do you ever have thoughts that keep coming into your mind that seem to come from nowhere and are difficult to get rid of? Are they the same thoughts each time? Do they bother you? Are there things you have to keep doing and redoing even though you know that it is not necessary? Like checking that you have locked the door or washing your hands repeatedly?

Excessive Guilt

Do you feel guilty (bad) about things that happened in the past? Do you blame yourself for things that aren't your fault? Do you think you should be punished more than you are? Do you feel that you aren't a good person, or do you feel worthless?

Concentration Difficulty

Do you have difficulty paying attention or keeping your mind on your schoolwork? Have your grades gone down? Do you have to make a much bigger effort than before just to keep up? Do you feel like your thoughts are slowed down?

Suicidal Ideation or Behavior

Do you think about death a lot? Do you ever think that life isn't worth living or that you would be better off dead? Do you think about killing yourself? Do you have a plan? Did you ever try to kill yourself or hurt yourself (e.g., cutting)? [See Part III for special issues.]

Sexual Symptoms

Has your interest in boys/girls changed recently? Have you had less sexual interest than usual? Are you interested in the same or opposite sex? Are you sexually active? If so, continue with questions. If not, go to next area. If so, are you using birth control? Do you have difficulty becoming excited? Sexual relations less often? Difficulty in obtaining an erection [boys] or reaching a climax?

Helplessness

Do you feel unable to change the situation? Do you feel like you don't know what to do to feel differently? Do you feel you need help to do things you normally could do for yourself?

Hopelessness

Do you feel that the situation will never be different? Do feel that there is little chance that you will feel better in the future?

Somatic Symptoms

Are you experiencing any physical aches and pains? Headaches? Stomachaches? Joint pains? Trouble going to the bathroom? Frequency of urination? Neck aches

Hallucinations

Do you hear voices when no one is around that no one can hear but you? What do those voices say? Do they speak to you or just call your name? Can you make them go away? Do you ever see things that no one can see but you?

The adolescents should be encouraged to describe the depression symptoms using their own language or set of beliefs. For example, some patients will see their experience in religious terms: "God is punishing me for not being a better daughter." Others will blame the problem on someone else—a mother for not listening to them, or a friend for not being understanding and tolerant of their behavior. The therapist will have the opportunity to explore these feelings further and put them in the appropriate context for treatment later in the evaluation process. The therapist should also obtain a description of how these symptoms are impacting the adolescent's general functioning such as relationships with family and friends as well as their schoolwork. This provides an opportunity to further discuss the impact of the depression on the adolescent's life in general and the need for treatment.

Task 2: Confirming Suitability for Treatment

An adolescent is felt to be suitable for treatment first and foremost if he is willing to acknowledge the depression and is willing to discuss the impact the depression is having on his relationships. The therapist must also confirm that the patient has the potential to be verbally engaged in the treatment. If the adolescent has comorbid disorders, a decision should be made confirming that the depression is the appropriate disorder upon which to focus treatment. The therapist also must feel that the adolescent would benefit from treatment on a once-a-week basis and currently is not in need of more intensive treatment.

Task 3: Education about the Nature of Depression

If the patient is in fact diagnosed with a depressive disorder, the first task should be to tell the patient explicitly that his symptoms indicate the presence of a specific disorder. If the physical exam results (conducted by a pediatrician) are negative, the therapist can inform and reassure the patient that any somatic symptoms are due to the depression rather than physical illness. It is important to reassure the patient that he does not have a serious physical illness, that the adolescent is not "going crazy," and that the psychological problems can be effectively treated.

The therapist should convey the diagnosis to the patient and family clearly by saying:

> *The symptoms you describe are all part of being depressed. Your appetite and sleep habits have changed. You feel sad the majority of your day, tired all the time, and have less interest in participating in your usual activities. You find yourself getting into more arguments or conflicts with your parents and friends and in general feel more irritable. You don't have the same amount of interest in your schoolwork, and you are experiencing concentration difficulties in school. These prob-*

lems along with your thoughts about death and feelings of hopeless-
ness are all part of the clinical picture of depression.

This discussion is most helpful when conducted following the therapist's meeting alone with the adolescent and then alone with the parent so that the therapist has a complete picture of the adolescent's symptoms and the role the depression may be playing in the home. If the parent has been unable to attend the session, the explanation and conceptualization should be discussed with the adolescent alone.

Task 4: Explaining Treatment Options

The fourth task is to impart some general information about the course of depression and its treatment. It is important for the adolescent and family to know that the prognosis for recovery is good. They also need to be informed that there are other treatment options available if for some reason IPT-A is not sufficiently effective for this adolescent. They need to be informed both about other psychotherapies as well as the possibility of treating the depression with medication. For example, the therapist might say:

> *Depression commonly occurs in children and adolescents as well as in adults. It is believed to be more common in girls than boys. Approximately 2–5% of adolescents may have a depressive disorder at any one time. Even though you feel badly now, depressions do respond to treatment. There is more than one way to treat depression. So, if the first approach does not work, there are other approaches to try. Most adolescents with depression recover rapidly with treatment. As a result of treatment you will likely feel better, your symptoms will decrease, and you will be able to function more normally at school and at home. Psychotherapy is one of the standard treatments for depression and has been proven effective in several studies. IPT-A is a specific therapy that focuses on the relationship between depression and problems in your relationships with significant people in your life. Therapy hopefully will help you understand what has been making you depressed and help you find ways to resolve the problem. If IPT-A doesn't seem to be helping enough, there are other therapies that can be tried, including medication. Let's see how you do with this treatment first.*

Task 5: Giving the Adolescent a Limited "Sick Role"

The goal of this task is to educate the adolescent and parent about the effects of depression on the daily activities of a teenager. This should follow the adolescent's completion of the review of his symptoms. The therapist explains to the adolescent and parent that commonly reported symptoms include fatigue, lack of energy, anhedonia (lack of pleasure in normally pleasurable activities), as well as difficulties in concentration. Therefore, it is not uncommon for the adolescent to be having difficulties with his grades and possibly attendance at school and for the parents to be complaining about how he never does anything around the house. The parents and therapist should be alert to the adolescent's tendency to withdraw socially as part of the depressive syndrome and to experience symptoms such as fatigue that are used to justify avoidance of social and school activities. The therapist's goal is to explain the effects of being depressed on one's actions and to assign the adolescent a limited "sick role."

The purpose of the limited sick role is to allow the patient some relief from the pressure of performing his usual social role at the same level as prior to being depressed and to receive some extra support for his efforts without punishment for the quality of the work in a time-limited way while he recovers. The adolescent is encouraged to think of himself as in treatment and as having an illness that affects his motivation and the quality of his performance. Nonetheless, the adolescent is encouraged to maintain the usual social roles in the family, at school, and with friends. Specifically, he needs to get up every morning and get to school, complete homework the best he can, and perform his chores around his house to the best of his abilities. The parent is advised to be supportive and to encourage the adolescent to engage in as many normal activities as possible, although it is recognized that the adolescent may have difficulty performing up to par. The assignment of the sick role and psychoeducation can help family members to respond more positively toward the adolescent. It is important to discuss the "sick role" with the adolescent's parents, stressing the need to be supportive and not punitive with their child. The psychotherapist might say something like:

> Your child does not feel like participating in many of his usual activities. This apathy and lethargy are symptoms of depression, not oppositional behavior nor laziness. It is important for you to encourage your child—without getting angry—to do as many of his usual activities as possible while treatment is going on.

To the adolescent the psychotherapist might say:

> You may not feel like going out with your friends or doing your schoolwork, but it is important that you try to maintain as many of your usual activities as possible. It is one of the steps that will make you feel better. Over the next few months together, we will be working

hard toward the goal of you feeling better. We expect that you will participate in your usual activities and that with treatment you will begin to feel much more energized. As time goes on and we begin to understand and cope with the problems related to your depression, we have every reason to believe that you will feel better than ever.

Task 6: Introducing the Basic Principles of IPT-A

At this point in the session, it is a good idea to introduce the basic structure of IPT-A to the adolescent. The therapist restates that the focus of treatment is going to be on trying to reduce the depression symptoms he is experiencing and to improve his important relationship difficulties that seem most connected to his depression. In order to do that, for the next several sessions, the therapist is going to focus on getting a thorough history of the positive and negative aspects of the adolescent's relationships. Therefore, the therapist will be asking many questions. The goal is to get an accurate picture of the adolescent's life and how his mood is affecting his relationships and how his relationships affect his mood. During the second phase of the therapy, the therapist and adolescent together will identify and practice strategies and skills to improve the targeted relationships and in turn improve his mood. Most of the sessions will occur with the therapist and adolescent alone, but they may talk about inviting parents or significant others into a session or two in the middle phase if it looks like it might be helpful.

Task 7: Obtaining Commitment to Treatment and Explaining the Goals for Session 2

When the therapist has confirmed in her mind that this is a reasonable treatment for the adolescent, it is important to openly discuss the decision to try this treatment with the adolescent. By discussing the decision with the adolescent, the therapist is showing respect for the adolescent by inviting his input into the decision. Hopefully, the discussion will help the adolescent be more engaged in the treatment process and feel as though he has input into the nature of his treatment. It is laying the groundwork for the collaborative relationship that the therapist hopes to have with the adolescent throughout the course of treatment, working as a team on the problem of the adolescent's depression and interpersonal difficulties.

Emphasizing that they are a "team" decreases the adolescent's sense of isolation with the depression. Discussion of recovery reinforces the adolescent's participation in the treatment as necessary to facilitate improvement in functioning. The adolescent needs to be educated that therapy will involve work by the adolescent as well as the therapist to understand the conflict precipitating the depression and to find ways to resolve it. The theme of recovery should continue to be an integral part of the treatment.

The adolescent is sent home from session 1 knowing that session 2 will focus on reviewing his significant relationships. The therapist informs the adolescent that she will call during the week to check on his mood before the next session.

PARENTAL INVOLVEMENT IN THE INITIAL SESSION

Parents should be interviewed during the initial session whenever possible. The parents should be integral to the initial session, as the therapist will discuss with them the adolescent's depressive symptoms and need for treatment. Specifically, the parents should be similarly educated about depression, the limited sick role, and possible treatments, including a discussion of whether there is a need for medication. As issues emerge, parents may need to attend again to be counseled regarding necessary changes at home or in school. The therapist will need to be educative and instructive to the parent. Ideally, one should give the parents the role of collaborative therapists—the ones carrying on the work at home. For example, one might tell them:

> I will be talking to your child once a week, identifying specific problem areas and discussing them. You are there with your child all the time, so your input will be as important as what I do. I want you to keep me informed as to how you see your child doing, any new problems that appear, and anything else you notice about your child. Don't be upset that I cannot tell you everything. We have found that the best way for treatment to work is if the child feels a confidentiality of his or her discussions with the therapist. In our experience, it is helpful for the adolescent to feel that the therapist's office is a safe place to talk and to facilitate trust in the therapist. I will not withhold information about any situation of danger to your child. I will keep you up-to-date on your child's general progress. If I feel your child's behavior poses a danger to him- or herself or others, I certainly will inform you and discuss the situation with you. In addition, I may suggest changes at home based on my sessions with your child.

Parents should be given information about how to manage the adolescent's depressive symptoms, such as encouraging the child to do as much as possible, identifying warning signs of the depression worsening, and planning strategies to deal with an emergency such as increasing suicidal ideation or a suicide attempt. The therapist should inform the parents that they might be asked to participate in future sessions if it seems as though it could be helpful in addressing a problem related to the depression. It is important that the parents be apprised of the specific parameters of therapy: frequency and length of sessions, fees, missed sessions, and length of treatment.

Some parents may be experiencing psychological difficulties of their own or may have need for greater guidance in handling their child than the IPT-A therapist can address. In such cases, it is useful to consider referring the parent(s) to another therapist for either a psychiatric evaluation or counseling.

Challenges to Parental Involvement

There are circumstances in which the parent may refuse to be involved in the treatment or the adolescent may refuse to have the parent be involved. If this occurs in the initial phase of treatment, it is important for the therapist to have a separate session with the parent to assess the impact of the refusal to participate on resolution of the interpersonal issue. The individual session with the parents is an opportunity to further educate the parents about how they can assist in the recovery of their child. The therapist may be the expert on treating depression, but the parent spends more time with the adolescent and has more specific knowledge of the adolescent. This information will be invaluable to the therapist in helping the adolescent to feel better. The therapist should try to directly address the parental concerns about participation and clarify any misunderstandings about the elements of treatment that may be contributing to parents' resistance to participation. Similarly, in cases where the adolescent refuses parental involvement, the therapist must assess whether the refusal is symptomatic of the interpersonal problem associated with the depression or whether it is a realistic assessment of the parents' dysfunction and inability to assist in recovery. If it is the latter, it is important for therapist and adolescent to identify another adult who could contribute to the adolescent's recovery through participation in treatment. If it is the former, a treatment goal may be to feel confident and capable of communicating effectively with a parent in a future therapy session.

Contact with School and Educator

In many cases the therapist also should establish an alliance with the school system. Prior to assuming a role in relation to the school system, the therapist should discuss school involvement with the parent and obtain parental and adolescent consent to discuss certain aspects of therapy with the school. Family refusal for school contact can impinge on recovery, especially when the adolescent is demonstrating impairment in the school setting. In such cases, the therapist needs to explicitly outline the contribution the school could have to recovery and negotiate specific parameters for contact, such as specific school staff to contact and particular types of information that may be shared. This negotiated agreement can be continually revised as needed during the course of treatment. The therapist can assume the patient-advocate role with the educational system, educating teachers about the effects of a depressive episode on school functioning. If school refusal is associated with the depression, it is important for the therapist to work out an appropriate plan with the school for making the child feel comfortable in returning. This may include such things as reducing the course load, assigning one teacher to look out for the adolescent, and helping the school staff to temporarily revise their expectations for the adolescent's performance while he or she recovers from the depression. The school should be encouraged to contact the therapist if any changes in the student are noticed and believed relevant to the treatment.

SUMMARY

By the end of the first session, the therapist will have accomplished the tasks of confirming the DSM-IV depression diagnosis and confirming that IPT-A is a potentially effective treatment method for the particular adolescent. Comorbid diagnoses, family structure and relationships, and individual characteristics of the adolescent as determined by clinical history, diagnostic assessment tools, medical examination, and the emerging therapeutic relationship form the basis of the therapist's recommendation for IPT-A. The work of the therapy has already begun by this time. The adolescent and his parents have been educated about the depressive disorder, and have received an explanation of the principles of IPT-A and an overview of the expected course of treatment. Both parent and adolescent have learned the construct of the "limited sick role" and its specific applicability to the adolescent's daily activities and responsibilities. The parents have been instructed on how to encourage participation without the criticism that can grow out of frustration with the depressed adolescent's lowered performance standards. The first session culminates in the adolescent and family making a commitment to the treatment orientation and expectations for the ensuing 12 weeks of treatment. The groundwork is set for initiating the review of significant interpersonal relationships in session 2.

CHAPTER 6

Initiating the Interpersonal Interview

THE INTERPERSONAL CONTEXT OF DEPRESSION

The focus of treatment shifts in session 2 to understanding the interpersonal context of the depression, particularly the event that may have precipitated the depressive episode; the reasons for seeking treatment now; and what has been happening in significant relationships that may be associated with the onset of symptoms. These are the tasks of sessions 2–4. This work culminates in the identification of one or more problem areas as the focus of treatment.

Prior to initiating the interpersonal inventory, the therapist explains the structure of the next month of sessions. The therapist tells the adolescent that each session will begin with a brief check-in on the adolescent's depressive symptoms that were endorsed the previous week, in addition to assessing suicidality. The therapist instructs the adolescent in the use of a mood rating, explaining that she would like the adolescent to rate his mood on a scale of 1–10, with 1 being the best he could feel (i.e., the happiest) and 10 being the saddest he could feel. The adolescent is then asked to rate his mood for the past week. The therapist should ask if there was ever a time in the past week when the adolescent felt worse than the global rating just given, what the rating was, and what happened at the time that the adolescent felt worse. It is the first opportunity for the therapist to begin to link the adolescent's mood with events that are happening in his daily life. The therapist must assess whether or not there was an increase in suicidality during this period of worsened mood and again assess patient safety to be enrolled in once-a-week psychotherapy. This process of linking a mood rating to a relationship event teaches the adolescent how to review his past week and evaluate how his symptoms impacted on his functioning and what events or people were able to influence his moods one way or another. These are important linkages to identify so that by the end of the initial phase the therapist and adolescent know which of these linkages need to be targeted in the treatment to improve the adolescent's mood.

THE INTERPERSONAL INVENTORY

It is necessary for the therapist to conduct a detailed review of the patient's significant relationships, both current and past. Although the emphasis is on current relationships, obtaining a complete picture of the nature of the patient's social relationships and interpersonal functioning is helpful in understanding his overall patterns of interaction and communication in his relationships. In IPT-A, this is referred to as an interpersonal inventory. The therapist can think of it as the diagnostic assessment of interpersonal symptoms to parallel the completed assessment of depression symptoms. Although the majority of the interpersonal inventory is conducted in these initial sessions, it may be updated as treatment progresses and more information is gathered.

The first task in conducting the interpersonal inventory is to obtain a complete list of the most significant relationships in the adolescent's life. To do that, it is helpful for the therapist to use the "closeness circle." The closeness circle is a series of circles, one inside of the next, with an × in the middle of the circles signifying the patient. (See Appendix A.) The therapist explains that the circles around the patient represent circles of closeness, and the goal is to place the adolescent's significant relationships within the appropriate circles of closeness. The result is a picture of the significant people orbiting the adolescent's life and the emotional valence associated with their position in the adolescent's life. The therapist says:

> Here on this paper we have a series of circles one within the other with an × in the center. You are the ×. What we are going to do is make a list of the important people in your life and place them in these circles to give us a picture of the closeness you feel with them. The people in the circles closest to the × are those people with whom you feel closest or most connected, even if sometimes it is not all positive. People in the

larger circles further away are people who are important to you but to whom you may not feel as close and/or people with whom you would like to change your relationship. We will be talking about what you like and don't like about your relationships with these people, how you get along with them, who you can confide in, and more after we finish placing everyone in the circles.

Once the closeness circle has been completed, the next step for the therapist is to begin to discuss the important relationships in some depth. It is helpful to ask the adolescent which relationship would he like to speak about first. The adolescent frequently selects a relationship that is not as problematic as others in his circle. This is fine because it allows the adolescent to warm up and get into the rhythm of exploring and talking in detail about the nature of the relationship and how it might change using a less stressful relationship. The therapist can begin the inventory process by stating:

I would like to talk to you about the important people in your life, people like your mother and father, sisters and brothers, best friend, girlfriend or boyfriend, other close friends. Has your depression affected your relationship with the people you are closest to? How? Do you think you have problems in your relationships with people? What are those problems? Which relationship would you like to talk about first?

Questions about the significant people in the adolescent's life including family, friends, and teachers may include the following:

Are you able to feel close to people, or is it hard for you to confide in people? Who in your family do you feel closest to, feel that you can confide in and go to for help? What makes that relationship so special for you? Who in your family don't you feel close to? What is the problem in your relationship with this person? What would you like to change about that relationship? Who outside of your family do you feel especially close to? What is it about that relationship that makes you feel close to that person? Do you have friends that you are not close to? What prevents you from feeling close to that person? Are there other people you are close with, like a teacher or a clergy person or a relative or a family friend? Of all the people we've been talking about, to whom do you feel closest? What would you like to change about yourself to help you have better relationships with the people in your life?

The therapist does not need to ask all of these questions of each adolescent. It is important for the therapist not to use these question guidelines as the basis for an interrogatory-like interview. The goal is to use these questions to facilitate the adolescent telling the story of his current life as played out in his significant relationships. The questions are there to keep the storytelling going, not to serve as a formal question-and-answer survey. As the therapist begins to get a sense of the adolescent's relationships, certain areas will be probed in more detail than others. See Appendix B for a list of questions related to specific potential problem areas. Generally, the therapist obtains this information largely from the adolescent.

Some information about problems in relationships has typically already been obtained from earlier meetings with the parent during the pretreatment evaluation and the first session of IPT-A. These discussions help the parent gain perspective on how depression can affect a person's relationship and may help the parent place recurrent problems in the relationship in the context of a depressive episode that can be expected to be resolved. The parental information and, when possible, any teacher information that was obtained in the pretreatment evaluation are used to supplement the information obtained directly from the adolescent. Clinical judgment applied by the therapist is used to correct distortions and misperceptions on the adolescent's part.

In session 2 and beyond, it is the adolescent who provides the bulk of the information about his relationships with significant others, such as grandparents, boy- or girlfriend, and anyone else. The information gathered about each relationship should include the following:

1. The person's interactions with the patient, including how frequently they saw each other, what they did together, what they do and don't enjoy doing together, and so on.
2. The terms of the relationship or expectations for the relationship, whether or not they were fulfilled or revised, and the perceived effect on the outcome of the relationship. Is the relationship ongoing? If not, did it end positively or negatively?
3. A discussion of the positive and negative aspects of the relationship with specific examples of both sides of the relationship.
4. Changes the patient might want to make in the relationship. Has the patient tried to make any of these changes already? What has he tried? How did it go? What worked or didn't work? What else could he do to try and implement these changes either in himself or the other party?
5. How has the depression affected the relationship with the ado-

lescent, and how has it affected the adolescent's other relationships?

It is important when conducting the interpersonal inventory to obtain information about relationships that illustrate interpersonal strengths as well as those that illustrate deficits or areas of weakness. In a short-term therapy, the therapist needs to build up the extant strengths of the patient in order to facilitate change in the targeted relationships. It is imperative not to give the adolescent the message that he is just an amalgam of deficits. A strategy of the treatment is to foster a sense of hope and optimism that change can occur, which is based upon giving the adolescent the message that he has strengths upon which to build and make his relationships, and consequently his mood, better.

Life Events Associated with Depression

Diagnosis of major depression according to DSM-IV criteria does not require the identification of a precipitant; however, through discussion one is often identified. Adolescents initially are not always aware of such an event, but often one can be elicited. The therapist should probe for (1) changes in family structure; (2) changes in school; (3) any moves; (4) death, illness, accident, or trauma; and (5) onset of sexuality and sexual relationships. The therapist can learn a great deal about the adolescent's interpersonal functioning through discussion of stressful events. Does the adolescent seek support in a healthy fashion, or does the adolescent provoke and alienate the people he can depend on the most? Does the adolescent convey his feelings to others in his life in an open fashion, or does he withdraw when upset? Does the adolescent deal directly with the people he or she is closest to, or do feelings emerge in misdirected and ill-conceived actions that are self-defeating and self-destructive? Does the adolescent socially and emotionally withdraw, thereby increasing the depression, when hurt and disappointed by a close relationship? What the therapist learns from such an exploration may not have been immediately apparent to the adolescent or may not be something the adolescent was capable of articulating. To establish a time frame and sequence of events relating a possible precipitant to the depression, the therapist might say:

> You told me before that you began to feel depressed 1 month ago. That seems to be around the same time you broke up with your boyfriend. Did you begin to feel sad around the time you broke up with your boyfriend?

By establishing this time frame, the therapist is also facilitating the connection between the depression symptoms and an interpersonal circumstance or event. This connection is a necessary precursor to identification of the targeted problem area.

When conducting the assessment of depressive symptoms and educating patients about depression, it is important for the therapist to stress, from the beginning, the relationship between the depression and interpersonal functioning. While patients may be aware of the role of problems in their relationships and subsequent influence on their mood, they still may be more inclined to see the problem as inherent in themselves, independent of the other person in the relationship, or they may blame the other person for causing them to feel badly. As a result, they perceive themselves as a failure or as somehow inadequate. Another possibility is that the adolescent's problems in his interpersonal relationships may not be readily apparent to him or he may be so withdrawn from relationships that the opportunities to see hope for change are no longer there. Therefore, making the connection between the relationships and his depression is even more difficult for him. In such cases, it is the role of the therapist to help patients begin to make the connection through direct explanation:

The specific causes of depression are unknown but include environmental and biological influences. Nonetheless, depression is commonly associated with difficulties in relationships, including problems with parents, friends, siblings, and teachers. It is not always clear which came first—the problems in the relationship or the depression—because the depression can cause interpersonal difficulties, exacerbate interpersonal difficulties, or be the outcome of interpersonal difficulties. Problems in relationships with significant people can cause depressed feelings. Similarly, a person experiencing a depression may have difficulty thinking of appropriate coping skills to address the problem. In this treatment we will try to understand your expectations for your relationships and yourself and will help you to fulfill the realistic ones and to cope with the unrealistic ones.

Adolescents appear to approach the interpersonal inventory from two different styles: those that speak only about feelings but can't link them to events or those that speak about events but can't link them to feelings. To work with the former, the therapist must work hard to find out what has happened to the adolescent on the given day when he may rate his mood as worse. Often asking an open-ended question such as "Did anything happen that day that might have affected your mood?"

may not be productive. The therapist may need to take the adolescent on a step-by-step journey through the day or part of the day when the mood is described as most depressed. The therapist may do this by saying:

> Let's trace your steps and activities that day to see if we can uncover anything that might have happened that could have affected your mood. Let's start with when you woke up that morning? What time did you wake up? Is that your usual time? Who did you speak to when you got up? How was breakfast? Did any conversations happen at the breakfast table? [etc.]

Often by guiding the adolescent through the review of the day, it is possible to uncover some conversation or interpersonal action that contributed or exacerbated the patient's depressed mood.

For the adolescent who has difficulty labeling his emotions, the therapist must re-create the interpersonal event that is reported and break it down into discrete components and encourage the adolescent to describe his affective reaction to the different event components. For example:

THERAPIST: So you told me you had a big argument with your mother about curfews on that day. How did you feel when that happened?

PATIENT: I didn't feel anything. I don't care what she says I can do.

THERAPIST: Really, you felt nothing? Let's try and re-create the conversation and look at how you responded at different points in the conversation. What kind of day were you having before the conversation happened? Was it a good or a bad day?

PATIENT: It had been an OK day up until then, and then my mother said, "Oh, by the way, you have to be home by midnight from that party you are going to Saturday night."

THERAPIST: What did you say or do when she said that?

PATIENT: I just got up from my chair, went into my room, and slammed the door shut so I could be by myself and not have to hear her nagging.

THERAPIST: Look at what you just said. You said you went into your room and slammed the door. What are people usually feeling when they slam the door?

PATIENT: Angry.

THERAPIST: Is it possible that you were feeling angry when you slammed the door and that your angry feelings often turn into feelings of sadness later on?

By breaking down the events and having the adolescent describe his actions, the therapist helps the adolescent to see the actions as indicative of specific moods or feelings. The goal in both of these strategies is to facilitate the adolescent's linkage of his mood with events that are happening in his significant relationships.

Challenges to Conducting an Interpersonal Inventory

What should you do if the adolescent answers reluctantly with little information about the relationships? In such instances, it is useful for the therapist to shift away from asking many questions to asking the adolescent to describe a memorable (good or bad) time spent with the person being discussed. Often the adolescent is able to be more talkative when describing a concrete situation than when having to respond about feelings.

What should you do if the adolescent states that he has no significant relationships? While this is rare, adolescents who eventually are formulated to have interpersonal deficits can have a paucity of relationships to discuss. In such instances, it is suggested to determine if there are more relationships to discuss from the past than the present. In addition, the therapist can discuss with the adolescent whom he would like to put in his closeness circle—in other words, who is missing from his close relationships but for whom closeness is desired.

How can the therapist elicit all this information in three sessions? As stated earlier, the inventory should develop into many narrative tales about the adolescent's relationship with different people in his life. The therapist can organize the narratives by beginning with some factual questions, then move into the adolescent's feelings about the person to information about situations that trigger these feelings, and finally to discussion of past attempts to resolve the problems and current hopes for change (see Appendix B). It is necessary for the therapist to keep the adolescent focused on salient information that will facilitate identification of the problem area rather than getting every detail about what has transpired in the relationship. One or two examples of positive and/or negative interactions are usually sufficient for providing an understanding of the significance of the relationship for the maintenance of the adolescent's depression.

SUMMARY

The therapist's primary goal in conducting the interpersonal review is to identify those interpersonal issues most relevant to the onset or exacerbation of the patient's depression. The therapist wants to identify any conflicts or interpersonal difficulties as well as identify potential areas for change. The problem area is a result of difficulty with a relationship that has become exacerbated by a chronic depression, or it may be an event involving an important person in the adolescent's life that has become problematic for the patient and thus a precipitant of the depression. By the end of session 4, the therapist will have completed a comprehensive interpersonal inventory and will conclude the session with an interpersonal formulation linking the adolescent's interpersonal situation with his depressed mood and placing the formulation within the framework of the problem areas.

CHAPTER 7

Selecting the Problem Area and Making the Treatment Contract

The final task in the initial phase of IPT-A is to provide the patient with an interpersonal formulation of his depression and make a specific contract for treatment. After completing a successful interpersonal diagnostic assessment, the problem area formulation should occur as a natural outgrowth of the recent discussions. The interpersonal problem area formulation will set the stage for the tasks of the middle phase.

CONNECTING DEPRESSION SYMPTOMS TO THE PROBLEM AREAS

Upon completion of the inventory, the therapist specifically explains her perception of the problematic interpersonal situation in the context of the depression to the patient. The therapist should begin with an overall summary of the important points that were made by the adolescent about his relationships during the past several sessions. It is helpful for the therapist to weave the narratives of each relationship into one larger interpersonal narrative for the adolescent, pointing out any noticeable patterns across relationships or relationships of meaningful proportions. While doing this, the therapist should continuously seek the adolescent's

opinion of her summary, giving the adolescent the opportunity to acknowledge the issues, to show understanding of the issues, and to disagree with the issues. The constantly changing nature of interpersonal
relationships should be stressed, but at this point in time, this is how his
relationships appear.

IDENTIFICATION OF MAJOR PROBLEM AREAS

Well-defined problem areas help the therapist formulate a strategy to improve interpersonal functioning within the context of the problem area.
Typically, it is best for short-term treatment to focus on one problem
area, but there are occasions when two problem areas may be identified.
In such a case, it may be helpful to prioritize the problem areas in terms
of which one to focus on initially. The four problem areas do not purport to cover all of the underlying dynamics of a depressive disorder. Instead, they serve to help focus the treatment on a specific circumstance
of interpersonal functioning that has potential for change and improvement and which may in turn generalize to other situations. The problem
areas that form the basis of establishing realistic goals for a brief treatment are (1) grief due to death; (2) interpersonal disputes with friends,
teachers, parents, and siblings; (3) role transitions such as changing
schools (e.g., elementary to junior high or junior high to high school),
entering puberty, becoming sexually active, birth of another sibling, becoming a parent, illness of a parent; and (4) interpersonal deficits such as
difficulty in initiating and maintaining relationships and communicating
about feelings.

PRESENTING THE INTERPERSONAL FORMULATION

It is important in these sessions to be more open-ended when talking
with the adolescent in order to enable him to describe the experiences in
his own words and to feel that he is being listened to and heard. The initial goal is to assist the adolescent in identifying the significant relationships, particularly the ones in which there are conflicts or difficulties.
Once the key relationships are identified, the therapist and patient can
more specifically address the actual difficulties, the potential to make
changes in the relationships, and possible strategies to facilitate these
changes. It is important to help the patient see the connections the therapist makes between situations, feelings, and functioning. These connections should be made explicit so that the focus of future sessions is clear.
For example, the therapist might say:

It seems from our discussions that you have been having conflicts with your parents. It is possible that these problems may be related to your feelings of depression, since these feelings emerged at the same time. Sometimes depression can make problems seem too large to handle. This is because you are depressed, not because you can't change the situation. As you feel better, you may find alternative ways to handle the situation. Over the next few weeks, we will meet once a week to talk about these problematic situations, and we will try to generate alternative ways to cope with the situation. At this time, medication does not appear necessary to relieve you of your symptoms but may be considered in the future if your symptoms continue.

CHALLENGES TO SETTING THE TREATMENT CONTRACT
Overlapping Problem Areas

At times it may appear that more than one problem area should be the target of treatment. This may occur, in part, because the majority of depressed adolescents appear as though they have interpersonal deficits. Despite that, all adolescents do not get identified as having the problem of interpersonal deficits. The deficits problem area is reserved for those adolescents for whom depression is associated with significant social withdrawal to the point that the adolescent no longer knows how to participate in his normal social milieu, receive social support, and establish friendships. For those adolescents who may be experiencing role disputes or transition problems, very often they are having these problems because of the need for better communication and problem-solving skills. However, these specific skill deficits underlying the dispute or transition problem do not require a secondary problem area of deficits. Rather, they become targets for enhancement and amelioration during treatment as part of the primary problem area.

It also is possible to perceive a specific relationship problem as both a dispute or transition or some combination of the two. In such instances, it is helpful to identify a primary and possibly a secondary problem area. To establish primacy, the therapist listens to how the adolescent describes the interpersonal problem and the framework within which the adolescent appears to place the events. For example, if the adolescent is most frequently emphasizing the conflict within the relationship, then it might be most logical to identify role disputes as the primary problem area. If the adolescent speaks of the difficulty of adjusting to a new situation that in turn has led to conflict, it might be more helpful to formulate the problem area as role transitions. The bottom line is that it will be most productive to work with the adolescent by using a language or perspective that is most consistent with the adolescent's use of language in describing the relationship. It is feasible to address the primary dispute and secondary transition effectively in the time-limited treatment because similar interpersonal strategies can be beneficial for both problem areas.

Disagreement about Problem Areas

There are circumstances in which the therapist and patient do not agree on the identified problem area and/or relevant interpersonal issues, or the patient and the psychotherapist may disagree about the appropriate focus. The disagreement may be due to a patient's denial of a particular problem's relationship to the depression or a minimization of the conflict. Four typical negative reactions include:

1. Denial of the psychological basis of the problems and attribution of the symptoms to a physical illness.
2. Unwillingness to acknowledge the possible connection between the symptoms, or functioning, and stressful life events.
3. Denial of the presence of symptoms altogether.
4. Blaming external circumstances or people, asserting, "If only my parents or my teachers were different, I would be fine," rather than assuming some responsibility for the problem.

We must preface the discussion of how to handle such negative reactions by reporting that such negative reactions are extremely rare in IPT-A. If a careful and comprehensive inventory has been conducted, the therapist and adolescent's formulations of the problem are usually quite similar. If different, there are several options for the therapist in such a situation:

1. Postpone identifying the specific problem area and goals until the patient gains a better understanding of the issue.
2. Begin with very general goals and increase the focus as the therapist gains an understanding of the patient's difficulties.
3. Agree to address the patient's concerns first with the idea that you will address your areas of concern afterward.
4. If the patient is correct, the therapist will need to revise the treatment plan.

If the therapist encounters a negative reaction to the interpersonal formulation and the adolescent refuses to engage in the treatment, it may be helpful to involve the parents in the treatment. Joint sessions should be held with the adolescent and parent to discuss each of their points of view in order to help the adolescent look at the problem from another perspective. The therapist's role at this time is not to argue with the patient or parent or to try to change anyone's mind. Rather, the therapist should acknowledge the patient's experience of the symptoms, acknowledge the patient's view of how it affects his or her functioning, and discuss how treatment may be beneficial. If the patient continues to disagree with the therapist's assessment of the situation, the therapist should try to engage the patient to come to the session next week so the therapist can again try to understand what is being experienced and how the therapist may be helpful. She might say:

> *I can understand that feeling sad a lot, having trouble sleeping, and having frequent headaches and stomachaches is unpleasant and uncomfortable. I know you want to find out what is causing them, and I want to help you try to do that over the next few weeks. Let's see how you are doing next week and discuss your concerns further then.*

It can often be helpful to review with the patient where you agree with the perceptions and where you may differ:

> *It seems we both agree that you are feeling sad almost every day, that you are having trouble sleeping, that you have lost your appetite, and that you don't feel like being with your friends the way you did previously. However, we have different views on what may be causing all these feelings for you. I suggested to you that conflict with your parents is related to your depression. Since you appear to disagree with that, I think we should continue to talk over the next few weeks and try to further understand what has been happening to you recently.*

If the therapist and patient are still unable to find common goals, then IPT-A may not be the appropriate treatment for this patient or at this particular time, and the patient should be referred for another form of treatment. It can be very frustrating for patients to feel that the therapist doesn't agree with or understand their point of view. This frustration may be manifested in acting-out behavior toward the therapy by not keeping appointments, arriving late, or stopping treatment. (The handling of such special problems is discussed in Chapter 15.) Again, keep in mind that disagreement on the problem area is a relatively rare occurrence, but these strategies will be helpful in the few instances in which this does occur.

TEACHING PATIENTS THEIR ROLE IN IPT

After identifying the patient's problem area and exploring the patient's goal for the problematic relationship, the therapist should explain to the patient the general techniques of the therapy. The patient actively participates in the treatment. Patients should understand that the focus of the sessions will be on difficulties that are occurring in the present, not the past. During sessions the patient should discuss the previous week's events or feelings that might be related to how the patient is currently feeling.

During the initial sessions, the IPT-A therapist is active and directive in conducting the review of symptoms, obtaining an interpersonal history, delineating treatment goals, and making the treatment contract. The therapist will be comparatively less directive and active during the middle phase of the therapy. It is necessary prior to beginning the middle phase of treatment to stress to the patient that he is responsible for selecting the topic of discussion for the ensuing sessions. The adolescent should be informed that the therapist will be less active than initially but will be there to ensure that the identified problem area is addressed. The therapist should explain that, although she will not ask as many questions as initially, it is not due to a lack of interest or involvement. Rather, she would like the adolescent to have the freedom to bring up topics and feelings related to the identified problem area that are most on his mind. To prepare the patient for the middle phase of treatment the therapist might say:

> In the past few sessions we have discussed your depressive symptoms and your significant relationships and have agreed upon a problem area of focus. In the sessions to come, we will be focusing on events and feelings related to this problem area. Your job will be to talk about these events and how your feelings may be affecting your relationships with others. We will discuss these situations in relation to the specific goals for change that we have identified. As we discuss these issues, other situations, feelings, or issues may come up that seem related to the problem area. You should feel free to discuss these topics as well so that we can explore their relation to the depression. It will be very important for you to talk about feelings as well as about the event itself. You are most in touch with your significant relationships and what is affecting you, so it is your role to monitor your feelings and select those topics for discussion that are most connected to feeling better. There are no right or wrong topics for discussion as long as they relate to your feelings. Therefore it is also important to share ideas or feelings that seem confusing or embarrassing to you.

This includes being free to discuss feelings about the therapy itself, me, and/or our relationship.

This discussion is considered part of the negotiation of the treatment contract, as it outlines the therapist's expectations for the patient's behavior in the session and acknowledges the patient's expectations for the therapist. This experience can be a good model of how to conduct such interpersonal negotiations within the context of other relationships.

Setting the Treatment Contract

Setting the treatment contract involves outlining the adolescent's and parents' roles in the treatment, identifying treatment goals, clarifying expectations for treatment, and outlining the "nuts and bolts" of treatment. Both the improvement in interpersonal functioning and reduction of symptoms are equally important achievements and most frequently will occur together. Therapist and patient should set goals that are likely to be attainable within the brief treatment so that the patient can feel the goals were achieved and can have a sense of progress throughout the treatment.

Case Example

A 12-year-old girl was brought by her mother for treatment with a depression of moderate severity. She was experiencing increasing academic difficulties, conflicts with her mother and siblings, and increasing social withdrawal. In addition, her father suffered from Alzheimer's disease and was taken care of by her mother and a full-time home attendant. During the course of the initial interview, it became clear that the girl was attempting to minimize the importance and repercussions of her father's illness and their impact on her life, denying that there were any problems to be worked out. She was reluctant to admit social isolation from peers and increasing conflict with her mother and sister.

In setting up the treatment contract, the therapist explained to the patient that she was dealing with many more difficulties than did most 12-year-olds. The therapist explained that her depression was in part precipitated by such stressful life events as living with a father with Alzheimer's disease, feeling different and isolated from peers due to the illness, and feeling neglected by her mother, who is preoccupied with caring for her ill husband. The therapist identified her primary problem area as role transitions. She was having difficulty making the transition from being a daughter in an intact family to being a daughter without a functional father and with a mother burdened by the care of her ill father. The therapist said to her:

> *You've had to make a transition from being a child to being someone who can take care of herself more. A second issue is how to make friends when it is not easy for them to come and visit you and how to explain to them what it is like at your house. A third problem seems to be how you handle your feelings toward your father: your sadness at his sickness, your anger at the burden he's become and his disruption of the house, and your anger at your mother for her preoccupation with your father so she cannot take care of you as she did before. There may be other problems you would like to add.*

The therapist provides the opportunity for the adolescent to disagree or add to the formulation of the problem. It is also helpful to have the patient repeat to the therapist her own version of the problem in her own words to ensure comprehension of the formulation and fuller integration with the patient's conceptualization of the problem. The therapist's view is that the stress of the transition was causing a significant amount of conflict with the girl's mother. After confirming that the adolescent was in agreement, the therapist stated to her that these resulting difficulties are problems that can be alleviated and conveyed optimism that she could feel better. Although the therapist cannot cure her father, she can help her find more satisfactory ways to deal with her changing role in the family and her feelings surrounding her father's illness and its disruption of her home and family relationships. Specifically, the therapist explains that by learning new ways to communicate her feelings in these difficult situations and to problem-solve alternative solutions to some difficult predicaments, the therapist believes that the patient's symptoms would decrease.

Emphasis on the Potential for Change

It is often helpful to identify different steps toward achieving the overall goal of recovery so that along the way the patient can realize several smaller achievements or signs of progress and change. For example, the therapist might tell the adolescent that over the next several weeks she likely will have more enthusiasm and energy to participate in her usual activities as she gains a clearer perspective on the problems in her interpersonal relationships and begins to feel better. The next step will be for the adolescent to try to make changes in her relationship so that the relationship is more mutually satisfying. The therapist and adolescent will explore practical ways of making these changes. Throughout the work of the therapy, the adolescent can expect to feel progressively less and less depressed as she resumes her previous activities and perhaps involves herself in new activities and relationships. This discussion should be very specific to an individual adolescent, keeping in mind what is realistic for the adolescent and what aspects of the adolescent and her circumstances may impose limitations on what can be achieved.

After discussion of the therapist's perception of the interpersonal problem and agreement on the focus of the treatment, discussion should turn to the practical aspects of the therapy. The therapist should educate the patient regarding expectations for involvement of family members, length of sessions, frequency of sessions, fee, management of missed or canceled sessions, the use of the telephone, and so on. The therapist states her expectations that the adolescent will attend regularly once a week for 12 sessions over 12 weeks. If the patient can't make the session, he needs to call and cancel and reschedule. The limits of confidentiality are again reviewed, as well as guidelines for telephone contact with the therapist and the importance of honesty in the therapeutic relationship. The culmination of this discussion is a specific verbal treatment contract. The points to be made in the contract include the following:

The Importance of Honesty

I would like you to feel comfortable with me and trust me, but I realize that it takes time to build these feelings. We've been working together for 4 weeks, and in that time I feel we have started to do that. I hope that as we get to know each other better you will be able to be open with me about all that you are feeling and thinking because in that way I can be of the most help to you. If you ever feel that you can't tell me what you're feeling, let's try to talk about that.

The Confidentiality Limits of the Interactions

What we talk about is confidential between the two of us, and I won't tell your parents unless I become concerned that your behavior poses a danger to yourself or others. If I feel the need to discuss things with your parents, I will tell you first before I do so. I will give you the opportunity to discuss it with me, and if I agree with your reasons for not telling them, I won't tell them. But if I don't agree, I will tell them, but we can discuss the manner in which I do so.

The Interpersonal Context of the Intervention

We have already agreed that your depression is affected by your relationships and, in turn, negatively affects those relationships. Over the next few weeks, we will continue to explore your depression in relation to possible stressors and/or conflicts in your daily life and relationships.

The Brief Nature of the Psychotherapy: Approximately 12 Weeks of Therapy Meeting Once a Week for About 45 Minutes

We will meet once a week for 12 weeks, for about 45 minutes each time, to talk about what is happening in your relationships and how the relationship difficulties might be related to your depression. Together we will try to find ways in which you can change your relationships and feel better.

Telephone Contact

During the first 4 weeks of treatment I will call in between sessions to check on how you are feeling. If at any time you feel the need to talk to me in between the sessions, please call. It also is important that you phone if you cannot make an appointment so that we can reschedule and at least make some contact by phone. There may be times when you call that I can't talk to you, but I will arrange a mutually convenient time for us to talk.

SUMMARY

These tasks complete the initial phase of therapy, the assessment phase. However, the therapy has already begun. The therapist has presented the adolescent with the interpersonal formulation of her depression, and they have agreed on one primary problem area as the focus of treatment. The specific treatment contract has been established in which the guidelines for therapy such as duration, cancellations, and confidentiality have been delineated. The adolescent's role in the therapeutic process has been outlined, and patient and therapist are poised to go forward into the middle phase of treatment. The middle phase will be discussed in depth in the chapter that follows and in the chapters on each of the specific problem areas.

CHAPTER 8

The Middle Phase of IPT-A

OVERVIEW OF THE MIDDLE PHASE OF TREATMENT

Following agreement on the treatment contract and the identified problem area, the middle phase of treatment begins. Typically this occurs by session 5 and continues through session 8. The middle sessions focus on the problem area identified in the initial sessions as a means towards achieving the goals of the treatment: alleviation of depression symptoms and improvement in interpersonal functioning.

The *objectives* of the middle phase of treatment for all adolescents include (1) further clarification of the problem area, (2) identification of effective strategies to attack the problem, and (3) implementation of interventions to bring about resolution of the problem. The tasks that target these objectives depend largely on the particular problem area being addressed, but there are some more general tasks that are appropriate for all problem areas. The general *tasks* associated with the middle phase of treatment are as follows:

1. Monitor depressive symptoms and consider adjunctive therapy such as medication if there is no improvement or a worsening of symptoms.
2. Enable the patient to discuss topics relevant to the identified problem area.
3. Monitor feelings the patient associates with the events discussed and with the therapeutic relationship. Facilitate the patient's self-disclosure of his affective state.

4. Schedule regular meetings and/or phone consultations with parents for counseling and education.
5. Maintain an alliance with the patient's parents so they will continue to support the treatment.

As stated above, there are more specific tasks for the middle phase associated with each of the problem areas. These tasks are discussed in the subsequent chapters that address the particular problem areas.

CONDUCTING THE MIDDLE PHASE OF TREATMENT

Before discussing the key components and issues involved in conducting the middle phase of IPT-A treatment, we want to highlight several characteristics of this phase of treatment. Although IPT-A is a manualized treatment, it differs somewhat from other treatment manuals in its degree of structure and proscribed steps for each session. The components of the therapy are intended to be somewhat more fluid; tasks can occur in multiple sessions, depending upon the progress the patient is making and the identified focus of the treatment. The initial sessions of IPT-A are more structured than the middle phase, requiring the therapist to accomplish specific tasks in the sessions while leaving some flexibility about the timing and flow of the sessions. During the middle phase of treatment, the treatment is less specific in its session proscriptions, as the tasks are implemented in varying combinations depending upon the particular patient and identified problem area. Although there are clear objectives and tasks for this phase and guidelines for accomplishing them, this phase focuses more on the process of working through interpersonal problems in contrast to the systematic gathering of symptom and interpersonal diagnostic information. As such, sequences of tasks and processes are explained in detail, but each patient is unique, and the sequences and patterns for recovery will differ somewhat from patient to patient. This work of the middle phase also differs to some degree depending on the particular problem area(s) being addressed. Consequently, the clinician must look to both this introductory chapter on the middle phase and relevant problem area(s) chapters to implement this phase of treatment.

Roles in Treatment

During the initial sessions, the therapist directs the treatment while assessing the patient's depression symptomatology and establishing its association with the patient's interpersonal relationships. Treatment focus now shifts responsibility to the patient to contribute ongoing information that is related to the agreed-upon problem area. The patient must take a more active stance in bringing in the relevant information related to the identified problem area.

In the middle phase of treatment, the role of the patient shifts from providing historical information to actively searching for solutions to the problem. By now, the patient should be feeling more comfortable with self-disclosure and be more at ease in discussing interpersonal relationships and feelings. The patient is encouraged to talk about events that occurred during the past week related to his problem area and to describe feelings associated with those events. This allows the therapist and patient to relate those events to the identified problem area and therefore to the patient's depression. The therapist then assists the patient in clarification of the problem and discussion of ways to improve the situation, or the patient's approach to the situation. The patient is encouraged in the discussion through the use of continuous feedback from the therapist regarding progress in the use of the strategies or techniques and decreases in depressive symptomatology. Changes in functioning are constantly being identified and reflected back to the patient. The positive feedback bolsters self-esteem and a sense of competence in changing the social interactions and/or adapting to circumstances.

The therapist's role in the treatment also changes in the shift from the initial to the middle phase. In general, the therapist remains active in the session: patient and therapist, together, decide the focus of treatment, discuss the preceding week's events or feelings, and clarify the conflicts and generate solutions. As always, the therapist monitors improvement of depressive symptoms. The therapist must continue to monitor the patient's self-disclosures to see if it is necessary to alter the focus of treatment. The therapist works collaboratively with the patient as a team facilitating the patient's engagement in problem formulation and clarification of feelings. The therapist's role gradually shifts at this time in treatment from the role of directing the session topics and systematically gathering information to partnering with the patient to hear about the currently identified interpersonal situation, analyzing the problems, and together generating solutions and new means of communication. As the patient takes on increasing responsibility for reporting events and feelings, the therapist's role becomes slightly less active. The degree of shift depends largely on the patient and his ability to take on the more active role.

Structure and Focus of Middle-Phase Sessions

The focus of the middle phase proceeds logically from the topics identified in the interpersonal inventory and in the delineated treatment contract. Discussion progresses from the general problems to the specific expectations and perceptions of the situation, to generation of alternative solutions, to the eventual efforts at changing behaviors and attempting new solutions.

During the middle phase of treatment, the therapist and patient continually assess the accuracy of the initial formulation of the problem in order to maximize the amount of change that can be accomplished in the treatment. The therapist must keep the patient's discussions relevant to the identified problem areas. If this proves increasingly difficult, it may be necessary for the therapist to review with the patient the reasons for choosing the particular problem area and to discuss the possibility of revising which problem area they will focus on.

The sessions generally begin with the patient being encouraged to select the topic of discussion as it relates to the problem area. The therapist begins the session by either waiting for the patient to initiate discussion or by asking a general question about what transpired since the preceding session, such as "What has happened in the past week since I saw you last?" or "How have you been feeling this past week?" The patient's silence and/or difficulty starting a session are not interpreted except as it relates to the problem area. For example, the therapist might begin the session by saying:

> *Last time we met we were talking about the fight you had with your mother over your boyfriend. We discussed ways for you to handle this kind of situation in the future. I am sure things have come up since I saw you last. Perhaps you can tell me about what has happened.*

The therapist will usually conclude the session with a synopsis of themes brought out in the session and their relationship to the identified problem area.

Much of the focus of the middle sessions is on what occurs outside of the treatment sessions. The patient is likely to begin to apply some of what is discussed to situations outside of the sessions. For example, after discussing negotiation strategies with the therapist, the patient may try the strategies out at home and then report the next week on their success or the difficulties encountered. The therapist should monitor the patient's outside functioning to obtain a better perspective on the problem and/or improvements. For adolescents, this may mean periodic school contacts with a guidance counselor to assess current school performance and family contacts to assess progress at home. The need for revision of the treatment focus may occur as new information about the patient's interpersonal relationships becomes available.

Use of the Therapist–Patient Relationship

During the middle phase, the therapist should pay close attention to his or her own feelings toward the patient and to the progress of the treatment. This is especially true if the patient's identified problem area is interpersonal deficits. By monitoring one's own reactions to the patient, the therapist may be able to better understand the patient's interpersonal difficulties. It is the therapist's role to relate interpersonal strategies used in session to those that may be used in relationships outside of the session. The therapist addresses the interpersonal style seen within the therapist–patient relationship only if it pertains to an interpersonal style and problem that is occurring outside the session. By working out the interpersonal problems in the relationship with the therapist, the patient is afforded a safe opportunity for role playing or communication clarification. These strategies resemble working with transference and countertransference; however, IPT differs from psychodynamic psychotherapy in its specific treatment of the therapist–patient relationship. While psychodynamic psychotherapy would encourage the development of the transference, IPT brings these feelings quickly into the open to be discussed in relation to difficulties within the identified problem area. Therefore, the feelings are discussed earlier and more overtly and are directly related to current interpersonal functioning.

Involvement of Others in Sessions

Other family members or significant others may be asked to participate in one or two sessions during the middle phase of treatment. For example, in the case of a role dispute, the therapist may ask the patient and the other person in the dispute to attend a session together in order to assist in negotiation or to clarify the other person's expectations for the relationship. This is particularly helpful in cases where the patient is having trouble negotiating a relationship at home. Family members have been prepared for this possibility during the initial phase of treatment when they discussed the depression and the process of treatment with the therapist. The therapist must be vigilant in these sessions to ensure that all participants remain focused on the identified problem area and that the discussions are constructive rather than destructive.

Maintaining a Brief Treatment Time Frame

One of the most important aspects of this phase of treatment is keeping the time frame of the brief treatment as a salient aspect of the treatment. The therapist should place the treatment plan, strategies, and goals in a time frame and make the patient aware of how many more sessions are remaining. Researchers have written about changes in the rate of a patient's progress as the brief treatment continues. They have found that the most important activities of brief therapy that result in some degree of change occur during the first 8 sessions of treatment (Garfield, 1986; Howard, Kopata, Krause, & Orlinsky, 1986).

To assist the patient in completing treatment, the therapist should emphasize the patient's role in making changes in behavior and/or understanding interpersonal relationships. Although the middle sessions are more fluid and process-oriented than the initial sessions of treatment, there are clear objectives, and these should be shared with the patient. It is important to make the treatment goals as unambiguous and overt as possible. The goal is to instill a sense of mastery and to maximize the patient's sense of competence to continue using these improved interpersonal skills. Each of the phases of interpersonal psychotherapy builds upon the preceding phase, and the therapist must help the patient prepare for the next phase of treatment.

ISSUES ENCOUNTERED DURING THE MIDDLE PHASE OF TREATMENT

Managing Peripheral Material Presented by Patients

If peripheral material is introduced in the session or significant topics are being avoided, the therapist must decide if what is being discussed is somehow relevant to the problem and then bring the situation to the attention of the patient. The perceived tangentiality of the material should be discussed with the patient prior to shifting the focus to more pertinent information. It is important to allow time to explore for relevance because it does not necessarily emerge initially. If the patient actually presents information that does not appear related to the identified problem area, the therapist might say:

> *It seems that today you are talking about* [topic]. *I'm not sure how this is related to the other issues we have been discussing in relation to your problem with* [identified problem area]. *How do you see the two topics as related? If they are not related, which issue do you feel is more related to your current depression? Let's focus on what appears most related to your current depression.*

To clarify relevance, the therapist should refocus on what the patient is saying and explore its relationship to issues that previously have been the focus of treatment.

It is not unusual for a patient to initially present minor issues and later in the treatment focus on more relevant issues. Conversely, it is not uncommon for a patient to withdraw from discussion and minimize a problem area that may be the one most related to their depression. Both reactions may stem from discomfort with intimate self-disclosure, lack of understanding about the problem, and/or distrust of the therapeutic relationship. In such instances, the treatment contract may need to be revised and renegotiated during the beginning of the middle phase of treatment.

Management of Crises

As a result of uncovering and identifying feelings associated with significant relationships, crises sometimes arise. Feelings can become intensified as a result of increased communication between the patient and a significant other. Concurrently, the patient's depression or anger may increase and result in acting-out behavior or suicidal ideation. It is important for the therapist to try to anticipate such a crisis by helping the patient to anticipate the consequences of the actions or discussion and the feelings that might be generated in the other person by the disclosures. The therapist should review with the patient possible reactions to the statements, how particular responses to the disclosures could be handled, and the feelings surrounding them. By preparing the patient for the possible outcomes, any expressions or behavior will be less shocking and disturbing and less likely to precipitate a crisis situation. When this fails and a crisis occurs, the crisis takes precedence and becomes the immediate focus of treatment. It is beneficial if the therapist can relate the crisis to the identified problem area, but this is not always immediately possible. In order to bring about a swift resolution of the crisis, sessions may be scheduled more frequently for a time. (Refer to the section on crisis management in Chapter 17 for further explication.)

Maintaining an Interpersonal Focus of Treatment

One of the most commonly reported challenges reported by clinicians is maintaining the interpersonal focus of the treatment. This is a challenge in part because of the slightly less structured nature of the middle phase of treatment. In our work with clinicians, particularly those in community settings, time and practical constraints often limit their opportunities for both supervision and processing of sessions. Take time prior to the sessions to mentally review the focus of the preceding session and think about what strategies you might want to introduce in these middle phase sessions so as to continue to maintain a focus on the interpersonal process. Ask yourself such questions as: (1) What tasks and objectives related to the problem area and the middle phase in general were accomplished today? (2) How did our discussion relate to the problem area? (3) What is the next logical step toward the relevant objectives? and (4) How can I help the adolescent accomplish this in the remaining sessions? Finally, presenting the patient with a summary of the session's focus and how it relates to the problem area and course of treatment is another important way to ensure that treatment adherence is occurring.

Managing Patients' Frustration with the Treatment Process

Treatment and change are not easy. We have often found that patients who were highly motivated and on-board during the initial phase of treatment can become frustrated by the pace of change, the necessity of small steps, and the hard work needed to bring about these changes. This also is true for patients' families. The therapist needs to highlight changes and improvements, as small as they may be, for the patient and family members. It is often necessary to repeatedly explain to patients that even very small changes in communication style can lead to more substantial changes in symptoms and functioning. Alternatively, the middle phase can often be the time when resistance to change becomes more apparent. The therapist should remain aware of this and explore any resistance as it occurs. This issue is discussed in more detail in Chapter 15, on clinical issues in treating depressed adolescents.

SUMMARY

During the middle phase of treatment, the therapist narrows the focus of therapy to a specific problem area, helps generate strategies, and suggests the application of techniques that will lead to clarification and resolution of the patient's problem. The therapist and patient play active roles together by collaborating on tasks that serve to provide support and direction for the adolescent. Formulated strategies may necessitate the involvement of significant others, such as parents, both in and outside of the sessions. The expectation of a 12-week treatment duration must be emphasized as goals are targeted and interventions are implemented. It is also important to continuously review the changes observed to increase the patient's feeling of competence. The patient's education continues throughout each phase of treatment, illuminating the process of identifying problems, clarifying the issues, generating strategies, applying strategies for problem resolution, and acquiring skills that result in increased interpersonal self-confidence and improved functioning. By reviewing these steps with the patient at the end of the middle phase and at the beginning of the termination phase, the therapist assists in fostering the patient's independent use of interpersonal problem-solving techniques in future situations.

Chapter 9 provides detailed descriptions of the techniques used in IPT-A as well case examples to further illustrate these techniques. Chapters 10–13 focus on the four potential problem areas of IPT-A: grief, interpersonal role disputes, interpersonal role transitions, and interpersonal deficits. Specific tasks associated with each of these problem areas are delineated and discussed.

CHAPTER 9

Therapeutic Techniques

It is important to keep in mind that the techniques employed in IPT-A are not unique. They are techniques that may be used in other treatment orientations. What is unique is the manner in which they are used in the IPT-A treatment framework of identified problem areas. In this chapter we will describe the various techniques employed as part of IPT-A treatment. The descriptions are aimed not only at giving the reader an understanding of the techniques but also at addressing the issues involved in employing these techniques specifically with adolescents. Examples of many of the techniques are provided.

EXPLORATORY TECHNIQUES

IPT-A employs a combination of nondirective and directive exploratory techniques. Simply stated, nondirective exploration involves the use of open-ended questions or nondirective statements with no specific endpoint in mind. Such techniques include, but are not limited to, supportive acknowledgment, extension of the topic being discussed by the patient, and receptive silence (Weissman et al., 2000). Each of these techniques constitutes a way in which the therapist encourages the patient to continue to explore an idea, insight, feeling, or theory without inserting the therapist's agenda into the session. Directive exploratory techniques include more targeted questioning and interviewing. Examples of directive exploration include a clinical interview focusing on a patient's depression symptoms and the interpersonal inventory. The therapist should keep the current treatment objective in mind to ensure that questioning leads in a productive direction.

When and with Whom to Use Exploratory Techniques

The therapist must consider the treatment objective she is trying to achieve, the stage of treatment, and the nature and style of the particular patient when deciding what type of technique to employ. Nondirective exploratory techniques are most helpful when the therapist is looking to explore an area for which she has limited information or no specific hypotheses. They are helpful techniques to use intermittently, early in treatment, to ensure that the patient feels heard and respected while working to develop the therapeutic relationship. Directive techniques are equally critical in a short-term treatment wherein only a limited time is allotted to reach specific goals and objectives. They can be used when specific types of information are required to accomplish a treatment objective, to ensure patient safety, or to clarify the clinical status of a patient.

Nondirective techniques are most effective with patients who are verbal, insightful, organized, and less apt to become overwhelmed. Patients who are more severely depressed or who have difficulty managing their emotions may find the lack of structure and guidance inherent in these techniques anxiety-provoking and overwhelming. Patients who are more disorganized or whose lives are chaotic can "get lost" in the lack of structure and spend unproductive time jumping from discussion of one stressor or crisis to another. These latter types of patients will most likely benefit more from the use of directive exploratory techniques.

Special Issues for Adolescents

Adolescents need the chance to be heard and to feel a sense of control and mastery over the treatment situation, as they do with all tasks and relationships in their lives. Nondirective techniques can provide this opportunity by allowing the adolescent an opportunity to direct part of the session, thereby helping the adolescent to feel respected and powerful in the treatment process. At the same time, adolescents clearly require structure. They live in the moment. On any given day, they may walk into your office with nothing to say or with a litany of events they wish to discuss that day. Although many of the events may be in some way relevant to the course of treatment, hearing each of these in detail can occupy the better part of any treatment session and leave the adolescent feeling as overwhelmed and depressed as he was at the start of treatment. The therapeutic process can feel extremely foreign and daunting to the adolescent. By providing structure to treatment and employing directive techniques, when appropriate, the therapist can help remove some of the mystery of the therapeutic process and diminish the confusion an adolescent may feel while in treatment.

Common Challenges to Implementation

> When I try to lead the way in treatment and ask direct questions of my patient, she just responds with one-word responses such as "OK" or statements like "I don't know." If I just let her talk, she can go on and on about whatever is on her mind. She seems to "get things off her chest," but she becomes more sullen and seems annoyed if I try to redirect her. How do I deal with this?

This is a common dilemma experienced, particularly by therapists who are accustomed to doing more nondirective supportive treatment. It is a delicate balance to establish a relationship with the patient by allowing him to be heard while moving the treatment along in a productive manner, but this balance is critical. Many of our therapists have commented that once they found a way to establish this balance, they felt like treatment was much more productive and that they actually accomplished something versus just managing the "crisis of the day."

In trying to find this balance with a somewhat resistant adolescent patient, there are a number of things that you can do. First, continue to use nondirective exploration and give the adolescent the time to share what's on his mind, while providing moderate structure to this discussion. For example, say:

> It seems that you have a lot on your mind when you come in here, and it is difficult to work on the goals we have made until you can say what you need to say. I suggest we take 5 minutes at the start of each session for you to air things out from your day and to let me know what is on your mind. Then, I will remind us what we are working on and see how what you talked about may or may not be connected to our goals.

It is important to pay attention to the types of questions you are asking and to continue to use open-ended questions within directive exploration. This makes it more difficult for the patient to shut down the conversation with one-word responses.

ENCOURAGEMENT OF AFFECT

Encouragement of affect refers to a range of techniques used to help the patient express, understand, and manage his various affective states. Encouragement of affect includes (1) facilitating acknowledgement and acceptance of painful affects about events or issues, (2) helping a patient use his affective experiences in making interpersonal change, and (3) encouraging the development of new, desirable affects that may facilitate growth and change (Weissman et al., 2000). In IPT-A, a key concept is connecting one's affective states with the interpersonal context in which they occur. This occurs throughout all phases of IPT-A treatment and is integral to the process of therapeutic change. More specifically, the IPT-A therapist is always listening for and commenting on the link between affective states and experiences and interpersonal events impacting the adolescent. When one or the other becomes the subject of treatment, the therapist works to relate it to the other dimension of interpersonal interactions.

This category of techniques takes many forms over the course of treatment. One specific IPT-A technique related to the encouragement of affect is the "depression circle." The therapist, in consultation with the adolescent at the end of the initial phase of treatment, creates a depression circle to illustrate a schematic representation of the connection between events in relationships and the adolescent's affective experience, specifically his depressed mood. The circle tells the story of the adolescent's specific experience and helps to illustrate places in which to intervene to break the depression cycle. This circle can then be used periodically throughout treatment to highlight repetitions of the pattern, to identify potential areas for change and to document improvements when they occur by making alterations in the circle. Figure 9.1 presents an example of a depression circle. The following is an explanation a therapist might provide to an adolescent.

> *Jerry, this circle represents the pattern we have been talking about over the course of our last few meetings. It shows how your depressed and angry feelings, as well as some of your other depressive symptoms, are related to interpersonal events that have occurred in your life. Starting at the top, your father left you and your mother 2 years ago. Your mother was very upset and depended on you for support and for doing a lot of things around the house. You were angry and sad about your father leaving and felt guilty that maybe you had done something, but you were also concerned about your mother being overwhelmed, so you kept your feelings to yourself and shut down.*

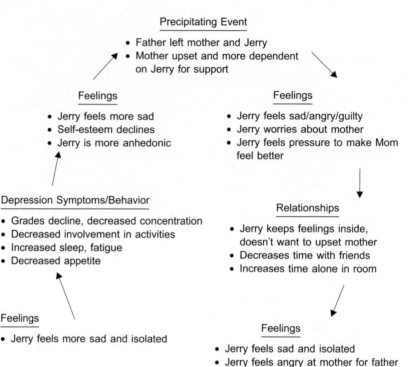

FIGURE 9.1. Jerry's depression circle.

You spent less time with your friends and more time alone. This time away from people made you feel more isolated and sad. You also started to feel angry with your mother because you needed to do so much around the house and you "had to worry about her so much." Your mother felt like you were pulling away, becoming more irritable and distant. Your friends stopped calling as much because you rarely seemed interested in spending time with them. This made you feel more sad and isolated. Your grades have dropped, and you have pulled out of activities that you used to enjoy, in part, because you are feeling so sad. Doing poorly in school has made you feel worse about yourself, and not doing the things you enjoy has made you feel more isolated. Do you see how things that happen in your life with friends and family are related to your depression? Is there anything you don't agree with? Is there anything you would want to add to the circle? What I also want you to see from this circle is that there are various places where we can try to make a change in this circle and in the pattern so that it does not keep going and so you can feel better.

In the same session and in subsequent sessions, it is advisable to have the adolescent describe the depression circle in his own words.

When and with Whom to Use Encouragement of Affect

There are several issues to consider in the timing of when to use techniques for encouraging affective expression. First, the therapist must have a clear idea as to her goal with respect to affective expression. IPT-A does not generally support the notion that simply expressing feelings with no structure or end goal is necessarily beneficial. Affective expression should lead to greater understanding of emotions and their impact on relationships. Second, the therapist must consider the adolescent's capacity to tolerate the expression of his feelings and the ability to modulate his affective expression as needed. Some adolescents may become overwhelmed and disorganized by this experience, particularly those adolescents who lack adequate support systems to help them manage their reactions to such affects. The therapist will need to proceed slowly in these cases and combine affective expression with training in skills that involve effective communication strategies to prevent the intensification of the affect.

In trying to help the adolescent develop and recognize alternatives, or more positive affective experiences, therapists may have to do what can be called "affect training." This training involves teaching the patient to identify his feelings in the context of his interpersonal experiences. Some therapists use "feeling cards," which depict various feeling states and discuss when people might experience such a feeling, as well as when the adolescent has experienced this feeling state and how he behaves when feeling this way. While some adolescents will need only minimal training, others will need more extensive training with some repetition from session to session.

Special Issues for Use with Adolescents

It is our experience that adolescents are often of two types with respect to affective experience. There are those adolescents who experience their affects intensely and can readily express them. They have limited understanding of the events in their lives—particularly interpersonal—that may be associated with those affective states. Such adolescents will walk into a therapist's office and readily express their feelings, but often experience those feeling states as coming out of nowhere. When asked about what may have happened related to their feelings, they often respond blankly. They have difficulty recalling events and even more difficulty understanding their association with their feelings. These adolescents experience feelings as "out of their control."

The other type of adolescent can give the therapist a detailed description of every event that has occurred over the past day or week with absolutely no mention of any affective experience. When asked about how they felt during an event, such adolescents might respond, "I don't know," "fine," or shrug their shoulders. For this latter type, it is helpful to ask how they responded behaviorally in the situation and then ask what emotion is most often associated with such a behavior. For example, when asked how it felt when he fought with his father, the adolescent said, "Fine, I don't care." But when asked what he did at the end of the argument, he reports that he went into his room and punched his fist into his pillow. The therapist then asks, "What do people usually feel when they punch a pillow repeatedly after an argument?" Either the adolescent will volunteer the feeling of "angry" or the therapist can assist in labeling it that way by saying, "Usually when people punch a pillow they feel angry and/or upset." "I wonder if you get angry after these arguments and if the anger eventually turns to sadness?" By distancing the emotion from the adolescent and talking about "people" it is sometimes easier for adolescents to initially acknowledge the affect. For both types of adolescents, encouragement of affect involves educating them in the identification and labeling of emotions as well as using standard therapeutic techniques to foster the expression of affect.

COMMUNICATION ANALYSIS

Communication analysis is aimed at identifying ways in which the patient's communication is ineffective and fails to achieve the goal of the communication. The goal of this technique is to teach the patient to communicate in a more effective manner by increasing his clarity and directness. The therapist helps the adolescent understand the impact of his words on others, examining the feelings conveyed by the words in comparison to the feelings that generated the verbal exchange.

Five categories of ineffective communication have been identified and constitute areas for intervention. Patients may be (1) using ambiguous, indirect, and/or nonverbal communication rather than using open confrontation; (2) holding incorrect assumptions, which are then communicated; (3) using unnecessarily indirect verbal communication; (4) using "silencing" (often described by teens and their parents as "the silent treatment") wherein they close off communication; and (5) using hostile communication, which leads to either hostile or passive responses from those with whom they are interacting (Weissman et al., 2000).

Communication analysis involves doing a thorough investigation of a specific dialogue or argument that occurred between the patient and another person. Of course, the therapist is not privy to the details of this interaction and must rely on the reporting and memory skills of the patient. As such, the IPT-A therapist must be skilled at helping the patient to re-create interactions in the therapy session. This involves helping him to identify a specific, significant interaction and encouraging his recall and reporting of the details including all dimensions of the interaction (e.g., verbal and nonverbal communications, feelings generated, and responses given). If the patient was automatically skilled at this, he would not need the assistance of communication analysis. Therefore, the therapist will need to do a considerable amount of prodding and cueing. Keep in mind that the goals of communication analysis are to help the patient understand (1) the impact of his words on others, (2) the feelings he conveys with verbal and nonverbal communication, and (3) the feelings that

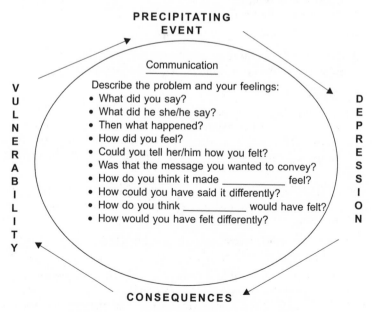

PRECIPITATING EVENT

Communication

Describe the problem and your feelings:
- What did you say?
- What did he she/he say?
- Then what happened?
- How did you feel?
- Could you tell her/him how you felt?
- Was that the message you wanted to convey?
- How do you think it made _____ feel?
- How could you have said it differently?
- How do you think _____ would have felt?
- How would you have felt differently?

VULNERABILITY

DEPRESSION

CONSEQUENCES

FIGURE 9.2. Functional analysis of communication.

generated the verbal or nonverbal exchange. The hope is that through the use of communication analysis the therapist can break the cycle of negative or ineffective communication that forms an integral part of the depression circle described earlier in this chapter. Figure 9.2 is a schematic representation of how effective communication can interrupt the cycle of depression.

Putting communication analysis to use involves teaching alternative communication strategies, including (1) communicating feelings and opinions directly, (2) using empathy (e.g., give to get), and (3) putting yourself in the other person's shoes to see their perspective. Communication analysis involves dissection of the communication into its separate statements and behavior change techniques discussed in the following section.

Case Example

This is an example of a communication analysis conducted in the middle phase of treatment.

THERAPIST: Mary, we have been talking about your relationship with your mother and how you feel that she just doesn't care about you because she doesn't let you do things like other teenagers, such as going to the movies and hanging out in the neighborhood. I was wondering if you and your mother had any difficulties during the past week.

PATIENT: We always have problems.

THERAPIST: Can you remember a specific time during the past week when you had an argument with your mother?

PATIENT: Two days ago.

THERAPIST: What I would like you to do is to tell me as much as you can about the argument you had with your mother. I want you to tell me things like who said and did what, when things happened, and how you were feeling. First of all, how did it start?

PATIENT: I was talking on the phone with my friend Julie and my mother walked in and just started yelling at me that I didn't do anything around the house.

THERAPIST: Had anything happened before your mother started yelling about that?

PATIENT: No. She had just walked in the house from work, and she starts yelling—always at me—no one else. She knew I was on the phone, and she just embarrasses me. She just doesn't want me to have any friends.

THERAPIST: So, what exactly did your mother say when she walked in the door?

PATIENT: She didn't even look at me. She just started yelling about how I didn't clean up the kitchen and my school stuff was all over the living room. And then she said to get off the phone.

THERAPIST: OK, what I want you to do now is tell me the different things you and your mother said to each other.

PATIENT: I don't remember exactly.

THERAPIST: I want you to do your best. Say it as best as you can remember.

PATIENT: Well, OK. My mom said, "Mary, what are you doing on the phone? The house is a mess—you didn't even clean up the kitchen, and look at your books and shoes lying on the living room floor. I want you to get off the phone and clean up around here!"

THERAPIST: And how did that make you feel?

PATIENT: I was mad because I was having this really good conversation and in this good mood, and she came in and ruined it. She always says I don't do anything.

THERAPIST: And what did you say in response to your mother?

PATIENT: I told her I would get off . . . but then I didn't . . . I wanted to keep talking.

THERAPIST: Can you remember exactly what you said and how you said it and tell it to me the same way?

PATIENT: I think I said, "OK, OK, I'll get off." But then I stayed on when she walked out of the room.

THERAPIST: And how do you think your mother felt?

PATIENT: Like I didn't care about what she wanted.

THERAPIST: What did your mother say or do next?

PATIENT: My mom gave me that look . . . and, well, I got off the phone, picked up my stuff, and went into my room.

THERAPIST: Did you say anything else to your mother?

PATIENT: No. We didn't talk the rest of the night. I just pretended she wasn't there.

THERAPIST: What we are now going to do is go back and see if there is anything you could have said differently that might have made the whole situation end differently and feel differently. When your mother came home and asked you to get off the phone, what could you have said that might have led to a different conversation and feelings?

PATIENT: I could have said OK, not sounding so annoyed, and then I could have gotten right off the phone.

THERAPIST: That is a start, but I am not sure that would change all of what happened. How would you have felt if you said that?

PATIENT: Probably the same as I did. Well, I wouldn't have felt as bad about stressing out my mom, but I would have been angry because she jumped all over me and made me get off the phone.

THERAPIST: So what else could you have said?

PATIENT: Well, I couldn't talk to her while I was on the phone.

THERAPIST: So what else could you have said to your mother after getting off the phone?

PATIENT: I guess once she calmed down, I could have told her that I know she had a long day and I am sorry that the kitchen wasn't all cleaned up, but that I did do a lot around the house already today and I just wanted to talk to my friend for a little while [EM-PATHY].

THERAPIST: Say it to me as if I am your mother.

PATIENT: Mom, I know you had a long day, and I am sorry you were upset by the mess in the kitchen when you came home [SEEING ANOTHER PERSON'S PERSPECTIVE], but I feel a little angry that you didn't notice all the cleaning I did do. I was going to clean up the kitchen after I got off the phone. I just wanted to talk to Erica for a few minutes. Can I please call her back and finish our conversation and then I will clean up some more?

THERAPIST: How would you and your mother have felt then?

PATIENT: I guess I would have felt a little better, and my mom might have felt better, like I understood her feelings a little.

THERAPIST: How do you think your mother might have responded?

PATIENT: Maybe she would have said that it was OK for me to call her back or at least said I did a good job on the other cleaning. Maybe she would have apologized for yelling.

When and with Whom to Use Communication Analysis

Communication analysis is a very useful tool for many adolescents. Most commonly, it is used during the middle phase of treatment when the therapist and patient are addressing the specific objectives of a given problem area. Communication analysis also can be useful during the interpersonal inventory while trying to clarify the problem area, particularly if a role dispute is in question. During the initial phase, however, the therapist is careful to use the technique to gather specific information regarding the adolescent's style of communicating his feelings and opinions without moving to the step of intervening in the communication. Intervention is saved for the middle phase once clear goals and objectives are set within the agreed upon problem area. Although communication analysis can be a useful strategy for all of the problem areas, it is particularly useful with role disputes since many difficulties between the patient and significant other are the result of ineffective communication, specifically poor negotiation skills.

Special Issues for Use with Adolescents

Communication analysis, which can be somewhat reminiscent of typical teenage "he said, she said," comes fairly easily to many adolescents and has an entertainment appeal. To others, however, the quest for specific details of the interaction can prove frustrating, particularly because they are not accustomed to paying attention to those details. This will take practice. For younger or more cognitively concrete adolescents, it can be difficult to track all of the information in their heads. It can be useful to draw a diagram (or even a cartoon for the younger adolescents) representing what was said by each person and his or her feelings in the situation.

Common Challenges to Implementation

My patient can never think of a specific interaction to discuss. Or when she comes up with something, it is vague and she can't provide any details. How can I do a communication analysis?

These patients can be difficult. Use your creativity and remember that you might have to step back and teach basic skills first, such as teaching them about the parts of an interaction (e.g., verbal and nonverbal) and how to attend to these details. You might need to devise a tracking method for the patient so that information can get recorded more immediately. (See the "Adjunctive Techniques" section later in this chapter.) You could create a list of questions, with the patient's help, that he would then answer more immediately following an interaction. Another alternative is to start by using an interaction between you (the therapist) and the patient. Here you have the advantage of knowing all the details of the interaction. You can use a relatively simple interaction to begin with as a teaching device so that they can learn to be better reporters of the events that happen during the week.

BEHAVIOR CHANGE TECHNIQUES

Directive Techniques

Directive techniques for behavior change include educating, advising, limit setting, and modeling (Weissman et al., 2000). These techniques are particularly important for use with adolescents, although they must be balanced with less active and more patient-driven interventions. The educational aspect of IPT-A is aimed at building knowledge, competencies, and skills in the adolescent. The therapist accomplishes this by identifying not only problems that the adolescent has in the conduct of relationships but also strengths that he has in interpersonal skills. Advising involves giving more direct suggestions to the adolescent. The IPT-A therapist is careful to use this technique sparingly so as to avoid encouraging any dependency on the therapist, which is particularly important in a short-term treatment. Modeling is used to encourage behavior change in a number of ways. Therapists can model affective expression, effective communication, and decision-making strategies, as well as many other useful interpersonal skills.

Case Example

Lana is a 16-year-old female with a 3-year history of dysthymia. Lana has a passive approach to her interpersonal relationships and, as a result, frequently leaves herself vulnerable to being mistreated. Early in treatment, the therapist learned that Lana was being influenced by her friends to take money from her grandmother, with whom she had a highly tenuous relationship. The therapist felt that more directive intervention was necessary at this time.

THERAPIST: Lana, we have talked a good deal in here over the last 4 weeks about your relationships. You have frequently talked about feeling as if you do not have any choices and as if you cannot do anything about the things that happen in your life. Part of this is your depression [EDUCATION]. If you remember back to our first sessions together, I explained to you that often when people feel depressed, particularly for a fairly long time as you have, they feel hopeless about changing anything in their lives. They feel as though everything will just have to stay the way it is and that whatever you do nothing will change. Is this the way you feel sometimes?

PATIENT: All the time.

THERAPIST: I also get the sense that you really want to have friends and you are not sure how to make those friendships. I think that maybe sometimes you think that you have to do things even if you are not comfortable with them because it's the only way people will be your friends. It seems like this might be what is happening with these new kids you have met here at school who are telling you to take money and things from your grandmother.

PATIENT: I don't know. Maybe.

THERAPIST: Well, do you really want to take things from your grandmother? I know that you said when you came in here that you would like her to trust you more and you would like to have a better relationship with her.

PATIENT: I don't want to take the things, but I don't know what else to do. I don't know what to say when my friends start talking about doing these things. Besides, it's not that big of a deal.

THERAPIST: [ADVISING] Well, I am going to encourage you to stop stealing from your grandmother and to instead work with me in here on finding another solution to this problem with your friends and grandmother. I know that you are having trouble seeing your options, but we will work on identifying them in here.

When and with Whom to Use Directive Techniques

Although directive techniques are employed throughout the course of treatment with IPT-A, they are used with greatest frequency early on in treatment. They are used across all problem areas and are particularly helpful with adolescents who have a limited support system and, therefore, limited guidance in their lives. These techniques are critical for those adolescents who come from more chaotic and challenging life circumstances. It is often necessary to guide them through the management of some practical problems, including transportation, housing, and financial needs if they are to have any possibility of benefiting from treatment. This is not to say that the therapist should become a case worker; however, it may be necessary for the therapist to assist the patient through the use of the techniques described above in accessing a case worker or reconnecting with family members who can help them address these pressing needs.

Special Issues for Use with Adolescents

Adolescents are encouraged to take an increasingly involved and active role in treatment as it progresses. Given that IPT-A is a time-limited treatment, it is critical that the adolescent take increasing control and responsibility for the changes he needs to make. The educational component of IPT-A is geared toward developing independence and interdependence rather than dependence. When educating and modeling specific skills, the therapist should ask questions that will lead the adolescent to arrive at the answer himself rather than supplying it for him. This takes more work initially on the part of the therapist, but will accelerate the adolescent's acquisition of these skills in the later sessions. A therapist who notices herself relying too heavily on the directive techniques and whose patient appears to be waiting for guidance at all times should re-evaluate the quantity and types of directive techniques she is employing. The pitfall of giving too much direct advice is that the adolescent will not learn the strategies to use on his own.

Decision Analysis

Decision analysis is employed when a patient is faced with a decision that is in some way related to the problem area. The therapist's role is to help the patient consider a range of alternative actions that he can take and to assess the possible consequences associated with each of those actions. The general steps involved in decision analysis are (1) to identify the decision that needs to be made, (2) to determine a goal, (3) to generate a list of alternative actions, (4) to highlight missing options and patterns in the patient's decision making, (5) to evaluate the options by thinking through the consequences, (6) to implement the "best" option, and (7) to evaluate the outcome and potential need to select a second option.

The first step, identification of the decision or dilemma, may seem obvious; however, one might be surprised by how difficult this can be for depressed adolescents. They often experience themselves as powerless, out of control, and helpless. With such a mind-set, it is difficult to consider that one has options in life. It also is a challenge to get adolescents to talk about a decision before it is made. The first step may involve highlighting decisions that the therapist notices the patient has already made and helping him to see how they were "decisions." The more skilled the adolescent gets at recognizing decisions, the more likely he is to bring them up in treatment before actually committing to an action.

The second step involves helping the patient to truly determine what the end result is that he hopes to achieve, prior to taking action. The patient needs to realistically assess this goal and to consider all components of the goal including his associated feelings. Steps three and four occur together. The therapist first encourages the patient to identify his alternative actions and then helps the patient to see alternatives that he has not yet considered. The therapist should pay close attention to patterns that emerge in the way the patient considers alternative actions and the types of alternatives he does or does not consider. These patterns should be highlighted for the patient in order to educate him so that he can make more effective decisions in the future. Next, the adolescent needs to consider the consequences likely to be associated with each alternative action and then choose the option believed to have the greatest likelihood of success in achieving the desired goal. The therapist encourages him to consider both the interpersonal and affective consequences likely to be associated with the various actions. The final steps are to carry out its implementation and then report back on its success and consider the need for changes to the solution or selection of a second option.

Case Example

José arrived for his sixth treatment session looking extremely angry and agitated. José has been having significant conflicts with a group of his peers with whom he had previously been friends. According to José, one of the boys, Terrence, had stolen a girl's music CD during gym class, and the girl accused José of taking it. The gym teacher sent José to the principal's office, and Terrence did not say anything. José was allowed to come to his counseling session because the principal was not available to speak with him yet. José is supposed to go back to the principal's office after his session.

PATIENT: I'm going to find Terrence after school and knock him out. They have to know that I am not someone to be messed with.

THERAPIST: José, I understand that you are very upset, but let's take a little time to think this through and consider your options.

PATIENT: I don't have any options. You have to show them you are a man not to be messed with. He lied about me, and that stupid girl believed it was me. I hate all these people!

THERAPIST: What are you going to say to the principal?

PATIENT: It doesn't matter. He never believes me. I'll just take the punishment, and then I will make Terrence regret it.

THERAPIST: It looks to me like you have a decision to make here. It may not feel like you have any choices, but I think that you do, and I would like you to think about them. Let's start by talking about what you want to have happen and how you want to feel in the end.

PATIENT: I want them to know I am a man and not to mess with me.

THERAPIST: Is there anything else you want to have happen?

PATIENT: I want people to believe me.

THERAPIST: Those are important things. How about in terms of your friendships? You have said in here during the past few weeks that you miss some of your friends and that feeling lonely is part of what is making you feel depressed. What do you want to see happen here?

PATIENT: I don't want to be Terrence's friend now. He should have told the truth.

THERAPIST: OK, I understand that, but what about the other people around you? Would you like to rebuild those friendships?

PATIENT: Yeah, I guess so, but I don't see how.

THERAPIST: Well, let's think about your options for how you can act in this situation. You have already said that you could not tell the principal the truth because you don't think he would believe you, and you could get into a fight with Terrence after school. Can you think of any other possible actions you could take, even if you don't think you would do them right now?

PATIENT: Well, I could tell the principal the truth, but then I would be a snitch, or I could just take the punishment and not fight Terrence, but there's no way that I am doing that.

THERAPIST: Those are a few options. Let's see if there are any others. You could tell the principal that you didn't do it but you are not comfortable telling who did. You could go to Terrence and ask him to confess what he did and take responsibility for it.

PATIENT: Yeah, I guess those are things I could do, but I don't know . . .

THERAPIST: It's a hard decision to make. There is no easy answer because you want people to trust you—both adults and the other guys. You want to have more friends, but you don't want to be punished for something you didn't do. You don't want the other kids to think you are a pushover and that they can just do this to you. I see how this is a tough situation, but I think that the next thing we have to do is to think about the possible consequences that could happen with each of your choices of action. Let's start with fighting with Terrence. What could happen if you fight with him?

PATIENT: Well, I could get suspended and I could get grounded, but they would know not to mess with me.

THERAPIST: Yes, but would you have gotten people to trust you or made friends that way? It seems like there are a lot of negative consequences that go with that option, especially given that you have been trying to get your parents to trust you more. How do you think your parents would feel?

PATIENT: They wouldn't trust me, and they would be really mad.

THERAPIST: How do you think you would end up feeling after that option?

PATIENT: Tough, but still lonely and kind of sad because my parents would be upset.

THERAPIST: So, you would feel lonely and sad. How would you feel about your relationships? One of your main goals in therapy is to have better relationships with your parents and friends. Would this option bring you closer to these improved relationships?

PATIENT: No, probably further away from them.

THERAPIST: Let's look at one of the other options. What about telling the principal the whole truth? What are the possible consequences to that?

The therapist would continue through each of the options, considering the whole range of decisions that José could make and the interpersonal and emotional consequences of each option. The therapist needs to help José keep sight of his treatment goals and how different decisions work toward or against his goals. The therapist wants José to see that his mood and depression are more likely to improve if he feels more effective in his relationships. Being effective in his relationships requires taking control over the decisions he makes and taking control over his life in general. As the therapist works through the various options José has, she ties these options back to these goals. Finally, the therapist would have José select a course of action for handling the situation. When this decision analysis is complete, the therapist should check in with José on what this process was like for him and highlight the steps that he followed to come to his important decision.

When and with Whom to Use Decision Analysis

This technique is most commonly used during the middle phase of treatment, although it is possible that a pressing and significant decision could arise in the initial phase that will need to be addressed. It also is helpful during the termination phase, when the patient considers options for other treatment if necessary after the completion of IPT-A. If treatment has been effective, a patient nearing the end of treatment should be fairly active in the decision analysis and in identifying the steps that he should follow.

More cognitively limited patients and patients lacking resources and support might benefit from a somewhat less expansive array of alternative actions. Too many options may appear overwhelming to the patient.

Special Issues for Use with Adolescents

Developmentally, adolescents often have a limited perspective on the future and underestimate the impact of their current actions on their future lives. Therapists must work with the adolescent to identify consequences that the adolescent believes are likely to be related to his current actions. Although a broader perspective on the ways in which decisions affect his future may be important, such consequences may not be seen as likely enough or may not be real enough to truly affect behavior. Some adolescents will be able to logically evaluate decisions with the therapist in the office, but will have considerable difficulty implementing these decisions in their real lives. It is critical that the therapist evaluate what factors might impede the adolescent from implementing a decision to which he has committed. In many cases it is important to practice the implementation of the decision in the treatment setting. For a more thorough discussion of behavioral rehearsal, refer to the discussion of role plays below.

Common Challenges to Implementation

Decision analysis with adolescents can be made difficult by what is commonly referred to as "black-and-white thinking." Some adolescents have considerable difficulty recognizing the "gray areas" when they consider options. Choices seem to be either all or nothing, or yes or no decisions. The therapist should try to educate adolescents about these gray areas in order to help them recognize that they have more options than they realize.

Another problem that can arise is that there are situations in which there are limited or no options that would be close to the ideal. In these cases, the decision to be made is more about what is the best way to live with the current situation, given the limited options and resources. In these cases, it is important to educate the adolescent as to the fact that there is always a decision of some type to be made. For example, in a situation where a negative consequence is inevitable, such as grounding or suspension, the main decision might be about *how* the adolescent is going to decide to receive this consequence or notify others about it.

A final challenge occurs with adolescents who are particularly hopeless and who feel that whatever they do they still won't be able to change anything. Although some of the bigger concerns that the adolescent has may not be possible to change at this time, small changes are always possible. The therapist should educate the adolescent that depression can improve even by making small changes. One small change can lead to another, and these small changes can lead to fairly significant shifts in the adolescent's mood and other depression symptoms.

Role Plays

Role playing is a behavior change technique that can be used to rehearse new ways of behaving with others and to explore the patient's feelings and style of communicating with others. It provides a safe way to practice the skills that the patient is learning in treatment and to receive feedback necessary to fine-tune his skills before trying to apply them outside of the therapeutic setting. Finally, it provides a way to identify and practice managing the obstacles that may impede the patient's use of his new skills and another opportunity to build the patient's self-confidence.

Role playing is an active technique. The therapist doesn't just talk about what it would be like to use a strategy or new skill; rather, the therapist and the patient actually act it out. Role playing makes most people nervous, including therapists, and the result is that people often talk through the role play instead of actually doing it. Patients will sense the therapist's discomfort, so it is important when necessary to practice with a supervisor or peer and to be prepared to coax the patient to try it initially. Another option is to talk through the scenario with the patient before actually conducting the role play. This is an effective strategy, though the goal is to take the next step of actually conducting the role play.

In conducting a role play, the therapist selects a relevant topic and a small, manageable task that will not be too difficult for the patient the first time. The next step is to establish the context for the role play. Make it as engaging and fun for the adolescent as possible. Some adolescents respond positively to presenting the role play as though it were a play. Almost all adolescents have had some form of drama in school. The therapist can tell the adolescent that they are going to put on a play in the session. They need to assign their roles in the play and then review the script. Oftentimes actors read through the script to make sure they understand their lines and feel comfortable with the wording. They can talk through their lines in the same way. After practicing their lines, the next step is a dress rehearsal during which they take on their roles and prepare to perform the interpersonal interaction of the play. The final show will be when the adolescent plays his role in the scene outside of the session. The main focus in the session is the preparation for the role play and the role play itself. It is common to role-play several times in the session before the adolescent feels comfortable and feels like he owns his new communication style. Following the role play (and sometimes during the course of it), the therapist offers praise and encouragement to the adolescent. The therapist asks the patient how he thinks it went and did he think that there was anything either of them could have done differently, as well as how he would have felt in the situation and how he imagined the therapist would have felt. After providing some constructive feedback, they should try the role play again. Once the adolescent feels comfortable in his role, it is necessary to identify and problem-solve how to handle any imagined or real obstacles to the adolescent enacting this interaction outside of the session.

Case Example

THERAPIST: Let's pretend you are in school and you would like to join two kids who are sitting and talking to each other. One of us will be the two kids and the other will be you, and then we can switch parts. Who would you like to be?

PATIENT: I will be myself.

THERAPIST: OK, let's think about what you could do to try to join the other kids. What could you say to them? Let's give it a try.

PATIENT: I don't know how to start.

THERAPIST: Just try something that comes to mind. We are just pretending in here, so just relax and see what comes to you. Now, I will be the two kids over here talking and joking around . . .

PATIENT: Hi. How are you? What are you talking about?

THERAPIST: Oh, we are just talking about something that happened today in science. I think you are in one of my classes, aren't you?

PATIENT: Yeah, I am in your math class. I sit two rows over from you.

THERAPIST: Oh, yeah, I remember. What did you think of that substitute teacher the other day? OK, let's stop there for a minute. How did that feel to you?

PATIENT: Kind of nervous, but it's just you.

THERAPIST: Sure, it is different when it is just me, but it's good to get the practice. You said you felt a little nervous. You still were able to come over and try to talk. You did a nice job saying hello and being friendly. How do you think the conversation went?

PATIENT: Pretty good. But I don't think they really would have talked to me.

THERAPIST: What do you think would have happened?

PATIENT: I think that they would have just looked at me and maybe laughed.

THERAPIST: What you said wasn't funny—it seemed just fine. When you asked, "What are you talking about?" I guess they could have felt like you were intruding. It really depends on the person. So, what else could you have said?

PATIENT: I don't know.

THERAPIST: Well, let's try switching roles and let me try a few strategies.

When and with Whom to Use Role Plays

Role playing is a highly useful technique, particularly in addressing the problem areas of role disputes and interpersonal deficits. With role disputes, role play is the mechanism for practicing more effective communication with the person with whom the patient has a dispute. With interpersonal deficits, role plays provide a forum in which to practice the skills that the patient is trying to develop. In-session practice is generally critical for these patients.

Although the technique can be used with all patients, it must be used with particular care with more socially anxious patients. For these patients, it is necessary to gradually lead into role plays. First, talk through the role play and provide him with adequate structure. Allow the patient to act out the role in which he is most comfortable. Often this involves not playing himself since he may feel that playing himself requires using newly acquired skills effectively, which makes him even more nervous.

Special Issues for Use with Adolescents

Many adolescents are inherently self-conscious. They are likely to initially scoff at or avoid the role play, as they may feel awkward trying to act it out. A good sense of humor and willingness to put herself on the line will be helpful if the therapist is going to expect the adolescent to do the same. An effective strategy for breaking the ice is for the therapist to greatly exaggerate the role she is playing almost to the point of absurdity initially. Give the adolescent the chance to laugh a bit and to experience success at providing the therapist feedback about what was ineffective about her approach.

Common Challenges to Implementation

I work with an adolescent who is really resistant to doing role plays. Every now and then he will agree to do one, but then he doesn't really participate.

It is not necessary to do role plays with every IPT-A patient, although it tends to be an effective strategy when employed well. With a resistant adolescent, the therapist should get a sense of whether this reflects a general resistance to treatment, social anxiety, or just a lack of comfort in this particular technique. The issue of more general treatment resistance is addressed later in this volume, and dealing with social anxiety has already been discussed. If the problem is solely with the technique, then use other techniques to achieve the same goal. Use work at home or just "talking through the role play" if these seem to work with this particular patient. Again, many times a patient can be sold on role plays through the use of humor and by the therapist putting herself on the line and modeling it for the patient.

The therapist also should closely evaluate her technique in implementing the role play. It could be that the topics being selected for role play are too big, too abstract, or too intimidating. The key is to start small and to pick something specific. For an adolescent who has a limited social network and has felt lonely and abandoned much of his life, the role play should not be about telling someone in his life how he feels about being alone or abandoned. Rather the role play could be to practice making plans to go to a movie or eat lunch with a friend. Always pick something that feels manageable and increases the likelihood that the adolescent will experience some success.

USE OF THE THERAPEUTIC RELATIONSHIP

As with any approach to psychotherapy, the therapeutic relationship is a key component to IPT-A. The description of the relationship was provided in the section on the initial phase of treatment. This is a discussion of the use of the therapeutic relationship as a technique. In IPT-A the therapeutic relationship functions as a minilaboratory and provides both an example of the patient's relationships and a forum in which skills can be practiced and feedback can be given. Throughout the course of IPT-A, the therapist asks questions and comments on experiences within the relationship, particularly as they relate to the goals and objectives of treatment.

In conducting IPT-A, negative feelings about the therapist are understood as transference phenomena but are not dealt with using a psychodynamic perspective. The therapist does not encourage the feelings in the patient or allow them to evolve fully (Weissman et al., 2000). Instead, the therapist will intervene and test the patient's perception of reality. The therapist might say:

> *It seems as though you are feeling angry today? Are you feeling angry? With whom are you angry? Has something happened in the session that has upset you? If so, I think it is important to talk about it. By*

talking about it together we can see how it occurred, uncover any misunderstandings that may exist, and improve our working relationship. I wonder if this situation ever happens with other people?

The therapist needs to encourage the adolescent to examine the negative feelings for the therapist in a supportive atmosphere. Such direct exploration of the adolescent's feelings will prevent misunderstandings that could lead to premature termination. This communication serves several purposes. It models direct communication between two people about their feelings. It also models an openness to hearing that one may have done something to upset another person without realizing it and it is OK to admit to making a mistake. It also helps to link what happens in the session to similar patterns that occur with other relationships. It gives the adolescent the opportunity to see that expressing hurt, anger, or disappointment within a relationship will not be disastrous, but in fact can lead to improvements in the relationship.

When and with Whom to Use the Therapeutic Relationship

This technique is particularly important for adolescents with interpersonal deficits as their identified problem area. Practicing skills can be extremely difficult for some adolescents, and their ability to report on their use of skills can be poor. Practicing open communication and the exchange of feedback with the therapist pertaining to their interactions can be extremely useful. This technique should not be employed too early in treatment, certainly not prior to the middle phase, since it is necessary that the fundamentals of the therapeutic relationship be well established and that a certain level of comfort be achieved in the relationship first.

Special Issues for Use with Adolescents

The therapist should offer feedback slowly and carefully since it is likely to be the adolescent's first experience with this type of feedback. Weave humor, when possible, into the initial feedback, and be sure to begin with giving more constructive advice for improvement based on strengths the therapist has observed in the patient in other situations. If the therapist emphasizes the adolescent's strengths and good qualities and helps the adolescent see how these can be used in other situations, the adolescent is more likely to feel receptive to the feedback.

Common Challenges to Implementation

For many adolescents, particularly those with histories that include trauma or abuse, establishing a trusting relationship with a therapist can be challenging. Being able to experience even constructive feedback in an open and accepting manner can be difficult. As such, the therapist should carefully gauge each adolescent's preparedness for and comfort in receiving this feedback to ensure that the process does not cause the adolescent to terminate treatment prematurely.

ADJUNCTIVE TECHNIQUES

IPT-A is generally most effective when the adolescent can carry out some of the work conducted in the treatment session in his outside relationships between weekly sessions. This increases the probability that treatment gains will be generalized outside of the therapy setting and into the areas of the adolescent's life where change is needed. IPT-A therapists generally assign work to be done at home (or school or other settings) in between sessions that typically involves practicing specific skills that were the focus of the session. The therapist should ensure that the assignment is reasonable for the adolescent, given his current level of skills as well as his emotional ability to manage such a task. Examples of assignments for "work at home" include initiating a conversation with a peer in the adolescent's class or talking to his mother about going to a movie with a friend on a Saturday night. In making an assignment, the therapist should take enough time in the session to discuss any concerns the adolescent might have about the task. The therapist and patient may make some necessary adjustments to the task, identify any obstacles to the adolescent's accomplishing the task, and devise solutions to those obstacles. When the therapist asks the adolescent to do something outside of treatment, she must check in with the adolescent on the outcome of the assignment during the subsequent session.

Case Example

Brandy is a 13-year-old female who developed depression 2 years ago when she entered middle school. During the summer before she began middle school, Brandy's parents separated, but she still was having regular contact with her father and continued to feel close to both of her parents, although it wasn't quite the same as before. Brandy had always had a number of friends in elementary school but has had difficulty establishing friendships in middle school. She was feeling sad about the changes at home and became overwhelmed by many of the shifts and changes in her peer group (i.e., increased cliques, interest in romantic relationships, etc.).

THERAPIST: Brandy, we have been talking a great deal about how you would like to have more friends in middle school. You told me recently about a girl in your science class who seems very nice and open to making friends. We have spent the last session practicing introducing yourself to her and asking if she wants to eat lunch together. You have done a very good job during those role plays and seem like you have gotten much more confident. How are you feeling about them?

PATIENT: Well, they were hard at first, but now it seems easier. I was kind of embarrassed when we first did it. But now I feel like I know some things that I could say. I guess I feel a little less nervous about doing it.

THERAPIST: I was thinking that this might be a good week for you to try introducing yourself to her. You don't need to ask her about having lunch if you don't feel ready. Maybe just start a conversation with her before or after class. How do you feel about trying that?

PATIENT: Oh, I don't know. It's different in here. I think I would forget what to say.

THERAPIST: I know it feels like that, and I know it makes you nervous to think about trying it, but you have really done a great job. And, remember, you used to be able to make friends. I know you still can do it. You just have been a little out-of-practice. You are very friendly and interesting, and you know how to ask questions and say things that make other people feel comfortable.

PATIENT: I guess so. But what would I say? Now I don't remember.

THERAPIST: What were some of things you thought about saying and asking her?

PATIENT: Well, I thought I could ask her where she lives, and I could tell her that I like her backpack because she has a really nice one. I also thought I could ask her if she likes our science teacher.

THERAPIST: Those are all great ways to start up a conversation. Do you think you could give it a try?

PATIENT: Yeah, I guess so.

THERAPIST: What do you think might get in your way of doing this?

PATIENT: Well, if I get really nervous, or if she is not there in school.

THERAPIST: Well, if she's not there, you would just have to wait for another day, right? What could you do if you get really nervous?

PATIENT: I could remember how I did the practices in here and that I will feel better if I try to talk to her.

THERAPIST: Those are all great ideas. I want you to give it a try this week, and then we can talk about how it went next session. Do you have any questions?

When and with Whom to Use "Work at Home"

Work at home is most appropriate during the middle phase of treatment, with any adolescent and for all problem areas. If a therapist has a sense that the adolescent is not particularly engaged in treatment and unlikely to follow through on a task outside of treatment, she should consider postponing the use of this technique until the adolescent is more engaged. Adolescents whose lives are particularly chaotic also may have difficulty following through on assignments. In these cases, the therapist should weigh the possible benefits and costs to encouraging this work. If the therapist still feels it would be beneficial, she should take care to assign something very manageable and to address the practical obstacles to doing it before proceeding with the assignment.

Special Issues for Use with Adolescents

Adolescents can have fairly negative and intense reactions to anything that reminds them of "homework," so the therapist should be sure to use a language and tone that is not at all reminiscent of their experiences in school, especially with adolescents who have had difficulty in school. "Work at home" should arise naturally from the content of the session and be framed more as an "interpersonal experiment" to make it more fun and minimize its negative connotation. It is analogous to doing an experiment in chemistry lab: it may or may not turn out the way you expected; but either way, it will be instructive. There is no right or wrong answer; instead, it is an exploration into how people may change their behavior and feelings if something is said to them or done differently. The goal is to have more information to discuss about the specific situation and relationship that will eventually lead to a solution that will help the adolescent to feel better.

Common Challenges to Implementation

When adolescents are depressed they often have difficulty following through on assignments and taking initiative. It happens sometimes that work-at-home assignments are not completed or not completed in the way that the therapist intended. Consistent with the "limited sick role" assigned earlier in IPT-A treatment, the therapist should encourage and support whatever attempts were made at a task. This sometimes involves praising the adolescents even for remembering what the task was or for considering trying it (even if they did not). Failure to complete such tasks should not become a source of anxiety that might drive an adolescent toward premature termination. These missed assignments should be taken in stride, discussed in a nonjudgmental way, and be included as additional information in the overall conceptualization of the adolescent's depression.

CHAPTER 10

Grief

Grief is selected as the problem area when patients describe the onset of depressive symptoms in association with the death of a significant person in their life. The death does not have to immediately precede the depression; the depression can be a delayed or distorted reaction to the loss. The significance of this relationship for the patient already will have been discussed in detail during the interpersonal inventory.

DEVELOPMENTAL ASPECTS OF GRIEF

Grief in Adults

Normal grief can resemble a depression in the nature of the symptoms experienced, such as sad mood, increased tearfulness, disturbance in sleep and appetite, disturbances in daily functioning, and feelings of excessive guilt. Normal, uncomplicated grief leads to only minimal disruption in normal functioning. In a normal grief reaction, symptoms and any impairment in functioning generally resolve without treatment within 6 months. When this does not occur, however, grief is considered complicated or pathological. Pathological grief is characterized by (1) inhibition, suppression, or absence of the grief process; (2) exaggeration or distortion of certain symptoms or behaviors that normally occur with grief; and/or (3) the prolongation of normal grieving (Raphael, 1983). Pathological grief also can lead to mood disorders such as depression.

Grief in Adolescents

The few studies of bereavement in adolescents (e.g., Osterweis et al., 1984) highlight several similarities in the mourning experiences of adults and adolescents. Horowitz (1976) identified themes in his research with grieving adults that are reported in clinical work with grieving adolescents (McGoldrick & Walsh, 1991). The most common feelings discussed by grieving adolescents include (1) sadness about having to cope with the actual loss of the relationship; (2) feelings of excessive guilt regarding activities or deeds they wish they had or had not done with the deceased; (3) anger at being left without the deceased; (4) feelings about not having a chance to say good-bye; (5) feelings of responsibility, that maybe if they had done something different the person would still be with them; (6) concern that the same thing may happen to them; and (7) overidentification with the deceased in order to maintain continuity of presence (Raphael, 1983). Still there are unique developmental tasks and transitions of adolescence that interact with the demands and effects of grief and can complicate the mourning process (Balk & Corr, 2001).

The most intense grief response in early adolescence appears to be associated with the death of a parent. Common reactions include withdrawal, depressed feelings, denial, pseudomaturity, identification with the deceased, and care-eliciting behaviors (Raphael, 1983). Adolescents may grieve differently from adults. Their grief may be more episodic than pervasive. They may continue with their usual activities while the grief is expressed in psychosomatic symptoms, angry outbursts, or school failure (Schoeman & Kreitzman, 1997). Boys and girls appear to respond differently: boys may turn to stealing, drugs, or social withdrawal, while girls may more frequently increase their closeness with their sisters or sexualize their peer relationships as a means of finding the comfort and attachment they have lost (Osterweis, Solomon, & Green, 1984). The socioeconomic loss accompanying the death of a parent can exacerbate the mourning process, especially for children from financially stressed families (Schilling, Koh, Abramovitz, & Gilbert, 1992). The adolescent may experience feelings of yearning for the parent, the intensity of which is determined by the former nature of their relationship and the degree of separation that had been achieved and the suddenness with which the death has occurred.

In assessing the impact of the death of a loved one in adolescence, one must consider (1) the adolescent's role in the family system or peer group before and after the death, (2) the nature of the relationship lost, (3) the remaining social and familial support network, and (4) the adolescent's psychological maturity and coping skills at the time of the death. Gray (1987) conducted a study of adolescent response to the death of a parent. He found higher levels of depression in those adolescents who experienced poor social support following the loss and in those who reported a poor prior relationship with the surviving parent. According to Raphael (1997), depression is the primary affect associated with loss and is frequently accompanied by anxiety, sadness, and loneliness.

The impact of the death of others such as a close friend, grandparent, or teacher, on the adolescent also is determined by the intensity of the relationship and the adolescent's preparedness for the death (Raphael, 1983). Sudden and unexpected loss may complicate the grieving process and increase the risk for chronic psychological distress (Raphael, 1997). Sklar and Hartley (1990) found that difficulties triggered by the death of a close friend might be as severe as—and in some cases more severe than—those found in the loss of a family member. This results from the adolescent being in a developmental stage where friends rather than family have become the focal point. In addition, the deaths of young people are more likely to be sudden, rather than from natural causes. Anxieties about the future play a prominent role in the adolescents' thinking, and death, separation, and loss only confirm their worst fears about what the future may hold (Rutter, 1979). Repression of the longing for the deceased may result in the adolescent's vulnerability to pathological mourning. IPT-A treats the depression associated with abnormal grief reactions, but also can be used to promote a successful grief process during a normal bereavement period. This is discussed in more depth later in this chapter.

ABNORMAL GRIEF

Incomplete or unresolved grieving can result in depression and/or dysfunction in daily living. Defining what is an abnormal grief reaction and when a grief reaction is true depression is complicated, although several researchers have worked to clarify these definitions (Weller & Weller, 1991; Brent et al., 1993; Geis, Whittlesey, McDonald, Smith, & Pfefferbaum, 1998). According to Clark, Pynoos, and Goebel (1994), pathological grief may have more to do with the frequency, intensity, and duration of symptoms than with the actual constellation of symptoms. Symptoms that have been identified as distinguishing between uncomplicated bereavement and bereavement complicated by major depression include a sense of worthlessness, psychomotor retardation, and functional impairment (Brent et al., 1993). Symptoms indicative of abnormal grief can appear during the normal grief period, or they may surface at a future date, perhaps triggered by the anniversary of the death or an encounter with a belonging of the deceased.

Pathological mourning of three general kinds is commonly noted in depressed adolescents: distorted grief, delayed grief, or a chronic grief reaction (Raphael, 1983; Middleton, Moylan, Raphael, Burnett, & Martinek, 1993). The types of mourning are the same as in adults; however, the manifestations are informed by development. For example, grief in adolescents may lead to truancy rather than job problems. The therapist's main task in addressing abnormal grief is to help the adolescent acknowledge and express the feelings surrounding the death. The therapist helps promote understanding of the impact of the loss on his other relationships and how to resume relationships in this new context.

Types of Abnormal Grief

A *distorted grief reaction* can take many different forms. It may be characterized by behavioral problems rather than sad mood (Raphael, 1983). It can occur immediately following the death or at some distant time in the future. Distorted grief can come from unresolved feelings of desertion and guilt that can result in angry aggression or in self-punishing behavior. It may consist of guilty ruminations, anger, or fantasies about the deceased. Drug or alcohol abuse, sexual promiscuity, truancy, and other maladaptive behavior changes may occur. If the symptoms are physical, it is necessary to rule out a physiological basis (e.g., a thyroid problem) to the complaints before proceeding to assess the psychological nature of the symptoms (as discussed in Chapter 4).

As implied in its name, a *delayed grief reaction* occurs at a time subsequent to the death and normal grieving period. The adolescent may have been unable to mourn adequately because the loss was too overwhelming or the associated feelings too frightening. Mourning also may be delayed until the adolescent is surrounded by secure relationships and feels supported (Raphael, 1983). When the feelings of sadness occur at a later date, the adolescent is unable to make the connection between the presenting depressive symptoms and the past loss. Many different types of experiences such as a second loss can trigger the delayed reaction. In order to determine the presence of a delayed grief reaction, the therapist must obtain a complete history regarding the relationship with the deceased and the events surrounding the actual death. Oftentimes when adolescents are excluded from the events of the death, such as the funeral, their mourning can become delayed.

A *chronic grief reaction* is a protracted, often recurrent, triggered emotion, such as sadness, that was previously experienced upon the death of the loved one. It is often the result of the patient's difficulty in expressing grief and its associated emotions or of unresolved feelings about the deceased. One type of chronic grief reaction is an anniversary reaction, in which the adolescent experiences significant sadness repeatedly at the same time of year as the original loss. The adolescent may experience chronic malaise, withdrawal, somatic symptoms, or frank depression without consciously connecting these symptoms to the previous loss.

Assessment of Abnormal Grief Reactions

The assessment of whether an adolescent is experiencing an abnormal grief reaction should begin with the detailed review of the adolescent's significant relationships during the interpersonal inventory. This review should include current relationships as well as past relationships with people who may now be deceased or who are no longer active participants in the adolescent's daily life. When asking questions about a relationship with someone deceased, it is important to obtain information on the adolescent's emotions surrounding the event (the death), the actual event itself, and the impact of the event on the adolescent's life. Some questions that might be asked in the process of the assessment are:

> Has anyone important to you died? Can you tell me about the death? When? Where? What circumstances? How did you hear about the death? What was your response when you were told? Did you cry? Did you miss any school? How much? When did you start to feel better? How did others in the family deal with it?

It is often necessary for the therapist to articulate some of the feelings before the adolescent is able to talk about them. The therapist might say:

> It is normal to feel tremendous sadness when someone you are close to has died. That feeling can last for months, sometimes longer. Expressing and talking about those feelings is an important part of the process of mourning for [name of person] and of coming to terms with living your life without [name of person] being part of your life. When you don't mourn for the person you have lost, many problems can happen, such as depression, anxiety, problems in your present relationships, and fears about getting close to people. By talking about your feelings, even though it may be difficult at first, you will be able to feel better again.

IPT-A Goals and Strategies for Treating Abnormal Grief

For adolescents identified with the problem area of grief, their specific goal in the treatment is to facilitate the delayed normal mourning process (see Table 10.1). As part of this goal, the adolescent must cope with the real loss (e.g., of a parent whose role was to provide nurturance and stability through the developmental process of adolescent separation and individuation), resolve the positive and negative aspects of the specific relationship with the deceased, and find or improve upon other relationships that can provide the support, nurturance, companionship, or guidance that has been lost.

Several strategies are used to accomplish these goals and objectives. Each of these strategies involves the use of a number of possible techniques. In the discussion that follows, the most relevant techniques are identified for each strategy. Chapter 9 provides details and examples regarding the implementation of these techniques.

Review in Detail the Adolescent's Relationships with the Deceased

The main strategy employed by the therapist is to review in detail the adolescent's relationship with the deceased in order to free the adolescent from the disabling attachment to the deceased. In doing so, the therapist must review with the adolescent both the positive and negative aspects of the relationship, conflicts in the relationship, and special qualities of the relationship. The adolescent may be reluctant to discuss or acknowledge angry or hostile feelings toward the deceased or may feel somehow responsible for the death, a reaction that connotes guilt and self-blame.

The adolescent will need to be encouraged, in a nonconfrontational manner, to explore and express these feelings. The therapist should help

TABLE 10.1. Summary of Goals and Strategies for Grief Problem Area

Goal	• Facilitate the mourning process
Strategies	• Review in detail the adolescent's relationship with the deceased
	• Provide reassurance regarding feelings and grieving process
	• Connect current behaviors to feelings surrounding the death (particularly for distorted grief reactions)
	• Improve communication skills (particularly for chronic grief reactions)
	• Develop other supportive relationships
	• Reintegrate into the social milieu

guide the adolescent in a gradual expression and discussion of these negative feelings so as not to heighten the adolescent's guilt and/or anxiety. It is important to educate the adolescent that this disclosure will be followed by more positive feelings and an understanding of the deceased, which will enable him to further examine the relationship and its impact on his life. Eliciting feelings about the deceased and exploring the interactions between the deceased and the adolescent can facilitate the disclosure. The therapist might say:

> *Tell me about your relationship with [name of the person]. What kinds of things would you do together? Can you describe what you liked about [the person]? Most people have good and bad times in their relationships. Were there times when the two of you had difficulty getting along? What would happen? How would you feel? Can you tell me about the time when you found out about the illness or death? What was it like for you? How did you feel?*

The therapist asks the adolescent to think about the loss, to discuss in detail the events surrounding the death and the emotional impact of the events on the adolescent.

The purpose of reviewing the relationship is to foster a better understanding of the complexity of their relationship in light of the difficult feelings experienced at the time of the person's death. It is an opportunity to clarify the relationship so that the adolescent can return to the normal mourning process. The adolescent can be helped to feel comfortable to express these feelings. The therapist might say:

> *It's normal to have both positive and negative feelings toward a person. Your feelings can vary with situations and different periods in your life. It is important to be able to recognize the different feelings you may experience toward [name of the person]. It also is important to learn that you can address these negative feelings within yourself even without [the person] so that they don't prevent you from developing other important relationships.*

The techniques employed as part of this strategy include exploration and encouragement of affect. How directive the exploration is and how active the therapist has to be in facilitating this process is largely dependent upon the presentation and interaction style of the particular adolescent. Typically, adolescents present initially as very reticent to talk, but with the therapist's support they begin to tell a narrative of their relationship with the deceased and engage in the therapeutic process of healing the wounds left by the loss.

Provide Reassurance

In exploring both the positive and negative aspects of the relationship, adolescents are often reluctant to mention events that have not been discussed in the family for a long time or that they were at one time advised not to speak about. They may fear punishment from another person for discussing them, hurting the other survivors' feelings, or losing control of their emotions in talking about the event. The therapist should reassure the adolescent that these fears are common, explore what it means to lose control of his emotions, and discuss the steps that would be taken by the therapist to prevent the adolescent from being overwhelmed by the emotions. These steps include monitoring the patient's affect in the discussion and guiding the speed or depth of disclosure accordingly. The therapist might say to the patient:

> *I know that talking about your mother's death and your relationship with your mother feels a little frightening. It seems like you are concerned about being able to control your emotions and afraid of getting overwhelmed and falling apart. It is common to feel this way, but I am going to help you with this. We are going to move slowly and talk about things as you are ready. I will watch to be sure that this does not become too overwhelming, and we will check in as we go to see you if you are feeling OK about continuing the discussion. If at any point it seems to me that you are feeling overwhelmed or you tell me that you need to stop, we will take a break from this discussion and only resume when you are ready. I assure you that, although it feels hard to talk about now, over time this will get easier and you will find yourself less anxious when talking about these things. Eventually, it will help you to feel better.*

Connect Current Behaviors to Feelings about the Death and Loss

In treating distorted grief reactions, the therapist also helps the adolescent connect current-acting out behavior with the feelings surrounding the death when relevant. For example, an adolescent whose academic performance began to decline and who became truant in the month just prior to the first-year anniversary of the death of his brother would be helped to see the association between the change in his school behavior and functioning and the resurgence of the accompanying depression. The therapist could say:

> *From what you and your school guidance counselor are telling me, it appears that you have been having some difficulty in school during*

the past month or so. Your grades on exams have dropped and you have skipped school on a couple of occasions. We have been talking about being just 1 month away from the one-year anniversary of your brother's death. This is often a time when people start to feel more sad and to experience some of the same emotions that they experienced when the person first died. I wonder if you have been feeling that way lately? Have you noticed any of your depression symptoms getting worse? I wonder if this may somehow be related to the increased problems in school around this same time? I wonder if you have been feeling not only more sad but also somewhat angry at either your brother or other people in your life. Sometimes, instead of talking about these feelings, people show these feelings through their behaviors. When you began treatment you were feeling really down on yourself and guilty about many things that happened in your life. I am concerned that you might start to feel this way again, given the trouble you are having in school. I know how important it has been for you to do well in school. It is important that we talk about the feelings and symptoms you might be having now so that we can stop them from interfering with how you are doing in school and help you to feel better.

By making these connections, the adolescent gains an understanding of the impact of the loss not only on his feelings but also on concrete behaviors that are likely to be causing more problems for himself and exacerbating his depression. Once the connection is established, the therapist can effectively target both emotions and behavior in the discussions of the deceased. Techniques that are helpful in facilitating this behavior–emotion connection are communication analysis of the problematic interaction as well as mood monitoring and linking affect to events.

Improve Communication Skills

Treating adolescents with chronic grief reactions will often include more emphasis on increasing communication skills and applying those skills to the significant relationships that have been impaired as a result of the chronic grief. The therapist should monitor whether the adolescent with chronic grief has developed maladaptive patterns of relating. This is accomplished through the application of communication analysis to current interactions and monitoring skills used in the session with the therapist. Through role playing, the therapist can assist the adolescent in practicing new styles of communication and can monitor for improvements over the course of treatment. Techniques used to promote better communication skills include communication analysis, behavior change techniques, such as role playing, and the use of the therapeutic relationship to provide feedback on observable communications occurring within the session.

Develop Other Supportive Relationships

The abnormal grief reaction may occur in the context of the loss of the adolescent's main support. The adolescent may be experiencing complications from losing a primary caretaker and/or source of support. The adolescent may experience a sense of isolation and the feeling that there is no one else to guide him through the normal process of mourning. Adolescents often feel unable to discuss the loss with peers because they feel peers may not understand their profound sense of loss, and they feel developmentally different from their friends. They fear their friends will perceive them as abnormal if they express what they are feeling (Baker & Sedney, 1996). Unaffected friends sometimes fear spending time with the grieving adolescent, finding the situation uncomfortable, and therefore avoid the adolescent (Balk & Vesta, 1998). The seemingly mundane concerns of their peers (e.g., girls, clothes, etc.) feel silly in light of their loss and the concomitant emotional turmoil.

The grief reaction also may be a result of a secondary loss of the surviving parent due to that parent's own depression, remarriage, or dysfunction. Osterweis et al. (1984) found that one significant risk factor for psychological morbidity following the death of a parent is the psychological vulnerability of the surviving parent, which may result in the surviving parent's excessive dependence on the adolescent. A conflictual relationship with the deceased or an ambivalent reaction to the loss of a primary caretaker can further complicate the picture. Therefore, in facilitating the mourning process it is equally important to aid the adolescent in developing or increasing the number of supportive relationships in his life. It is hoped that these relationships can provide some of the practical and emotional support that may have been lost with the death. Behavior change techniques, such as using the therapeutic relationship and conducting "work at home" are often helpful in the work to develop more supportive relationships.

Reintegrate into the Social Milieu

As adolescents begin to engage in the normal mourning process, frequently they feel as though they would like to resume more social interactions. They also may be vulnerable at this time to attaching to the first person who comes along to fill the empty space left by the deceased. The therapist can assist the adolescent in considering various ways to meet new people and in evaluating new social contacts for the potential to become significant participants in his life. The therapist can help the adolescent assess surroundings for new social opportunities such as after-school activities and religious or youth groups by asking:

> *What kinds of activities did you enjoy before the death of [name of deceased]? How has your involvement changed? How would you like to get back involved with people? What kinds of activities could you participate in? Where do you feel you would be most comfortable? What would be your concerns, if any?*

THE ROLE OF THE FAMILY IN TREATMENT

The role of the family in treatment for a grief problem area largely depends upon the circumstances surrounding the death and the adolescent's current family situation. In general, surviving family members can be very helpful in providing details surrounding the adolescent's relationship with the deceased and events surrounding the actual death. The therapist may ask a parent:

> *What was your [son's/daughter's] relationship like with [name of deceased]? How did [he/she] find out about the death? What had [he/she] known about the illness?*

Significant family members also can play a critical role in the development of supportive relationships and reintegration into the social milieu. In working with the family, either during in-person meetings or by telephone, it is very important to keep in mind that they too may be grieving and that this process follows a very different course for each individual. Sometimes family members need additional supports (such as their own treatment) in order to be able to be emotionally available and supportive of the adolescent's grieving process.

TREATING NORMAL GRIEF REACTIONS

IPT-A also can be used to help an adolescent negotiate a normal grief process. Intervention in these cases is particularly useful for adolescents who have previously been depressed and who are thus at increased risk for recurrence, given the addition of a new stressor: the loss. It also may be useful for adolescents whose support network is particularly limited; who have a lack of understanding of death; or who have experiences involving multiple or sudden deaths. A conflicted relationship with a deceased person, an overly dependent surviving parent, or a death by suicide or homicide also have been identified as risk factors for more complicated bereavement and the potential onset of depression (Clark et al., 1994). Treatment during this time can facilitate the processing of the grief emotions and prevent emotional and social isolation from occurring.

Specifically, the therapist facilitates the adolescent's movement through the grief process by providing support and guidance on how to address the accompanying and often intense emotions. Education about normal bereavement patterns can be very beneficial for the adolescent. An example of such education is as follows:

> After the death of someone you care about it is common to have certain kinds of feelings and experiences. This is part of what we call grief. Although everyone grieves somewhat differently, there are some things that many people experience. You might feel sad or angry and sometimes even numb. You might cry a lot or have trouble crying. Some people have trouble sleeping or eating. A lot of times, teenagers feel somewhat guilty about the death. They feel in some way responsible for what happened. You might notice that it is harder for you to concentrate, that you are less interested in things you usually like doing, and that you have a harder time doing your work at school. These are all a normal part of grieving. Sometimes you will have these feelings and experiences right away, and sometimes you will notice them after a little time. It is very important that you try hard to keep doing as many of the things that you usually like to do. Most of the time, your interest in these things and your ability to do your work will get better with just a little time. The different feelings you are having will last a while, but over time they will get a little less strong. You will probably have some days where you feel better and then have moments in those days that feel worse. This is all a normal part of grieving. It is very important that you talk about the feelings you are having (both positive ones and negative ones) in our therapy sessions and also with family and friends. One of the things that I can do as your therapist is to help you to figure out who in your life you can best talk to about these feelings.

The therapist also addresses the conflicts that may arise between the bereaved and other relationships as a result of the grief and the associated depression symptoms. The therapist might say:

Everyone grieves somewhat differently, and the stress that comes from grief can put some added pressure on other important relationships in your life. It is important to realize that problems in those relationships may be due in part to the grief you, and maybe the other person, are experiencing. We can talk about the problems you are having in these relationships and try to find solutions since these relationships will be important in helping you to feel better.

The emphasis is on learning to use current relationships as support for the grieving process. This support will be accomplished through better expression of emotions and better understanding of the link between the feelings of grief and the overt behaviors such as conflict or withdrawal within other significant relationships.

The strategies employed to treat normal grief are similar to those for treating abnormal grief. The therapist assists the adolescent in discussing the relationship with the deceased, the feelings surrounding the death, and the impact of the loss on his life. The therapist may discuss the adolescent's transition back to being more socially active and participating in normal activities after a period of withdrawal. Together they can address concerns about how to share the experience with others, for example, what to tell friends about a prolonged absence from school due to the death. Overall, the main focus is on identifying and exploring the adolescent's feelings about the relationship with the deceased and the death, and how his current functioning is being affected.

SUMMARY

IPT-A is used to help adolescents who are coping either with a normal or an abnormal grief reaction. The main objectives for the therapist are to assist the adolescent in a review of the relationship lost, the associated feelings, and the impact of the loss on current functioning. Following a resolution of feelings about the loss, attention can turn to establishing new interpersonal relationships and/or reestablishing relationships that had been interrupted by the reaction to the loss.

The following case example illustrates the use of IPT-A for the treatment of a chronic grief reaction complicated by significant family disruption.

CASE VIGNETTE: THE CASE OF HELEN

Helen, a 17-year-old girl, was living with a cousin of her grandmother since her mother's death 3 years ago. Helen's parents had divorced right after she was born, and she had never met her father. Immediately following her mother's death from a terminal illness, Helen lived with her grandmother, but they did not get along and she left her home after a year. She went to live with her grandmother's cousin and had been there ever since. She was attending a small private school, where she had developed a close relationship with the school guidance staff.

Helen presented to the clinic with a major depression. She said she had been feeling depressed since her mother had died. She reported sad mood, irritability, increased fatigue, concentration problems, decrease in grades, feelings of hopelessness and helplessness, mild paranoia, and derealization. She denied any sleep or appetite disturbance but reported that she felt too lazy to prepare any food, so she had been eating less. A child psychiatrist had recommended medication, but Helen had refused to take the medication on a regular basis.

Initial Sessions (1–4)

During the initial sessions, discussion focused on the circumstances of her mother's death and the unstable home life that the death had precipitated. She spoke with disbelief about her mother's death and her grandmother's lack of understanding of teenagers. She cried as she told the therapist that she thought of her mother's death throughout the day every day. She felt alone in the world despite living with this cousin. Although it was better than living with her grandmother, she still felt like a guest or boarder in her cousin's tiny apartment. During this time her uncle who lived in Texas invited her to come live with him. As much as she longed to be part of a family and have her own room, changing high schools for her senior year to live with an uncle whom she didn't know very well presented her with a significant conflict. The need to make this decision exacerbated her anger at her mother for dying and leaving her with this difficult decision. The therapist speculated that a substantial part of Helen's difficulty coping with her present situation was due to Helen's failure to grieve over her mother's death appropriately and to address the myriad of feelings toward her mother and the rest of her family. Helen and the therapist agreed by the end of the initial phase that the focus of the treatment should be on the relationship between the death of her mother and her current depression.

Middle Sessions (5–8)

A pressing decision for Helen at this time was whether or not to move to Texas to live with her uncle or to stay in her current living situation and at her school with the school staff who had become like a family to her. By focusing on Helen's feelings of abandonment and anger, she was better able to sort out her feelings and thoughts about this issue. Helen and the therapist spent their time discussing Helen's feelings toward her mother, both positive and negative, in addition to the feelings about her relationship and interactions with her grandmother, grandmother's cousin, and uncle. She expressed much anger at them for not supporting her more in dealing with her mother's illness. She talked about the guilt she felt about her own difficulties spending time with her mother when she was near death, and her absence from her mother's room when her mother eventually died. She felt that she had not been loving enough in her mother's time of need and, as a result, had felt badly about herself.

Psychoeducation regarding normal reactions to death and illness helped relieve her of some of the guilt. In addition, the therapist helped her to focus on the strengths she had demonstrated in coping with such a difficult situation. Helen worried that her mother's death and conflict with extended family were going to mar her future relationships. Treatment focused on how her fears of being abandoned and losing significant relationships could make her hesitant to enter new relationships or to be less open in her relationships, so that if she lost these new relationships the pain would not be as great. They were able to examine this in the context of her relationship with her grandmother's cousin and in her initiation of a new relationship with a male friend. By the end of the middle phase of treatment, Helen was able to talk about her mother more easily with less visible distress, and was reporting a decrease in irritability, anger, and feelings of guilt.

Termination Sessions (9–12)

At the beginning of the termination phase, Helen reported that she had made the decision not to move to Texas to live with her uncle. She stated that over the past few weeks he had shown through various unfulfilled promises that he might not be able to deliver on all that he was promising her. She had been able to discuss her feelings about this with him. She reported that at the same time she had tried to talk more to the family with whom she was living and was feeling more comfortable there. She loved her school and the teachers who cared so much for her. She was feeling happier and reported better concentration in school, improved eating and sleeping habits, decreased tearfulness, and fewer feelings of guilt and self-blame. She still thought a lot about her mother, but without the anger she previously felt. She also felt proud about the way she was handling her life, making decisions, and taking care of herself in the absence of her mother. She was much more comfortable in talking about her feelings in interactions with family members and the school staff. She discovered that people responded positively toward her when she shared her feelings, which made her feel more cared for and supported. At the time of termination, Helen completed the 11th grade and was eagerly awaiting her senior year, preparing to apply for college, and feeling more confident that she would be able to develop good relationships in the future and achieve her academic goals.

CHAPTER 11

Interpersonal Role Disputes

An interpersonal role dispute is a situation in which the patient and at least one significant other person have "nonreciprocal expectations about their relationship" (Klerman et al., 1984). Nonreciprocal expectations refer to disagreements about the terms and/or guidelines for behavior within the relationship. It is chosen as the identified problem area when adolescents describe their depression in relation to conflict within a significant relationship. This chapter will focus on how depression can distort expectations within a relationship and how IPT-A addresses the resulting problems.

The significant relationships in an adolescent's life usually include relationships with family members, teachers, best friends, and romantic attachment figures. The quality of these relationships can be significantly affected by depression as well as be a precipitant of depression. Family adversity and poor perception of their role within the family predict adolescent depression in longitudinal studies (Fergusson, Horwood, & Lynskey, 1995). For example, depressed children frequently have persistent interpersonal problems with parents, siblings, and friends even after the depressed mood has been successfully treated (Puig-Antich et al., 1985b). Good family relations lead to a better outcome of depression for adolescents (Sanford et al., 1995). Disputes with families and friends also can contribute to the development of a depressive episode (Schocket & Dadds, 1997; Lewinsohn et al., 1994b; Vernberg, 1990). An example of a peer dispute is the teenage girl who expects a best friend to be supportive of the time commitment inherent in her newfound love relationship; however, the best friend expects the friendship to take priority over romance. The girl is disappointed, feels rejected, and sad. Role disputes in families can occur when parents expect their adolescent to confide in them fully about intimate feelings and details of life, while the adolescent feels the need to separate more from the parents and uses friends more than family as confidantes. One particularly common interpersonal dispute that occurs between adolescents and parents is the conflict between a conservative parent and the adolescent who is trying to behave consistently with his generation of peers. Often these conflicting values lead to different expectations for the adolescent's behavior.

Interpersonal role dispute becomes the identified problem area if the adolescent's depressive episode coincides with such a conflict. The type of dispute that is most likely to precede a depressive episode is one in which the adolescent feels helpless to resolve the conflict and the dispute keeps being repeated in the relationship, generating feelings of increasing helplessness. Since the adolescent feels misunderstood with no hope of mutual communication, self-esteem decreases, which can result in social withdrawal and poor communication. An example is the adolescent who is having a dispute with a parent over permission to go out at night with friends. The parent, worried about safety, doesn't want to let the teen out of the house after dark. The teenager wants to be able to socialize with his peer group. They are unable to agree on a reasonable activity and/or curfew. The discussions escalate into yelling matches and end with each of them withdrawing, leaving the problem to reoccur at the next invitation. The adolescent expresses the feeling that the parent is never going to change and is never going to let him out of the house. As a result, the adolescent begins to withdraw from friends so that the inability to join them will not be noticed and invitations will not need to be rejected.

Nonreciprocal expectations and disputes seem particularly acute in children of immigrant parents who are unfamiliar with the ways of their new country and even more acute for female children. For example, with female Latina adolescents, the culture shock after immigration frequently results in increased parent–adolescent tensions about appropriate female roles and behaviors (Hardy-Fanta & Montana, 1982). In traditional Latino families, the male and female roles are strictly defined; however, in the United States the roles are not so clearly demarcated or similarly conceptualized. As a result of a fear of the unknown, parents often become very rigid and overprotective of their children. The children attempt to rebel against this rigidity, viewing their parents' way of life as inferior to the American way (Ghali, 1977). Although specific disputes occur in immigrant families, similar ones also can be seen in the traditional adolescent rebellion against parental authority when the adolescent attempts to separate from the family.

Problems in resolving the disputes can be the result of an inability to see the other person's point of view, significant differences in expectations for the relationship, inability to communicate about feelings and expectations, or the feeling of pervasive helplessness that results in withdrawal from attempts at resolution. Parental communication also may have a significant role in adolescent depression (Slesnick & Waldron, 1997). In comparison with nondepressed children, depressed children perceive their families as more hostile and less nurturant (Slesnick & Waldron, 1997; Harold, Fincham, Osborne, & Conger, 1997). The perceived or real threat of the loss adds to the isolation and loneliness the depressed teen feels.

DIAGNOSING INTERPERSONAL ROLE DISPUTES

To determine whether a role dispute is the problem area, the therapist conducts a thorough history of the adolescent's significant relationships. Information to look for in diagnosing disputes includes conflicts with significant others that may elicit emotions such as anger, sadness, and/or frustration. Often the most salient feeling is the adolescent's sense that the situation will never change and that he is misunderstood. Sometimes, however, the conflict may not be as overt. In such cases, the therapist needs to observe for nonverbal signs of repressed or denied emotions and to be alert if relationships with significant others are briefly mentioned. If the adolescent shies away from discussion or appears to portray an ideal relationship, these may be clues that the adolescent is experiencing negative feelings that are uncomfortable to express. It is often helpful at this time for the therapist to educate the adolescent about the acceptability of having ambivalent and even negative feelings in relationships and how difficult relationships can often make a person feel sad and precipitate a depression.

Case Example

Liz presented with a major depression, but was unable to identify what was making her so upset. In conducting the interpersonal inventory, the therapist asked her about her relationship with her mother. She reported that her relationship was great and that they got along very well. The therapist responded to this enthusiasm about their relationship by stating that most teenagers have some conflicts with their parents, and she wondered if the patient did too. Gradually the patient revealed conflicts with her mother about her restrictive rules and her inability to talk with her mother about her desire for more freedom. The therapist then reflected to Liz that it sounded as though she was experiencing significant conflict and feeling much anger toward her mother that might be contributing to her depression. The exploration of the initially idealistic relationship led to a more accurate accounting of the role dispute between mother and daughter.

A critical part of diagnosing the problem area of role disputes is pinpointing the stage of the dispute. There are three possible stages the dispute may be in when presented to the therapist (Klerman et al., 1984):

1. *Renegotiation.* In this stage, the adolescent and significant other are still communicating with each other in attempts to resolve the conflict and are being open about the presence of a disagreement. If they are seeking treatment, however, it is likely that their attempts at negotiation have been largely unsuccessful.
2. *Impasse.* In this stage, the adolescent and the significant other typically are no longer attempting to discuss the conflict. Communication has often ceased, and social distancing between the two, known as "the silent treatment," commonly occurs.
3. *Dissolution.* In this stage, the adolescent and significant other have already decided that the dispute cannot be resolved and have chosen to terminate the relationship.

GOALS AND STRATEGIES FOR THE
TREATMENT OF ROLE DISPUTES

The goal for treatment of interpersonal role disputes depends on the stage of the dispute (see Table 11.1). For those adolescents whose disputes are in the renegotiation or impasse stages, the goal for treatment is to help the adolescent define and resolve the dispute. At times, the goal may be complete resolution of the conflict, and at other times the goal may have to be more limited to understanding the nature of the dispute and/or revising expectations for the relationship. Attaining these goals involves identifying the conflict and the significant people involved and modifying communications and expectations to help bring about some resolution to the dispute. If the relationship is in the dissolution stage, on the other hand, then mourning the loss of the relationship becomes one of the primary goals. This again involves identifying the conflict and the

TABLE 11.1. Summary of Goals and Strategies for Interpersonal Role Disputes
Problem Area

Goals	*Renegotiation and impasse stages* • Define and resolve the dispute by modifying communications and expectations *Dissolution stage* • Mourn the loss of the relationship
Strategies	*All stages* • Explore dispute • Identify dispute patterns • Conduct decision analysis • Improve communication skills

people involved in the conflict as well as understanding what occurred in the relationship and feeling competent and ready to establish new relationships. Regardless of the stage of the dispute, there are several common strategies to the treatment. As discussed with other problem areas, each of these strategies involves the use of a number of therapeutic techniques.

Identify and Explore the Dispute

Based on the interpersonal inventory, the therapist is likely to have some understanding of the nature of the dispute and the participants involved in the dispute. In order to decide on a plan of action for addressing the dispute and to confirm the stage of the dispute, however, the therapist needs to facilitate further discussion. This discussion should focus primarily on two areas: expectations for the relationship and communication patterns that may be contributing to the dispute.

The therapist needs to determine, regardless of whether or not the expectations are realistic, how they differ from the expectations of others in the dispute and how the adolescent has tried to resolve the dispute. The adolescent learns that disputes often arise because the people in the relationship have nonreciprocal role expectations and that exploration of the expectations may reveal some areas of agreement that can be starting points for resolution or negotiation of a compromise. In exploring role disputes the therapist may ask:

What do you and [name] fight about? How do your fights end? How do you feel when that happens? How would you like [name] to re-

spond to you when you have these fights? How do you think [name]
would like you to respond? Then, how would you both feel? What are
your expectations for this relationship? In what ways have you been
disappointed? Do you think you have disappointed [name]? How do
you think your relationship with [name] can be helped or improved?
If [name] can't change, how can you handle it? What other options or
resources are available to you?

The therapist and adolescent also explore communication patterns that may be complicating the resolution of the dispute. Disputes often are difficult to resolve because the participants are reluctant to approach each other about the conflict, they do not know how to express their negative feelings in a nondestructive manner, they are stuck in their repetition of complaints and/or they are unable to move into the reconstructive stage due to fear of having to confront their role in the dispute.

THERAPIST: It sounds like you and your mom had a pretty common argument about whether or not you could go out with your friends.

PATIENT: Yes, it happens almost every weekend. I know that no matter what I do she is never going to let me go to any parties with the guys.

THERAPIST: What have you tried to say to her when you ask permission?

PATIENT: I just tell it like it is: "Mom, the guys have invited me out to a party on Saturday night, but I know you will never let me go, will you? I mean, I am the only one who is never allowed to go out to these kinds of things. I hate it!"

THERAPIST: How do you think those statements made your mom feel?

PATIENT: Well, she got pretty angry and said, "I don't care what anyone else is allowed to do. I only care about my son, and you're not going."

THERAPIST: What did you do then?

PATIENT: I went into my room and threw some stuff around my room— just pillows and clothes and stuff, but I was really angry.

An adolescent often acts out with disruptive, antisocial, or self-punishing behavior rather than expressing his feelings directly. The therapist might say to the patient:

When you and [name] fight, it's clear that aside from becoming angry,
you also feel very sad and disappointed. These feelings have been hard

for you to acknowledge to yourself, let alone talk about with [name]. Instead, you become angry and act like [list behaviors]. Have you ever tried to tell [name] what you are feeling? What do you think would happen if you told [name] how you really felt? How do you think [name] would respond? Would you be willing to try to tell [name] how you feel?

The aim here is to help adolescents recognize their complex, mixed feelings of anger, fear, and sadness and the ways in which their difficulties in communicating these feelings effectively have contributed to their dispute and, in turn, their depression. This understanding will enable the adolescent to make choices about modifying communication techniques and negotiating the actual details of the dispute.

Identify Patterns within Disputes

The therapist also needs to look for similar patterns of nonreciprocal expectations or communication problems in previous or other relationships to better understand the nature of the adolescent's difficulties. Such parallels include repeated conflicts with friends and earlier conflicts with parents that were difficult to resolve. Sometimes the similarities to other experiences may be more covert, such as the adolescent who describes many people having similar negative reactions to him. To better assess the scope of the particular dispute the therapist might ask:

Have you ever had similar conflicts with other people? Have other people ever reacted to you in a similar manner? Would you say you get into disputes with people frequently? What happens? Do you feel this way often?

When the dispute is discovered to be part of a larger pattern, it is important to explore what is happening to the adolescent as a result of these disputes. Is there any positive outcome for the adolescent? Is there a common misconception about the conduct of relationships underlying the disputes? What keeps leading the adolescent to similar disputes?

Make Decisions Regarding Solutions to the Dispute

After achieving an understanding of the issues or nonreciprocal expectations underlying the dispute, the therapist and adolescent move to the second stage of the treatment where decisions are made regarding specific solutions to the dispute.

Renegotiation or Impasse Stage

For the treatment of disputes at the renegotiation or impasse stage, the latter sessions focus on the specific negotiations and concomitant decisions about the issue in question. At this stage the therapist might say:

> *Now that we understand the connection between your depression and your relationship with [name] and how your feelings have led to behaviors and actions that are ultimately self-defeating, let's see what things you can do to change this pattern in your life. What other options do you see for yourself? How would you feel if you handled the situation in these different ways?*

The length of time and steps needed to make decisions regarding a plan of action for resolving a dispute vary with the nature and complexity of the dispute.

If the therapist and patient determine that the role dispute is in the state of renegotiation, it might be handled as follows:

> *You and [name] are fighting frequently. It seems to me that the underlying reason for your fights is that you expect something from [name] that [name] isn't giving to you and vice versa. No matter how hard the two of you try, you get stuck in the same battle, and neither one of you can find a solution. You both care about each other and want to find a solution. I'd like to help you clarify what it is you want from the relationship and find new ways of communicating with [name] about these goals. To make this work easier, we may ask [name] to come in to a later session to see how together we can practice some skills and try to decrease the conflict.*

In the case of an impasse, the therapist might say:

> *You and [name] are at odds with each other. Neither one of you understands the other, and you each feel there is no solution to the problem. Now you don't even talk to each other. Maybe you're right that there is no solution, but I'd like to try to get the two of you to talk to each other again to see whether you can work out your problems. Maybe talking to someone outside the immediate situation will help you feel differently and help you find a better solution to your problems with [name] than not speaking. At first you and [name] may be fighting again and it will feel like before. Once you understand your own feelings better and have tried everything you can to resolve the problem between you and [name], you will feel better and can then*

make a clear decision about whether this relationship can be helped or not.

It is important that the therapist doesn't direct the adolescent to one or another of the solutions. Rather, the therapist's job is to guide the adolescent to see options that he has and to evaluate those options. The technique of decision analysis is very useful at this point in the treatment of a role dispute. The therapist might say:

> *It seems that you are at a crossroads in your relationship with your brother. The two of you have very different expectations for your relationship, and you are having considerable difficulty communicating your feelings about the conflict. Recently you have chosen to pull away from the relationship, and although you have said to your mother and to me that you don't care anymore about it, you seem very upset and bothered by the distance between the two of you. It seems that your decision to withdraw from the relationship has actually led to your feeling even more depressed. I think you may have other options, and I would like us to consider those together. Can you think of any other options for solving this problem?*

The therapist helps the adolescent identify his options for solving the dispute and evaluate those options for their advantages and disadvantages. In doing so, the adolescent explores how different decisions are likely to make him and his brother feel and how that might relate to his depression. These therapy discussions are likely to lead to changes in the adolescent's view of the dispute. These changes can take the form of revised expectations for the relationship, improvements in their ability to communicate with each other, identification of other resources to fulfill certain needs that may take the pressure off this relationship, or, if necessary, an informed decision to end the relationship.

Since many of the disputes occur between the adolescent and the parents, there are times when less-than-optimal outcomes have to be accepted if the parent is resistant to change. For example, the adolescent may need to understand the parents' difficulties that may be preventing them from meeting some of the adolescent's expectations for their relationship. In this instance, the adolescent's expectations may be reasonable and those of the family may not be. The therapist helps the adolescent find strategies for coping with the unreasonable and immutable expectations of the parent and the feelings of anger and sadness engendered. It is helpful for the adolescent to have another person verify his perceptions of the dispute, in addition to finding ways to cope with the situation. It must be stressed that this is a less-than-optimal goal, but one that sometimes must be adopted when dealing with a resistant parent or any second party.

Case Example

John presented with a major depression precipitated by conflicts with his father, who was described both by John and his mother as very rigid and short-tempered. John's depression stemmed from his father's severe restrictions of his activities, so that he was unable to participate in extracurricular activities and had very limited opportunities to spend time with friends. John's mother felt there was little she could do to influence the father, and the father refused to come for treatment with his son. Since the therapist was unable to assist in negotiations with the father, the goal of treatment was to identify methods of coping with the situation, realistic expectations of the father to eliminate repeated disappointments, and pleasurable activities that John could engage in with minimal contact with his father. Another goal was to identify an alternative family member to provide him with the nurturance, support, and interest in his activities that his father was unable to provide for him. This proved to be very beneficial for John. He was able to identify an uncle with whom he could talk and spend time. His depressive symptoms gradually dissipated, and his self-esteem and school performance improved.

Dissolution Stage

In working with adolescents, it is more common for relationships in the dissolution stage to be with peers, nonfamily members, or extended family members. Although the adolescent's relationship with his parent can be determined to be in the dissolution stage, whenever possible the therapist attempts to preserve workable family relationships. The therapist needs to consider whether direct intervention with family members will help alleviate the problems and whether outside social service resources are required. Social service resources may be helpful by sending a home health care worker to relieve an overwhelmed mother, a visiting nurse to provide services for an ill family member, or public assistance to provide necessary material goods or housing. If a resolution within the family is not possible, then the therapist may need to assist the adolescent in accessing alternative care, such as arranging for the adolescent to live with a relative.

If the therapist agrees with the patient that the relationship is irretrievably disrupted, the therapist's task is to help the patient successfully mourn the loss of the relationship and move on to other relationships. At this point, the strategies employed by the therapist resemble those discussed in the chapter on grief. The therapist helps the patient to review the entirety of the relationship, to explore the impact of the loss of the relationship, and to identify ways to move on to new relationships from this experience.

Improve Communication Skills

For most adolescents identified as having a role dispute, improving communication skills is an important strategy for resolving the dispute. These adolescents need to develop more effective communication skills regarding both their feelings and their expectations for the particular relationship that is at the core of the dispute. The communication problems of adolescents with role disputes differ from those of adolescents with interpersonal deficits in that their difficulties with communication often center on one particular relationship. This is not to say that they don't have difficulties in other relationships as well, but it is equally likely that a therapist will find that these adolescents do communicate more effectively in other relationships. This is important to determine so the therapist can use the adolescent's experience and skills from the other relationships as building blocks for improving his communication in the relationship of concern. For example, the therapist might say:

> *From our discussions about your relationship with your mother it is clear that you have considerable difficulty telling her directly when your feelings are hurt and talking to her about your desire to be closer with her. It is my sense that this is an area that we need to work on to help you to resolve your dispute with your mother. We also have talked about a number of other relationships in your life, including your relationship with your aunt. You describe her as being very important to you and someone with whom you can really talk. You described a time when you were upset with her because she shared information with members of your extended family that you had wanted her to keep in confidence. I was struck by how well you told her of your disappointment and frustration. It sounds to me like she was really able to understand how you were feeling and to behave differently in the future. How did that make you feel? Do you think that is something you might be able to try doing with your mother? What do you anticipate would be hard about doing that? What might help you to be able to use that skill with your mother?*

The goal is to help the adolescent learn effective strategies for managing the interactions in a particular relationship. These strategies can include expressing feelings more directly, avoiding situations that will lead to disputes and anger, and reducing impulsive behavior that results from failure to verify one's understanding of the behavior of others. This strategy is equally important for adolescents in the dissolution stage of a dispute, as they need to clarify and express their feelings directly and to constructively facilitate their ability to develop other successful relationships. In addition to interventions like the one described above, IPT-A relies on a number of therapeutic techniques to specifically target adolescents' communication skills, including modeling, communication analysis, and role playing.

THE ROLE OF PARENTS IN THE
TREATMENT OF ROLE DISPUTES

When the dispute involves one or both parents, it is often helpful to involve them in treatment. Early in the middle phase, the therapist explains to both the adolescent and the parent how interpersonal role disputes contribute to depressive symptoms and how resolution of these disputes can alleviate the symptoms. For example, the therapist might say to the adolescent:

> *The fights you are getting into with your father make you angry at first, but then leave you with a feeling of hopelessness and helplessness. You feel powerless to change his attitudes and see no way out for yourself. As we talk about your relationship with your father, we will try to find other ways for you to relate to him. You may find that your father will change toward you, but if he doesn't, then you may come to accept him as he is and find other ways of getting what you want.*

The therapist might say to the parent:

> *The fights you and your child are getting into make him feel worse about himself, and I am sure they are upsetting to you as well. Your relationship with [name of child] at this point seems more than either of you can handle on your own. Perhaps I can be more useful to you and your child by meeting with you together. That way, I can coach both of you to communicate differently with each other so that you both will feel understood. As this happens, your child will feel less depressed, which will be a relief to you, your child, and the rest of the family.*

For disputes in the renegotiation or impasse stage, one or two joint sessions later in the middle phase often are helpful in specifically addressing the expectations and communication difficulties that are at the core of the dispute. Prior to initiating a joint session, the therapist should carefully assess the adolescent's and parents' willingness to address the dispute and to work on the skills needed to improve their relationship. Preferably this should be done in person, but if necessary this can be done with the parent(s) by telephone. The joint session then focuses on clarifying expectations for the relationship and possible solutions to the dispute with the mediation, coaching, and support of the therapist. For disputes in the dissolutions stage, it still may be beneficial to have both parties meet with the therapist to discuss their feelings about ending the relationship so they can achieve a more successful good-bye and mutual acknowledgment that the relationship is over. The therapist helps the two people involved end the relationship with better knowledge of what went wrong so that they hopefully won't make the same mistake in the next relationship.

SUMMARY

Successful resolution of a role dispute occurs when the adolescent is able to communicate more openly, to engage the other person in direct nonconflictual discussion of the dispute, and to consider the other person's perspective in the renegotiations. In less optimal circumstances, successful resolution of the dispute may consist of developing more realistic expectations for the relationship that effectively remove the adolescent from the conflict by shifting his focus to other more rewarding relationships. Either strategy should contribute to a decrease in depressive feelings.

The following case illustrates the course of treatment addressing the identified problem of a role dispute in the renegotiation stage of the dispute.

CASE VIGNETTE: THE CASE OF ALICE

Alice was a 15-year-old girl who was living with both her parents when she began treatment. She was attending a girls high school. Her chief complaints were a lack of interest in her friends and school activities as well as increasing moodiness. Additional symptoms included sad mood, anorexia, insomnia, and difficulty sustaining attention in school. Her relationship with her parents had deteriorated over the preceding year. She found her parents to be intrusive and restrictive. They were vigilant about her schoolwork and were restricting her activities to ensure academic improvement. There was a great deal of tension and fighting between her and her parents, and she began to withdraw more and more into her room. She vacillated between directing anger at herself for being angry at her parents and directing anger at her parents for their lack of understanding and their restrictiveness. She related her depression to her relationship with her parents but had little hope that this relationship would change. She dated the onset of her difficulties to the middle of this current school year and the increasing tension and pressures she felt from her parents. She felt as though they did not trust her and had little consideration for her feelings and little understanding of a 15-year-old's world.

Exploration of her interpersonal relationships revealed a paucity of social supports and close friendships. This was associated with her inability to express her needs and get them met in her relationships. She was an only child, born in South America, and had lived there with her mother and her mother's parents until joining her father in the United States at the age of 6 years. Alice felt close to her mother but very estranged from her father. The tension of her relationship with her father had adversely affected Alice's relationship with her mother.

After gathering information about the current depression and the surrounding events as well as her perception of the difficulties in her relationship with her parents, the therapist tried to explore what Alice's goals were for therapy. She reported that she wanted (1) to better understand her mood changes and stop fighting so much with her parents and (2) to learn how to express herself better so that she could negotiate better with her parents.

Although the interpersonal history made it clear that the patient had some role transition difficulties, the most pressing problem appeared to be an interpersonal role dispute with her parents regarding rules about socializing outside the house and general adolescent culture.

Initial Sessions (1–4)

In the early sessions, Alice focused on her ambivalence regarding her parents' treatment of her as a young child. A part of her enjoyed times when she would look upset and she would be hovered over as if she was a young child. Another part of her was craving for some privacy. She expressed having the most conflicts with her father. She described a history of resentment for his strictness and an increasing sense of being hurt by his expectations and rigidness. She felt unable to please him. She felt her only options were withdrawal, secret disregard of his rules, or denial of her own interests and desires. An interpersonal inventory of her relationship with her parents revealed conflict with her parents, consisting of frequent disagreements over house rules, friends, and social activities. She felt they should be able to understand her feelings from looking at her and then reacting accordingly. The focus of these sessions was to elucidate her expectations for her relationship with her parents and how she thought things would have to change for the situation to improve. Since she needed to live with her parents and finish school, her goal needed to be to find a way to improve communication with her parents, particularly her father.

Alice's pattern of communication was discussed first. She described a conflict they had recently about whether she could participate in an after-school activity. She described a situation in which she had asked permission to participate in an activity, and when met with parental reluctance she did not pursue the issue but instead withdrew into her room upset and disappointed. She acknowledged that her withdrawal made it more difficult for her parents to understand what it is that she wanted to do and why. Her anger toward her parents frightened her and she feared expressing it, so instead she withdrew. She began to discuss a bit more about her dissatisfactions in her relationship with her parents and her unhappiness over their lack of trust in her. She said she would try to express her feelings more when in discussions with her parents, but she still believed that "it wouldn't change anything."

Middle Sessions (5–8)

Alice began to explore solutions specifically in regard to a dispute she was having with her parents over their suspicion that she was smoking in her bedroom. She discussed how she told them it wasn't true. Despite their scanty evidence, they were still convinced that it was true and lectured her extensively about her behavior. She did not respond to their lectures, although quite angry, because she felt that they wouldn't change their mind no matter what she said. She felt one of the fundamental problems was their basic lack of trust in her. Alice and the therapist began to generate other possible actions she could take when confronted with these lectures, including ways to state her feelings and demonstrate that she was being truthful. After role playing different options in a session, Alice and the therapist decided it might be helpful to have her parents join them for a session. Both Alice and her parents agreed to do so.

Prior to meeting jointly, the therapist met briefly alone with the parents first, and their communication difficulties were readily apparent. Alice's mother was very quiet throughout the meeting, leaving discussion of the rules to her husband. Alice's father was very dogmatic in his discussion of Alice's behavior in terms of what he felt was appropriate or not, and he appeared to mistrust her ability to be more independent. Before inviting Alice to join them, the therapist coached the parents on how to be more open to listening to the message Alice was trying to send and thinking of possible compromises for their disagreements. Alice joined the session. In anticipation of her father's punitiveness, she initially refused to respond to her parents. The therapist encouraged Alice to respond to her father and tried to help her father allow her to express her feelings without belittling her. They were able briefly to experience a different way of listening and speaking to each other that provided a spark of hope for Alice that things could change.

In the following session, Alice began to discuss things she would like to say to her parents, and she and the therapist rehearsed them in session. She reported that she was feeling more motivated in her schoolwork and having less trouble concentrating in class. She still expressed some fear about what her father's reaction might be to her new assertiveness. However, she had begun talking more with her mother, who also was encouraging her to express herself, so she was feeling some added support. Much time was devoted to improving her communication skills in a manner that could be received positively by her parents.

Termination Sessions (9–12)

In the final sessions, Alice began to explore her communication patterns in other settings such as school and identifying more effective means of communicating both at home and at school. Alice was still having conflicts with her parents about the time spent in her bedroom, but she was feeling better able to respond to them and assert her position. She still wished that she didn't have to put any effort into her relationship with her parents, that they could just intuit what she was feeling and thinking, but the therapist helped her to realize that this wish was unrealistic.

During one of the sessions, she again appeared more reticent and withdrawn. The therapist discussed what this behavior felt like for her in the session and its impact on the therapist's ability to help her with her problems as well as other people outside of therapy. She learned how her behavior affects the responses she receives from people and how she can help change these responses through her own facial expression and tone of voice. The final two sessions were spent discussing her recovery and how to recognize a reoccurrence. A major focus also was on recognizing her achievements in therapy and the application of these skills to other relationships and situations.

Alice was becoming more involved in the therapeutic process and while she had improved greatly, she would have benefited from follow-up continuation treatment to consolidate her improvements and new skills. Unfortunately, her family felt strongly about trying to work things out on their own. They were encouraged to return for treatment if there were any more difficulties.

CHAPTER 12

Interpersonal Role Transitions

A problem of role transition is defined as a difficulty adjusting to a life change that requires a modification of the old role or a new role (Klerman et al., 1984; Weissman et al., 2000). Role transitions mark the turning points between the major stages of life—from childhood to puberty, high school to college, single to married, student to worker, couple to parenthood, and married to widowed. Some transitions are biologically determined, while others are influenced by society and culture. When such transitions occur in a generally expected pattern, they are a normative part of development that one can anticipate and prepare for both psychologically and physically.

In addition to these more normative and predictable transitions, time and circumstances can place people in different social roles more unexpectedly. Events such as a sudden death, illness, or changes in one's family structure due to divorce or separation are unexpected and may be more unsettling and difficult to accept. The impact of such changes is strongly affected by the social context of the event and the other people involved in the person's social system.

Success in carrying out new roles affects a person's self-esteem and can affect personal, social, and professional relationships. Even positive life changes (e.g., graduation, acceptance to college) can trigger depression since they involve a loss of familiarity and comfort with the current stage of life. Depression can impair a person's ability to successfully negotiate a role transition. Conversely, difficulties in making the transition from one role to another can result in depression. These problems may

143

arise because (1) the role is thrust upon the person unexpectedly, (2) the role is an undesired one, (3) the person is not psychologically or emotionally prepared for the new role, or (4) the old role is missed. The social impairment and sense of loss experienced in an unsuccessful role transition can contribute to feelings of depression.

ADOLESCENT ROLE TRANSITIONS
General Transitions

Adolescents encounter role transitions as a normative part of their developmental process. Erikson (1968) delineated the normative transitions associated with the stages of adolescent and young adult development including (1) passage into puberty, (2) the shift from group relationships to dyadic relationships, (3) initiation of sexual desires and relationships, (4) separation from parents and family to achieve increased independence, (5) having to find a first job to support oneself financially, and (6) taking responsibility for one's future through such things as work, career, or college planning. These expected transitions are usually anticipated by adolescents and their family as rites of passage and typically handled successfully.

Problems, however, can occur during these transitions. Complications arise when parents are unable to accept the concomitant changes to the transition (such as their child's desire to spend more time with friends and less time with family) or when the adolescent himself is unable to cope with the changes. For example, adolescents who become depressed in the latter years of high school are commonly troubled by the increasing pressure and responsibility to make decisions about their future. They may have been more comfortable in the earlier grades where they were still protected from making such decisions.

Role transitions also can be thrust upon adolescents as a result of unanticipated circumstances. Unforeseen or imposed role transitions include (1) a change in family role due to illness in the family, an impaired parent, or separation from parents and (2) becoming an adolescent parent. The ability of adolescents to cope with unforeseen circumstances rests on prior psychological development and current social supports. Problems that occur with imposed transitions often are a result of the adolescent feeling overwhelmed by new responsibilities associated with the changed family structure and feeling unable to cope with the added pressures. Frequently there is confusion about what the new role involves and what desirable aspects of the old life can continue.

Difficulties with role transitions, both expected and unexpected, can present in a number of ways. These problems can be seen in the adolescent's (1) loss of self-esteem, (2) inability to meet expectations set by oneself or one's family such as increased demands to achieve, (3) difficulty managing peer pressure to fit in with the peer-group behavior, (4) inability to let go of dependence on the family due to lack of self-confidence, or (5) the family's reluctance to separate or inability to let go. Failure to cope with role transitions also can result in feelings of decreased social support and associated feelings of sadness, anger, fear, and disappointment. Difficulties with transitions occur for several reasons: (1) impairment in social functioning, possibly as a result of depression; (2) psychological and social immaturity; (3) adolescent–parent problems; and (4) changes caused by an unexpected event. Therefore, depression can contribute to role transition problems and vice versa.

Transitions Specific to Family Structural Change

When the adolescent's role transition is precipitated by a change in the family structure through divorce, separation, or simply interparental conflict years after the event, these events can set off a chain reaction of other changes as well as familial disputes. Many teens living in single-parent and stepfamily situations manage the transition with only minimal difficulty and disruption in functioning. For vulnerable teens living in particularly challenging family systems, however, the conflicts and complexities of this transition and the resulting family structure may trigger depression as well as other related difficulties.

Many models have been proposed to explain the association between family structural changes and difficulties in child adjustment. Hetherington, Bridges, and Insabella (1998), in a review of the literature in this area, have found support for the role of parental distress, stress, socioeconomic disadvantage, family composition, and individual risk for adjustment problems contributing to the association between family structural change and emotional and behavioral problems in children. The quality of the relationship among the parents and between the child and each parent affects the child's ability to cope with the family structural changes (Brody & Forehand, 1990). Children from both divorced and remarried families are at higher risk than those from nondivorced families to experience a number of difficulties, including internalizing and externalizing symptoms, academic problems, lower self-esteem, and difficulties in relationships (Hetherington et al., 1998; Amato & Keith, 1991; Cherlin & Furstenberg, 1994; Hetherington, 1989, 1997).

Adolescents whose depression appears most proximally related to a change in family structure are distinguished from other teens with the identified problem area of role transitions. In the previous edition of this book, these adolescents were identified with the problem area of single-parent family. Based upon another decade of treating adolescents, it seemed that the challenges were really of a transitional nature, compli- cated by disputes, and these would be best conceptualized as a subtype of transition. The problem in these families typically involves the adolescent's parents and only peripherally involves the adolescent, although it still af- fects the adolescent significantly. Problems occur in situations where there has been a change in the family structure or when an event has occurred that has stressed the functioning of the existing structure. The parents' dif- ficulties and sense of helplessness frequently cause an age-inappropriate shift in the adolescent's role in the family. This results in both role conflict as well as problems in making the transition to a different stage of life or family structure. The changes and disputes created by the stress of this transition often place conflicting and developmentally inappropriate de- mands on the adolescent that often lead to depression.

Since many of these adolescents have a secondary problem area of role disputes, their treatment involves an integration of the two problem areas with a primary focus on the relationship conflict that is complicat- ing the transition. Since the locus of the difficulty tends to reside in the parental relationship or the parents' handling of the dissolution of the relationship, different strategies may need to be used. Some key differ- ences in treatment will be highlighted throughout this chapter. For ex- ample, in divorce situations, the adolescent can get entangled in issues of parental compliance with the custody agreement. It is important to ex- plore any instances where the adolescent feels responsible for enforcing such issues. The adolescent may feel a need to stand up for the custodial parent who is perceived as helpless, but at the same time the adolescent will find this a very stressful and unpleasant role to play. In these situa- tions, the therapist needs to empower the parents to relieve the adoles- cent from the role of family mediator or verbal messenger and reassure him that it is a matter for the parents to work out themselves.

DIAGNOSING ROLE TRANSITION PROBLEMS

A therapist is likely to diagnose role transition as the identified problem area if the interpersonal history and review of life events suggests that the onset of depression coincides with some type of social or role-change event. The transition specific to family structural change is targeted when the adolescent's depression appears to be the result of family stress specifically caused by a change in family structure (e.g., a shift to becom- ing a single-parent or stepfamily structure), or stress event (e.g., failure to comply with a child custody agreement). It may be that the structural change occurred several years ago, but the problems have arisen more recently due to increased or decreased contact with a parent. The adolescent often is able to identify such an event as being associated with decreased self-esteem that later impairs social functioning. In order to gain more information about the nature of an expected transition, the therapist might ask:

> *What was it like for you to [leave school, have your first romantic relationship, first job, etc.]? Was it different than what you expected? How did it make you feel? Did your life change in any way? How? How did you feel about these changes? Did the important people in your life change? In what way? How did you like being in this new role [as student, employee, boyfriend/girlfriend]? How did your mother react to this change in your life? Your father? Your brothers and sisters?*

Role transitions for adolescents affect and are affected by the family. It is important to question the parents as well as the child about the transition. Therefore, the therapist might ask the parent:

> *Could you tell me about the changes you see occurring with [name]? Are you comfortable with these changes? What do you like about the changes you see? What do you not like about the changes you see? Are there changes you would like to see in [name], new responsibilities you would like [name] to assume that you don't see happening? How do you feel about [name] [becoming more independent, or spending more time away from home, having a boyfriend/girlfriend, or working at his/her first job]? What are your concerns? How have these changes affected your relationship with [name] or the rest of the family?*

At times, it is family members that are having trouble accepting the changes in the adolescent's role in the family. Their lack of acceptance can result in depression in the adolescent. At other times, the family may be pushing the adolescent to make a transition faster than is comfortable, for example, sending the adolescent away to school before the adolescent feels ready to leave home.

TREATING ROLE TRANSITIONS

Common goals and strategies are employed for the treatment of depression that is associated with the different types of role transitions experienced by adolescents: general transitions and transitions specific to fam-

TABLE 12.4. Summary of Goals and Strategies for Role Transition Problem Area

Goals	• Relinquish old role and accept new role
	• Develop sense of mastery over new role
Strategies	• Educate about the transition
	• Review old and new roles: Feelings and expectations
	• Assess and develop social skills
	• Develop social support

ily structural change. The main goals of the treatment are (1) to help the adolescent relinquish the old role and accept the new one and (2) to enable the adolescent to develop a sense of mastery and competence in his functioning in the new role (see Table 12.1). Although goals for the treatment of family structural change as a transition are essentially the same as for general transitions, they differ in their focus on both the adolescent's role associated with the old and new family structures as well as relationship conflicts occurring in those structures. In order to accomplish the general treatment goals for both types of transitions, the therapist uses a number of strategies, many of which are illustrated in the following case example.

Case Example

Sally was a 14-year-old who presented with a major depression. Her depressive symptoms coincided with her graduation from middle school and her entrance into high school. While in middle school, Sally had been a good student and had a small group of friends with whom she spent her time. She was involved in one or two activities at the school but would typically come home after the end of the school day and spend time with her younger sister. Sally presented for treatment midway through the ninth grade, her first year in high school. She was no longer doing well academically and had withdrawn from her friends. She would complain that she didn't feel well and frequently left school early or did not go at all. She described feeling as though she no longer fit in with her friends and other peers. She felt they had changed a lot in ways she didn't like. The therapist's goal was to explore what Sally had liked about middle school, what was missing in high school, and what Sally might need to do in order to make herself feel more comfortable in high school. The therapist used several strategies: reviewing the positive and negative aspects of the old and new roles; identifying skills needed to feel more competent in the new role; and practicing new social skills, improved communication techniques, and new problem-solving skills. Sally and the therapist role-played skills for different interpersonal scenarios that might present in high school so that Sally could feel more confident with her peers. They practiced how to communicate more clearly and confidently about her opinions on whether or not she liked a particular activity or was comfortable participating in it.

As seen in the above illustration, Sally needed to mourn the loss of her old role as a middle school student and identify the difficulties she was having in the move to high school. To do this, Sally needed to review the feelings associated with the old role that were comforting and to express her fears associated with the new role that were making the transition problematic. Some of her difficulties stemmed from her reluctance to talk about her feelings with her parents and friends and to obtain their support during the transition. Specific strategies for addressing general transitions as well as transitions specific to family structural change are discussed in more detail in the following sections.

STRATEGY 1: EDUCATING PATIENTS
AND PARENTS ABOUT THE TRANSITION

General Transitions

Continued education about the impact of transitions and the association between the transition and the patient's depressive symptoms is critical early in the middle phase. Frequently, parents must be educated about normal developmental tasks for an adolescent, the feelings such tasks may elicit in the parents, and ways to cope with their feelings. The therapist might say to the parents, in a separate session:

> *Your child is growing up, having new experiences. Even though you realize the importance of these changes and are proud of your child, it can sometimes be hard for parents to see their child growing up and growing away from them. Is there anything that makes you uncomfortable about letting your daughter have these new experiences? What concerns you? You may feel a certain sadness and loss about these changes. Kathy needs to feel your support for these changes, and it's all right for Kathy to know that you feel sad as long as she knows you basically want these changes for her. Kathy needs to have your support and know that you are there for her. Without the feeling of support and permission to move on she will feel conflicted about making the transition, and this can lead to feelings of depression.*

In educating parents, the therapist should remain sensitive to and respectful of the familial and cultural differences among families. The process of negotiating a role transition within the family system involves a compromise; it is about helping the parents see the adolescent's point of view and, in many cases, helping the adolescent better understand his parent's perspective. The therapist must keep the cultural context and its set of expectations for behavior in mind when assisting in finding a compromise solution. By encouraging effective communication, the therapist helps the family find a compromise that is likely to lead to improvement in the adolescent's symptoms and functioning without undermining the family's cultural framework. For example:

> An adolescent girl had a great deal of difficulty managing her separation from her parents and involvement in peer activities since she felt it was culturally expected of her never to challenge her parents' restrictions. She knew it was normal for an adolescent to actively participate in activities with friends after school. At the same time, such participation was not acceptable to her parents, whose native culture restricted such a shift in focus from family to peer activities. She tried to ignore the extent to which their restrictions made her unhappy and prevented her from pursuing activities, such as dance and theater, which she would have enjoyed. In this case, it was the parents' inability to accept a normative role transition that was contributing to the adolescent's inability to move forward developmentally and subsequent depression. However, the therapist needed to put the parents' stance in its cultural context. The therapist addressed the parents' concerns as well as those of the adolescent by meeting with the parents to understand their fears and to provide psychoeducation about normal adolescent separation and individuation from parents, including the cultural norms of the United States that differ from those of their culture.
>
> Armed with knowledge of both parties' concerns and the cultural context of the parents' expectations, the therapist assisted the family in negotiating a compromise that would acknowledge the importance of both points of view. In this case, the family was able to agree to allow their daughter to participate in certain activities with guidelines for setting curfews.

Prior to conducting such negotiations, the therapist needs to ask the adolescent:

> *How do your parents feel about your interests in these activities? How do you feel when your parents express their concerns and restrict your participation? What do you say to them? When you see the other students staying after school, how do you feel? Even though we love our parents, sometimes they make decisions for us that make us*

unhappy. It is all right to love your parents and be angry at them too. Ideally, what would you like your parents to say when you ask to do these activities? Do you sometimes feel like doing them anyway? How else do you feel? Do you ever feel guilty about feeling angry or feeling like you want to disobey your parents?

In circumstances where the adolescent is engaging in objectively inappropriate behavior, the therapist discusses these behaviors with both the adolescent and the parent(s). Together they must negotiate guidelines for more socially acceptable behavior. Necessary groundwork for the negotiation includes clarifying the adolescent's expectations for his parents' behavior toward him, educating the adolescent about appropriate and/or safe behavior, correcting the adolescent's misperceptions about his behavior, and assisting the adolescent and the parents in finding activities that will be acceptable to each of them. This set of negotiations will involve sessions alone with the adolescent as well as joint sessions with the parents.

THERAPIST: It sounds like you are doing some things that may be dangerous to you, like staying out in the park until 3:00 A.M. Can you understand your parents' concerns?

PATIENT: Yes, but I am hanging out with my friends—other kids are there. Why do they have so many rules?

THERAPIST: It is important to understand why your parents are making these rules and then think about how you can respond to them. Can you tell me what is the purpose of your parents' rules?

PATIENT: I guess my parents want to make sure I am safe and keep me from having a good time.

THERAPIST: And what are your goals?

PATIENT: I want to have fun like the rest of my friends.

THERAPIST: I am not sure that your parents want to stop you from having fun. The question is can you find a way to have fun and be with your friends while respecting your parents' real concerns for your safety? Being out in the park all night is not safe. What other activities might be fun as well as meet the safety concerns of your parents?

Some parents have difficulty accepting developmental changes such as their adolescent wanting to spend more time with friends than with family, wanting later curfews, or not sharing as much information about herself with the family. The parents need to be educated as to what is appropriate behavior for an adolescent so they can recognize what behaviors to accept and what behaviors to be concerned about. The therapist can tell the parents:

> Your child is going through changes that you find hard to accept. This is part of growing up and is perfectly normal. These changes don't mean Kathy doesn't love you or care about the family any more. Sometimes children react with anger or pull away from the family because they love their families so much it is the only way they can become independent. Can you remember when you were Kathy's age and what you felt like and wanted for yourself? Well, Kathy is now feeling those same things and needs to feel your support through this change. You have given your child ideas about life and a sense of values that are part of who she is, and you need to have faith in Kathy that she has learned well from you.

The therapist evaluates their concerns and fears, normalizes them, and puts them in the appropriate context. Asking the parents to recall their own experiences can help them empathize with their children.

Transitions Specific to Family Structural Change

In treating this specific transition, psychoeducation proceeds in essentially the same manner as general transitions. Education focuses on helping the adolescent and parents recognize and understand the association between the adolescent's depression and the change in family structure. Part of this work is acknowledging that a parent's departure or that the parents' separation/divorce was indeed a significant life disruption. Particular emphasis must be placed on educating all parental figures including custodial, noncustodial, biological, and stepparents, whenever appropriate, about the effects of their conflictual behavior on the adolescent. It is important to gain as many perspectives as possible on the changes that have occurred and the complex relationships between the parents, the adolescent, and the other parental figures. In many cases, effective treatment depends on facilitating critical changes within the parental unit of the family system.

STRATEGY 2: REVIEWING OLD AND NEW ROLES
General Transitions

The task of evaluating the adolescent's old role resembles the task of reviewing the positive and negative aspects of relationships—a strategy that is used to treat grief reactions as well as interpersonal deficits. The review helps the adolescent to develop a more realistic view of the old role. This enables the adolescent to relinquish the idealized version of the old role, mourn its loss, and begin to accept aspects of the new role. The therapist should elicit feelings associated with the change, including fear of associated expectations or challenges, sadness about the loss of the old role, anger at the change if it is unexpected, and/or disappointment if the changes are more limited than desired. To get a better sense of what the transition means to the adolescent, the therapist might say:

> *Sometimes people feel a sense of loss when they give up their place in a comfortable situation, even when they feel good about the changes. When this change occurred in your life, how did you feel about it? What did you worry about? For yourself? For your parents? For your friends?*

It is critical to consider both the adolescent's and the parents' reaction to the change. In many cases, it is a combination of both of their reactions that is ultimately leading to the adolescent's difficulties. This is illustrated in the following case example.

Case Example

Paige was having difficulty with her parents, making the transition from being dependent on her family for her social needs to being more independent and spending more time with friends. She felt her parents were not supportive of her transition, and she experienced feelings of guilt when she thought about asserting herself and joining more extracurricular activities in school. She felt guilty about challenging her parents' notions of what might be appropriate behavior at this age. In addition, she revealed concerns about her self-image and feared rejection if she tried out for the extracurricular activities and did not get accepted. Therefore, not only was she hindered by her parents' reluctance to let her be more independent, but she also had anxiety about becoming more involved in peer activities and risking rejection.

The therapist needed to first address Paige's interpersonal anxieties and review the necessary social skills for entry into these peer activities prior to identifying an appropriate compromise to discuss with her parents.

Transitions Specific to Family Structural Change

Due to divorce, remarriage, and abandonment, the review of social role expectations is necessary when addressing the stresses associated with family structural change. In contrast to general transitions, there are multiple layers of expectation associated with multiple parental figures. Consequently, the therapist needs to (1) identify all the key adults with expectations for the adolescent, (2) identify the adolescent's varying expectations for each relationship, (3) assess the adults' ability to work together to come to an agreement regarding expectations for the adolescent, and (4) explore and resolve the adolescent's feelings about any lost relationships or significantly changed relationships. This exploration of relationship expectations must be center stage in working through transitions specific to family structural change. The therapist addresses the adolescent's feelings of rejection, the loss of the previous family life, the guilt the adolescent may be harboring about the ruptured relationships, and the change in the adolescent's expectations about the role he would play in the parents' relationship (e.g., bringing them together, punishing the abandoning parent).

The therapist and adolescent need to be clear as to what each parent would like out of the relationship with the adolescent. In situations in which the noncustodial parent maintains an intermittent relationship with the adolescent, it would be ideal to have the parent come for a joint session with the adolescent. After clarifying their expectations, the therapist can either assist them in making the transition to a new type of relationship or can assist the adolescent in mourning the lost opportunity for a more consistent relationship. The therapist might ask the adolescent:

How do you feel about not seeing your [father/mother] very frequently? What is it like when the visits don't occur regularly? How has it changed your relationship? The way you talk to [him/her]? What do you miss about the relationship? What do you still enjoy about the relationship? What type of relationship would you like to have with your [father/mother] if [he/she] were available to you? Who makes the decision about how much time you two spend together? Have you ever told anyone how this visit schedule makes you feel and what ideally you would want?

In session, the adolescent may explore his wishes for his relationship with the absent or intermittently present parent. The therapist assists the adolescent in putting his sense of abandonment or loss in a perspective from which he can move on to other interpersonal relationships with the capacity for trust and mutual intimacy. If the parent is not available, then the therapist can try to engage the custodial parent to clarify the absent spouse's expectations and to help the adolescent develop more realistic expectations for the relationship. The therapist needs to understand the custodial parent's ideas about what type of relationship the adolescent could or should have with the noncustodial parent. It is necessary to consider whether the adolescent's relationship with the noncustodial parent may be contaminated by the custodial parent's feelings toward the departed spouse.

The therapist also needs to clarify whether the parental absence is permanent or temporary. If the noncustodial parent is not available for even intermittent contact and the absence is believed to be permanent, the main task is to achieve a realistic appraisal of the relationship (i.e., to help the adolescent to accept that the parent may no longer play an active role in the family) and to mourn the loss of the desired relationship. If the absence is possibly temporary, it is necessary to discuss reactions that might arise if or when the parent reappears. The adolescent should be prepared to handle a variety of encounters with the parent. The therapist might ask:

> How do you think you would feel if your [mother/father] returned home in a few months or a year and wanted to be involved in your life? What do you think you might want to tell [him/her]? What do you think you would be worried about? What would you like to do when you saw [him/her]?

Discussions also might focus on how to reconcile the desire to have the parent return with the fear that the loss would be repeated.

Another stressor arising from these structural changes is the change in the adolescent's relationship with the custodial parent and, at times, the adolescent's perception of the parent's role in the separation. The therapist could ask:

> What type of relationship do you have with your [mother/father] with whom you live now? Would you like the relationship to be any different? How would you like it to be different? Do you ever blame your [mother/father] for your [mother/father] leaving your home? If so, how do you think [he/she] was involved in your being separated from your [mother/father]? Do you feel anyone else had a part in causing this separation? How so?

It is important to try to uncover any misconceptions and/or incorrect assignment of blame for what has occurred in the family. There are some instances, particularly in circumstances of drug abuse allegations or incarceration, where the adolescent does not know the reasons for the parent's absence from home. The therapist must work with the parent to find a way to properly inform the adolescent of the reasons for the absence, to end the adolescent's incorrect self-blame or inappropriate anger at the remaining parent. Parents need to be reassured that it is better to help the adolescent address feelings about the truth than to worry about the adolescent hearing the truth inadvertently from someone else or having mistaken notions of responsibility. If the absence is a result of incarceration or drug behavior, the therapist and parent should address the adolescent's feelings of demoralization and stigma that can be associated with these behaviors (Lowenstein, 1986). The goal of this therapeutic work is to enable the adolescent to be emotionally prepared for the parent's possible or eventual return.

The clarification of role expectations in stepfamily situations is equally important. Stepfamily situations are uniquely challenging for all members of the family. Very often roles and responsibilities (e.g., who will function as the disciplinarian) are not negotiated. Here, too, there are often several parenting figures involved, including custodial parent, noncustodial parent, and stepparent. Expectations and feelings related to each of these relationships need to be clarified to resolve the transition difficulties.

STRATEGY 3: ASSESSING AND DEVELOPING SOCIAL SKILLS
General Transitions

Frequently the difficulty in making the role transition stems from a lack of self-confidence due to a secondary problem of skills deficits. The adolescent either may not have the necessary skills or may have fears or unrealistic expectations about the role that prevents effective use of the skills. The therapist should assist the adolescent in assessing which skills might be necessary to perform competently in the social role. Together they can review whether the assessment is realistic and compare the identified skills with those that the adolescent possesses and those he wishes to acquire. It is important to clarify whether the adolescent is overestimating or underestimating his potential to perform within the new role. Some of the skills may be on a very practical level, such as how to apply to college or how to find a first job. Others may be more abstract, such as developing the self-confidence and communication skills needed to ask another person to go out on a date.

Often, performance of the social role is adversely affected by anxiety about being successful or not. To relieve such anxiety, the therapist and adolescent can role-play difficult situations associated with the anxiety and problem-solve ways to handle the situation that can be practiced within the safety of the therapeutic relationship. The therapist might ask the patient:

Are there any social situations in which you feel more uncomfortable than others? What are they? What feels difficult when you are in the situation? Is it hard for you to talk to people you don't know very well? If you need help doing something, are you able to ask for help or do you struggle with it alone? Is there a situation you can think of that didn't go the way you wanted and made you feel badly? Is it hard to start a conversation with another person? What feels awkward? In this situation [on first date, first job] what do you worry will happen? How would you feel if this happened? What could you do or say in such a situation that would make you feel better?

Transitions can be made difficult if the adolescent clings to stereotyped assumptions about the new role. These assumptions may be the result of peer discussion and/or observation and identification with another individual in a similar role. The therapist's task is to broaden the adolescent's thinking by together identifying other people who have made similar transitions and discuss the skills they used to master the situation. For example, Beth was a 15-year-old girl who presented with major depression. She identified as a precipitant her difficulty in making the transition to a new coed school and having male as well as female friends. Prior to this school change, she had attended an all-girls school. She was encountering considerable difficulties in her relationships with young men in her class, feeling awkward and uncomfortable. She was envious of how the other girls appeared so comfortable around the boys. She had heard her mother talk about how boys her age would be out to take advantage of her and how she should always be careful, but it didn't look to her as though the other girls were feeling that way. She wanted to be able to feel comfortable around boys and have friendships with them as well as the girls in her class. The therapist tried to address her concerns and understand what skills she needed to be able to feel more comfortable in her new school, saying:

What are your relationships like with boys you know outside of school? How do you feel when you are around them? How do you feel when you are in a group of boys and girls in school? When do you begin to feel nervous? Are you able to start a conversation? How do you feel if a boy approaches you to talk? How does it feel different than when you try to speak to a new girl in the class? How could you feel more confident?

The therapist helps the adolescent recognize what skills she needs to feel more confident in communicating and interacting with boys as well as girls in her new school. The adolescent identifies her feelings that arise in this new situation as well as what she could do to change them for the better. The therapist tries to focus on relevant skills and strengths that the adolescent brings to the treatment to identify building blocks for the capabilities she needs to acquire to manage the transition. Drawing parallels between her stronger skills in talking to girls and the skills needed to talk to boys will facilitate building upon her existing social strengths.

Transitions Specific to Family Structural Change

The skills most vital to the treatment of adolescents in this type of transition include communication and negotiation skills. Learning to communicate one's feelings effectively to all parental figures is critical to ensure that the adolescent will be able to manage the inevitable challenges that will develop in these family structures. In situations in which a parent is sick or injured, thereby altering the family's way of functioning, the adolescent needs to be prepared to negotiate perhaps with another adult who may enter the system to help with the unexpected situation. The therapist generally helps the adolescent improve his negotiating skills by together generating and evaluating various options or solutions to identified problems in the family relationships. For example, in a single-parent family situation, the therapist might say to the adolescent:

> *Since you know you can only see your [mother/father] on weekends, what type of arrangement would you like to make for activities during these visits with [him/her]? How do you think this would work for your [mother/father]? What might be some of the difficulties? What are the things you like about this plan? How do you think this arrangement would be for [custodial parent]? How does your relationship with [custodial parent] make you feel? How can you help improve the feelings in that relationship while not sacrificing what you want in your relationship with your other parent? What may be some other possibilities to consider? How would you feel if you could make that plan work? How can you present this plan to your [mother/father]?*

The therapist helps the adolescent examine the proposed solution from the perspective of everyone involved before presenting it to the other parties. The proposal can be discussed in a session with the parents present, or the adolescent can try it at home on his own. The following week the adolescent can discuss why the communication either failed or succeeded either in an individual session with the therapist or joint parent–adolescent session. As the patient moves from the clarification to the negotiation phase, symptoms tend to decrease and the adolescent usually experiences relief.

Case Example

Sam, a 16-year-old male, is an only child who lives with his mother. His parents have been divorced since he was 8 years old. He presented with a major depression. He reported feeling depressed every day, crying frequently, suicidal ideation, difficulty falling asleep, waking frequently during the night, feeling tired, and difficulty concentrating in class since his parents began to have problems with the alimony agreement and visitation. The identified problem area was role transitions, specifically related to the family structural change.

Sam reported that he was having difficulty with his father's visits in part because he knew that his father wasn't helping with the child support. In addition, when his father visited he would expect Sam to drop all of his activities and plans with his friends and spend time with him, even when he did not give Sam and his mother advance notice. When he would express reluctance to cancel his plans, his father would say, "You don't love me as much as you love your mother," or "You prefer your friends to your father, right?" In addition, when they spent time together, he would still treat him like a little boy, trying to wrestle with him.

Sam knew that his mother was under financial stress, since his father wasn't helping. He could hear his parents yelling at each other on the phone late at night. So when he would see his father and see that he was spending money on himself and his friends, he would get angry and get into arguments with his dad. Sam observed that these stresses also were making his mother depressed. He began to try to convince his father to make the payments and told him to stop being so selfish. However, he became depressed and angry about their relationship and felt that maybe his father really didn't care about him if he didn't want to help them with money. He also didn't like when his father tried to send messages to his mother through him, making him an intermediary.

The therapist began by helping Sam to express his feelings about the living and visitation arrangements, about feeling caught between his two parental relationships, about his need to make his father help out and give him the message that he is important to him. His father refused to participate in treatment, so he and the therapist practiced in the session telling his father about how he would like to be treated. Simultaneously, through a joint session with the mother, the therapist helped the mother communicate to Sam that she appreciated his efforts on their behalf but it was no longer his job to pursue the father for money. His mother was able to discuss her feelings about Sam's relationship with the father and listen to Sam's desire to make some of his own choices about how to conduct his relationship with him. With her mother's permission, Sam chose to renegotiate his visits with his father, explaining to him the importance of being with his friends. Sam discussed with him his need to make dates with him in advance so he could give him the time without it interfering in his participation in sports and other activities with his friends. His proactive approach to negotiating the parameters of their relationship resulted in a decrease in depression symptoms.

If the mother was unable to arbitrate instead of her son in the above case, the therapist would need to help the adolescent tell his mother that he can no longer play this role and that they would have to make a plan to live without the father's contributions until the mother could resume her role in enforcing the financial agreement. Some new roles, like this one, are not desirable at all. In these instances, the goal is to remove oneself from this role and find other options. Negotiations tend to be more successful if the adolescent first defines his expectations for his relationship with both the custodial and noncustodial parent. The therapist should encourage the adolescent to continue to have an ongoing dialogue with the custodial parent to enable future negotiations about their familial roles.

STRATEGY 4: DEVELOPING SOCIAL SUPPORT FOR TRANSITIONS

General Transitions

The presence of support from family and/or friends is an important component of a successful role transition. While the adolescent may have anxiety about forming new attachments, the new role will appear more attractive if the social rewards are desirable and visible. The adolescent needs to identify the source of the anxiety and practice skills to reduce the anxiety that often accompanies the prospect of new relationships and new situations. Anxiety of this sort commonly occurs in the transition to high school. Although the student may have been successful in junior high school, the increase in the size of the school, the amount of work expected, and the change in fellow students and teachers may make the adolescent feel unprepared for the new environment. The adolescent may feel apprehensive about making new friends and participating in school activities, although the adolescent is likely also to desire acceptance by a new social group. The therapist can suggest that the adolescent get involved with students by joining an extracurricular activity of interest, using the skills they have been practicing. This is an important task because depressed adolescents frequently lose interest, withdraw from activities they ordinarily enjoy, and miss opportunities to make friends. To help generate new opportunities the therapist might ask:

> *Are there any activities going on in your school or community that you might enjoy? What kinds of things do you enjoy doing after school? Is there a club or class that you could join where you could do this with other people and meet people with similar interests? It is often enjoyable to meet people with similar interests as a start for forming friendships and having someone else to talk to about the ups and downs of daily life. Would you feel comfortable joining any of these activities? What would make you feel prepared to join?*

Once again, role playing often is an effective technique to help facilitate the adolescent's involvement in new activities or with new friends. The in-session practice can help instill a sense of confidence and mastery of needed skills that will enhance the possibility that the adolescent will succeed in his interactions outside of the therapeutic setting.

Transitions Specific to Family Structural Change

Increasing social support should be emphasized for adolescents coping with this type of transition. Even when the quality of family relationships improves over the course of treatment, it is likely that the relationships will be somewhat different, and the adolescent may need or benefit from other sources of support. Building a network of supportive relationships outside of the immediate family who can function as additional supports is important to enhance the adolescent's resilience in the face of future familial stress and transition.

SUMMARY

The goal of IPT-A in treating transition problems is to help adolescents feel more prepared to accept the new role, to feel they have options, and to feel confident by correcting any unrealistic expectations about the social role and/or family transition that may make the transition undesirable or threatening. Strategies include expressing their feelings about the loss of the old role and clarifying confusion and ambivalence about the new role. By addressing anxieties and sadness about the transition, the adolescent prepares emotionally to accept the transition. Learning communication and negotiation skills provides the groundwork for establishing new relationships and improving current ones. The following case vignette illustrates the work that often must be conducted with both the adolescent and the parents in order to improve the adolescent's adjustment to the role transition.

CASE VIGNETTE: THE CASE OF PAM

Pam is a 13-year-old girl who presented to the clinic complaining of depressed mood, irritability, tearfulness, early and middle insomnia, increased fatigue, decrease in appetite, decrease in concentration, decline in grades, and frequent headaches. Pam was the only child of parents who had divorced when she was an infant. She had lived with her mother in North Carolina until she was 8 years old, when she moved to New Jersey to live with her father. She still spent the summers with her mother. Her father had remarried a year ago, shortly before her half-sister was born. At the time of treatment, she was living with her stepmother, father, and half-sister. Pam's depression worsened as conflict between her and her stepmother increased. They would argue about doing chores around the house, her relationship with her father, and her desire to spend time with him alone. To avoid arguments, she was spending the majority of her time alone in her room.

Initial Sessions (1–4)

Pam did not like her stepmother. She did not like the way her stepmother spoke to her, describing her as very critical and disapproving. She wished her stepmother would just go away. She stated that her stepmother was crazy if she thought she could interfere with her relationship with her father. She also did not like the way her stepmother and father related to each other, feeling that her stepmother was always yelling, putting him down, or bossing him around. It was apparent during the initial phase of treatment that Pam was having difficulty with the transition from being just her father's daughter to being a stepdaughter, having to share her father and acquire a sibling. It was unclear at this point how much her dislike of her stepmother was influenced by her difficulty in sharing her father or whether she genuinely did not like her. She agreed that this transition was difficult for her and that she wished it was just she and her father alone together, when everything was good.

Middle Sessions (5–8)

The focus of this phase of treatment was to examine the strategies Pam was using to adapt to this transition and to identify ones that might be more helpful. It became apparent that Pam did not communicate her feelings about the adjustment she was trying to make to having a step-mother to anyone, nor did she communicate her concerns about her role in the new family composition. Instead, she would keep it all inside until she exploded in anger, which only exacerbated her problems with both her stepmother and father. To help her, she and the therapist first had to discuss what her relationship had been like with her mother, how it had felt to leave her mother and move in with her father, her feelings toward her mother for letting her go, and what it had been like living with her father before the stepmother arrived. They discussed what she did and didn't like about these relationships, including her feelings toward her stepmother. The second step was to examine her expectations for her role in the family—whether or not they were realistic, and whether or not her fears about what her stepmother would do to her relationship with her father were realistic.

To facilitate the work with Pam and to better understand the family situation, the therapist also met with her father to discuss his perceptions of the problems that had occurred in the transition that accompanied his remarriage and the new baby. It appeared that part of Pam's problem in making the transition was that her father had never worked out with his new wife what roles she would have in Pam's upbringing—specifically, what she was able to do in terms of discipline or setting house rules. The therapist explained to him that it was necessary for him and his wife to clarify together what were reasonable responsibilities for Pam, what were acceptable punishments if she was remiss, who was to enforce the discipline, and generally how they wanted the household to function. Without clarifying Pam's and the stepmother's roles, Pam was going to continue to have difficulty making the transition.

While the father was working out these negotiations with his wife, the therapist helped Pam to think about what she might be able to keep from her old role of living alone with her father into the new family situation. For example, perhaps there was a way for her and her father to have some special time to themselves every week to keep that strong connection between the two of them. Also, maybe they could identify something she enjoyed doing with her new sister that would also be helpful to her stepmother and that could be one of her responsibilities in the house. By identifying different aspects of the transition that were positive, Pam was more willing to settle into her new role with less anger and sadness. She also learned to communicate her feelings to her parents so that they could better understand her needs and how she felt when treated a certain way. She practiced being able to tell her father and step-mother when something was upsetting her and to listen to their perspectives prior to negotiating a solution.

Termination Sessions (8–12)

Pam began to feel much better as she began to carve out special time with her father and to see that she wasn't being replaced but that the relationship was just being reshaped. Her parents' clarification of each of their responsibilities in regard to Pam's behavior facilitated her ability to accept large parts of her new role in the family and to negotiate with both of them the aspects of her role that she did not like. She reported feeling that she had a more secure place in the family and that she could still maintain a close relationship with her father, despite his remarriage. She decided that she still didn't like her stepmother very much but that it was possible to have a more peaceful relationship with her and not let her "get to her" so much. Her improved communication skills resulted in a significant decrease in irritable and angry outbursts, an increase in her ability to concentrate, and improvement in her grades, mood, sleep, and appetite. During termination, she and the therapist discussed other problems that might arise with the transition, such as increased attention toward her little sister and how she might handle the situation. She was able to apply the strategies she had learned (i.e., expression of feelings, review of the positive and negative aspects of the new situation, clarification of expectations) to address possible future challenges and changes in the family relationships.

CHAPTER 13

Interpersonal Deficits

Interpersonal deficits refer to a lack of social and communication skills that impair the conduct of interpersonal relationships (Klerman et al., 1984; Weissman et al., 2000). Examples of interpersonal deficits include inability to initiate relationships, inability to maintain relationships, inability to express one's feelings verbally, and/or difficulty eliciting information from others to establish communication. The area of interpersonal deficits is selected as the problem area for IPT-A when the deficits either contribute to or result from the adolescent's depression.

Typically the patient's interpersonal inventory reveals a history of mild social withdrawal with apparent difficulties in initiating and maintaining interpersonal relationships. These deficits, although apparent in some form prior to the depressive episode, are exacerbated by the depression and appear more severe at presentation for treatment. Erikson (1968) identified the primary task of adolescence as that of establishing a unique identity or sense of self. This task requires one to interact with others to establish a set of personal values, attitudes, and goals. As a result of interpersonal deficits, the adolescent may be socially isolated from peer groups and relationships, a situation that can lead to difficulties with identity formation and subsequent feelings of depression and inadequacy.

Interpersonal deficits also may be identified as a problem area when it appears that a depression has caused the adolescent to withdraw socially. The social withdrawal may result in a developmental lag in interpersonal skills that further perpetuates the depression by impairing social relationships. Puig-Antich et al. (1985b) found that, while the symptoms of depression may be transient in children, the accompanying interpersonal impairments tend to persist even after the depression resolves. The persisting interpersonal deficits place the adolescent at risk for future episodes of depression. Adolescents with a smaller social network and without close, positive peer relationships are less likely to receive emotional and physical support during stressful times (Sandler, Miller, Short, & Wolchik, 1989), making them more vulnerable to difficulties such as depression.

Social isolation may be more problematic during adolescence than during other life stages because establishing social relationships is the focus of many developmental tasks of adolescence. Peers dominate the social focus of adolescence, and difficulties in establishing and maintaining peer relationships are associated with internalizing symptoms as well as other negative adjustment outcomes (Hussong, 2000). Appropriate social behavior may become retarded or impaired by the isolation. Specific important developmental tasks of adolescence include making same-aged friends, participating in extracurricular activities, becoming part of a peer group, beginning to date, and learning to make choices regarding exclusive relationships, careers, and sexuality (Hersen & Van Hasselt, 1987). Adolescents tend to place greater value on self-disclosure and loyalty in their friendships than do their younger peers (Furman & Buhrmester, 1992). Withdrawal from social contacts may result in failure to learn and develop age-appropriate social skills. An adolescent with interpersonal deficits will find these tasks difficult to master.

Interpersonal psychotherapy, due to its time-limited nature, is better suited to address those interpersonal deficits that are primarily a result of the current depressive episode than those that are of a more chronic nature. As such, indicators that IPT-A is an appropriate treatment for a particular adolescent include the presence of deficits that are a consequence of either the adolescent's depression or a specific stressor and are less pervasive and less chronic.

DIAGNOSING INTERPERSONAL DEFICITS

An adolescent who is functioning well socially has a network of close relationships with family members and friends as well as a satisfying number of acquaintances, and typically feels comfortable socially in school. In contrast, the adolescent who is not functioning well reports a paucity of relationships or a history of disrupted relationships, uneasiness in social relationships, and/or discomfort in social situations such as school. As with all of the problem areas, the therapist must perform a thorough interpersonal inventory in order to diagnose the interpersonal deficit problem area. To obtain a complete picture of the adolescent's social functioning, the therapist should conduct a thorough review of positive and negative aspects of past relationships. Later, during the middle phase of treatment, the therapist should further investigate the adolescent's interpersonal problems, their chronicity, and their duration, focusing on patterns and trends in the relationships and interactions that were uncovered during the inventory and subsequent sessions. Questions the therapist might ask during this process include:

> *Who are your close friends? How long have you been friends? How did you meet? What makes [name] a good friend? How do you define a good friend? Have you had more difficulty being with friends since you have been feeling depressed? How did your friendship end? What is difficult about making friends for you? What is it like for you to begin conversations? Is it difficult to initiate friendships? Do you feel like you don't know what to do in a relationship once you have gotten past the initial meeting? What do you do to get to know someone better? What happens when you are with your friends? How do you feel? What was it like to be with your family and friends before you were depressed?*

The therapist should initially focus on the most current relationships and then progress to a discussion of the past:

> *How do you find your friends and activities now? Have your relationships with them changed at all recently? How so? Are they less enjoyable, more enjoyable? How do these present relationships differ from relationships you had in the past?*

In reviewing the relationships, the therapist should be alert for evidence of similar problems in multiple relationships, such as difficulties in deepening relationships or maintaining an ongoing relationship. Interpersonal deficits differ from other problem areas in that the interpersonal problem is usually present in the majority of the adolescent's relationships, while the dispute or role transition problem may be limited to one.

GOALS AND STRATEGIES FOR THE TREATMENT OF INTERPERSONAL DEFICITS

The specific treatment goals for interpersonal deficits are to reduce the social isolation and improve the relationships the patient currently has

TABLE 13.1. Summary of Goals and Strategies for Interpersonal Deficits Problem Area

Goals	• Reduce social isolation
	• Improve relationships
Strategies	• Review current and past relationships
	• Explore interactions with the therapist
	• Identify repetitive patterns and problems in relationships
	• Highlight strengths and skills
	• Build interpersonal skills

and the new ones he is developing (see Table 13.1). To do this, the therapist must directly address the deficits through a treatment focused on improving communication skills, increasing the adolescent's social self-confidence, improving the quality of existing relationships, and increasing the number of satisfying relationships.

Several strategies are used to accomplish the goals and objectives for this problem area. It is important to keep in mind the adaptability of the middle phase of this treatment. Although several strategies are suggested below for addressing this problem area, not all will be necessary or useful with all patients, and the order in which these strategies are employed will vary considerably from one patient to another. It is up to the clinician to determine the most appropriate manner in which to use these strategies to accomplish the treatment goals with each particular patient. As with the other problem areas we have discussed, each strategy involves the use of a number of possible techniques. Some examples of the techniques that can be used are provided in this section.

Review Current and Past Relationships and Interactions

In order to obtain a complete picture of the adolescent's social functioning, the therapist should conduct a thorough review of positive and negative aspects of the adolescent's relationships. Initially the focus should be on current relationships, as these are most salient to the adolescent and most relevant to his current interpersonal functioning. If an adolescent presents with few current significant relationships, the therapist should review past significant relationships, looking for and labeling patterns of difficulties. For example, the therapist might say:

> *Carl, as we talked about your relationships with your friend Lyle and your cousin Brad, I noticed some things that are similar about what happened in both of those relationships. You described both of them*

as people to whom you felt close at one time and really trusted but who hurt you by not keeping things you said in confidence. You also seem to feel as though they both turned their backs on you and abandoned your friendship. It seems to me that in both of those relationships your feelings were hurt and you were angry at them for telling other people your private business. But it does not seem to me that you ever really talked to them directly about how their actions made you feel. It sounds as if when your feelings were hurt you shut down and pulled away. Your friend and cousin may not have understood what you wanted in the relationship. They may have thought you were not interested in their friendship. Then, when they pulled away from you, you felt even more hurt. It seems that one of the things we should work on in your relationships is communicating your feelings more directly so that people will be more likely to understand your feelings and try to work out their differences with you.

In reviewing the interpersonal interaction patterns, the therapist encourages the patient to connect feelings and depression symptoms to events in the relationship. Techniques employed as part of this strategy include exploration and encouragement of affect.

There are particularly challenging cases in which the adolescent does not have any current supports or relationships and has a dearth of past relationships as well. For these adolescents, a critical target of IPT-A treatment is to help them identify existing relationships and support and to help them build new relationships and a support system. For example, the therapist might say to the adolescent:

One of the things that we should focus on in treatment in order to help you feel better is identifying people who can be a support to you emotionally as well as with practical issues that you are facing in your life. We have talked in our past sessions about how you don't feel that there is anyone you can talk to about things that are on your mind or who you can go to for help with things such as problems at school. I want us together to identify several people with whom we can work on developing a relationship so that you will have this kind of support. Can you think of any friends in the neighborhood with whom you would like to try to form a friendship? Is there anyone you have met in your classes or activities who seems like someone you would want to know better? Have any school staff ever been helpful to you in the past? Any teachers or counselors?

The therapist would continue along these lines and then, once some potential supports are identified, begin the work of building the necessary skills for making meaningful connections with these people, using the strategies discussed in this chapter. When no individuals can be identified, it may be necessary to help the adolescent get involved in a group or organization that could provide potential support.

Explore Interactions with the Therapist

If the adolescent is extremely isolated, the therapist will have to use her own relationship with the patient to explore the adolescent's interpersonal deficits. The therapist should observe whether any interpersonal or communication problems are evident in their relationship. The therapist gives feedback to the adolescent regarding his interpersonal style and its impact on the therapist, assisting the adolescent in practicing new skills. The adolescent also is encouraged to discuss the positive and negative aspects of the therapeutic relationship and how it might be possible to make more positive changes within the relationship. With specific patterns and deficits identified, the therapist can engage in education and role playing to expand the adolescent's interpersonal repertoire. The therapist–patient relationship can act as a model for how to establish a more appropriate or satisfying relationship (i.e., what the appropriate expectations and conduct in particular types of relationships are and how to communicate emotions and expectations more accurately).

Case Example

Dana is a 16-year-old girl who presented with a major depression and the identified problem area of interpersonal deficits. She had a history of having friends in school and getting along with others until the preceding year, when she became depressed and more withdrawn. Her symptoms were depressed mood, suicidal ideation, increased fatigue, anhedonia, decreased appetite, low self-esteem, and feelings of helplessness and hopelessness. When questioned about her relationships with peers, Dana described her discomfort around males, stating that they were impossible to talk to and never treated women well. In conducting an interpersonal inventory, it appeared that Dana's depression was precipitated by a problematic relationship with a boyfriend. Dana did not know how to initiate and deepen friendships gradually and/or how to remove herself from relationships (particularly with males) that were not satisfying for her. She did not know the appropriate boundaries in friendships and/or how to set limits for the relationship that were comfortable to her. For example, she would become sexually involved with boys even when she did not want to or feel comfortable doing so because she did not know another way to communicate that she wanted to get to know them better. The focus of the treatment became the explo-

ration of how to develop friendships, improve her self-image in relationships, and assert herself appropriately in relationships. The
therapist provided education about different types of intimacy and
appropriate ways to achieve them. In session, Dana practiced expressing her feelings clearly by discussing the therapist's perceptions
of her comments and whether or not these were the messages Dana
had meant to convey. Dana and the therapist practiced more effective communication, such as how to say "no" to sexual advances
and how to tell someone that you would like to get to know him
better and spend time with him through an in-session role play. For
this role play, Dana practiced meeting a new boy while the therapist
guided her in appropriate self-disclosure. This exercise helped Dana
clarify her communications, thereby decreasing the misperceptions
in her relationships and increasing the number of successful interactions outside the therapy.

In using role-play techniques, the therapist is able to stop an interaction in progress and discuss what the adolescent is feeling at the time in
relation to the behavior (see Chapter 9). In addition, the therapist is able
to facilitate a discussion of the impact of the behavior on the other person in the relationship. In this way, the therapist can identify unrealistic
expectations for a relationship, help the adolescent understand the
meaning of the words he is speaking, and correct any problems in communication. Where appropriate, the therapist relates issues in their own
relationship to other relationships outside therapy to foster broader social confidence and social skills.

In conducting IPT-A, the negative feelings about the therapist are
understood as transference phenomena but are not dealt with in a psychodynamic way. The therapist does not encourage the feelings in the
patient or allow them to evolve fully. Instead, the therapist will intervene
and test the patient's perceptions of reality. The therapist might say:

> *It seems as though you are feeling angry today? Are you feeling angry?*
> *With whom are you angry? Has something happened in the session*
> *that has upset you? If so, I think it is important to talk about it. By*
> *talking about it together, we can see how it occurred, uncover any*
> *misunderstandings that may exist, and clarify our relationship so we*
> *can continue working together effectively. I wonder if this type of mis-*
> *understanding ever happens with other people?*

The therapist needs to encourage the adolescent to examine the negative feelings for the therapist in a supportive atmosphere. Such direct exploration of the adolescent's feelings will prevent misunderstandings that
could lead to premature termination. The experience also provides a

model, for the adolescent, of how to address negative feelings or problems in other significant relationships through similar types of open discussion.

Identify and Explore Repetitive Patterns and Problems in Relationships

Patterns and problems in relationships are revealed during the interpersonal inventory. During the middle phase of treatment, these patterns and problems are labeled and clarified by the therapist. If a deficit such as maladaptive communication is found in one relationship, a subsequent session may explore the presence of the pattern in the patient's other relationships. While the focus of treatment often is on one particular relationship, therapy also will address how the use of these new interpersonal skills can generalize to other relationships.

Comparing problematic relationships to successful relationships and analyzing verbal exchanges as they occur inside and outside the session helps the adolescent learn to alter relationships through more effective communication. Adolescents may be reluctant to talk about relationships that have left them feeling badly, but they should be encouraged to do so to prevent future relationships from going awry.

Case Example

Working with Dana also revealed that she had a similar problem in initiating friendships with girls in school. For example, she would not talk to classmates unless they initiated the conversation. She felt she did not know what to say after "Hello, how are you?" The therapist helped her to connect her difficulties to her transition to a new school and her anxiety over meeting new people. She frequently described how her difficulties in negotiating relationships made her feel badly about herself and depressed. She felt helpless to make people understand what kind of person she was. A focus of discussion was on the issue of self-disclosure—how much is appropriate and to whom. To assist in understanding levels of self-disclosure, patient and therapist role-played various interpersonal exchanges. A recurrent theme was how to establish boundaries in relationships and how these boundaries vary with different types of relationships. Comparisons were made between relationships with family members, friends, teachers, acquaintances, and even her therapist.

Highlight Strengths and Skills

Although the name of this problem area is interpersonal deficits, treatment focuses as much on strengths as deficits. The therapist may help the adolescent recognize how skills used in other interpersonal contexts can be used in or adapted to the area with which they are having difficulty. For example, the therapist might recognize a skill that the patient uses in the session and label that skill for the patient.

> *I don't know if you noticed what you just did when we were talking, but I want to point it out to you because I think it is a skill that you can use in your other relationships. When I was reviewing what you just had told me about your hard day yesterday, I made the assumption that you were feeling sad. You stopped me in a very appropriate way and clarified that you were not really feeling sad, but rather frustrated and angry. You helped me to understand your feelings and your behavior. This is not always an easy thing to do with people, but you did it and you did it very well. It made me feel better to know what was really going on for you. If you had not stopped me and clarified your feelings, I would have had the wrong impression. I wonder if we can think about how you can use that skill in your other relationships so that people in your life have a better understanding of how you are feeling.*

As discussed elsewhere in this manual, IPT-A is aimed at building competencies and skills in adolescents. Such a competence-driven educational approach is critical with adolescents, as treatment is geared toward developing independence rather than dependence and a sense of mastery rather than defeat. It is particularly important to focus on skills and strengths in a time-limited treatment since it increases the probability of improvement within the time frame of the treatment.

Build Interpersonal Skills

The final strategy employed for this problem area is building interpersonal skills in the context of ongoing and developing relationships. The techniques that are most helpful in implementing this strategy are communication analysis and role playing. Through communication analysis, the therapist helps the adolescent understand the impact of his or her words on others and the feelings conveyed by the words in comparison to the feelings that generated the verbal exchange. Role playing provides the adolescent with a safe way to practice the new communication skills and get feedback prior to applying what is learned to outside situations. Successful role plays can increase the adolescent's social confidence. To initiate the role play the therapist might propose the following, for example:

> *Let's pretend that you have just come home from school and your father says to you that he needs you to work in the store all day tomor-*

row, but you have just made plans to go to a movie with your friend in the afternoon. How could you talk to your father about this? When would you try to talk to him? How would you start the conversation?

Or, in conducting communication analysis, the therapist might say:

How do you think the other girl felt when you said _____? How did you want her to feel? What had you wanted to say? How could you say it differently? How did you feel when she said _____ back to you? What do you think she was feeling?

More detailed examples of how to conduct both the role-play and communication analysis techniques are provided in Chapter 9. Because of the brief nature of the treatment, the therapist must be careful to focus on a circumscribed interpersonal deficit, such as how to initiate a specific social interaction, in order to make progress in a limited time. One of the most common mistakes that therapists make in trying to build skills is not selecting a specific relationship or specific situation upon which to work. It is more difficult to effect change if the work stays too general. The therapist must appreciate and convey to the patient that, although what they are working on may seem very small, it is the best way to build skills. Once the adolescent begins to gain confidence with this specific problem, then he will address other problematic situations using the same skills.

THE ROLE OF THE FAMILY IN TREATMENT

Family members may be involved in treatment, particularly when the adolescent's interpersonal deficits affect family relationships. In these cases, it is often helpful for a key family member to participate in one or two middle-phase sessions. In these joint sessions, the therapist should focus on very specific interaction processes and skills rather than addressing content issues. After working on a specific skill, it should be related to the larger patterns in the interactions between the adolescent and the family. A focus on the process of communication and problem solving will help to keep the session more manageable and more positive.

Even when family relationships do not seem particularly affected by the adolescent's deficits, the family can play a critical role in supporting and encouraging the adolescent as he develops skills in the pertinent areas. In these situations, the family members act as coaches, encouraging the changes and praising them when they occur. The parents are reminded of what an important role they play in helping the adolescent generalize any treatment gains to situations outside of the therapy setting. Sometimes the family members need a little coaching themselves in order to function as effective supports for the adolescent. In these situations, we recommend meeting briefly with family members (preferably parents or guardians) alone, or at least working with them by telephone, in order to prepare them for this supportive role. For an adolescent with whom the therapist is trying to help communicate more directly and effectively about his feelings, the therapist might meet with the parents separately and discuss this treatment goal. The therapist can then ask the parents to point out to the adolescent times when they notice the adolescent using this skill. The therapist may have to give the family examples of what would be considered direct and clear communication of feelings and help them think about what specifically they could say to the adolescent. For example, the therapist might say:

> *As you know, I have been working with Robby on developing some skills that will help him to have more satisfying relationships. It is my belief that, if Robby's relationships improve, his depression is likely to subside and he will feel better about himself. One of the things that I have learned about Robby through discussion, both with you and with Robby, is that he has a lot of difficulty letting people know how he really feels in a way that people can truly understand. For example, when he is hurt or angry he tends to become sullen—or, as you described it, "pout"—and he isolates himself from people instead of saying "What you just said to me hurt my feelings."*
>
> *Robby has been trying to work on communicating his feelings more directly and has done a nice job in our sessions, but it is even more important that he learn to do this in his relationships with his family and friends. I need your help with this. I need your help in pointing out to him when he does a good job of communicating his feelings directly and encouraging him to open up more when he shuts down. I would like him to be able to express himself in an assertive but not aggressive way. Does this make sense to you? Have you seen him doing this at all at home? Can you think of an example? I am wondering if, when we meet together with Robby in a few minutes, you could help me to point these things out to him as he tries to work on them in the session. I thought that we would focus the session on an issue that is a source of conflict for you and Robby, Robby's curfew, and see if we can help him to practice these skills.*

The therapist often asks the parents to try to act as coaches, pointing out to the patient when they notice him using this skill and how clear communication helps them to understand how he is feeling. By first doing this in the context of the therapy session, the therapist can coach the parents and the adolescent and can increase the likelihood that both will experience success. The prediscussion with the family is critical before attempting this type of intervention to ensure that the parent is able and willing to be supportive and to encourage this communication. If the therapist determines that the parent is likely to sabotage the intervention, then the therapist can change the treatment plan with respect to involving family members.

SUMMARY

The therapist's primary focus is on interpersonal deficits that have been exacerbated by the adolescent's depression and that may additionally be playing a role in the perpetuation of the depression. Conducting a thorough interpersonal inventory is crucial to the identification of the problem area. The goal of the treatment is to reduce the adolescent's social isolation and to improve existing relationships. Strategies employed to achieve these goals include improving communication skills, increasing social confidence, and encouraging participation in more social activities. The therapist uses the therapist–patient relationship to illustrate difficulties in interpersonal functioning that may be apparent in the actual treatment sessions as well as in outside relationships. The specific techniques of communication analysis and role playing are employed to practice new social skills that will facilitate the development of new and/or improved relationships.

The following case example illustrates how a life stressor can lead to interpersonal deficits, such as difficulty in communicating feelings and subsequent depression, and the use of interpersonal psychotherapy techniques to treat the depression.

CASE VIGNETTE: THE CASE OF CARMEN

Carmen is a 14-year-old female who lives with her mother, father, and younger brother. Her mother was very worried about Carmen's withdrawal from family and friends, and brought her for treatment. Carmen had been feeling depressed since her parents began to have marital problems resulting from her father's extramarital affairs approximately 2 years earlier. Three months ago, prior to her evaluation, she began to feel worse after her parents began to fight more and her father disappeared for 1 week. Around the same time, she broke up with her boyfriend, whom she had been seeing for several months. Carmen's parents did not know she had a boyfriend, so she was feeling both sad about the breakup and guilty about having the relationship without her parent's permission. Carmen presented with a major depression. Her symptoms included depressed mood every day for most of the day, decreased appetite, early and middle insomnia, increased fatigue, suicidal ideation, headaches, tearfulness, feelings of guilt, and low self-esteem.

Initial Sessions (1–4)

It was immediately apparent to the therapist in the initial sessions that Carmen had a very difficult time talking about her feelings. She confided in no one, even though she reported having two close friends who were concerned and interested in her. Carmen's inability to talk about her feelings began when her father's affair disrupted the household. She felt caught between her parents, embarrassed about the affairs, angry with her father for the affairs, and angry at her mother for staying with her father. She stopped talking to her father altogether and stopped confiding in her mother because she did not want to add to her problems or worry. By not talking to her father, she was hoping he or the problem would just go away.

As a result of withdrawing from her family, she turned to a boyfriend to provide her with a feeling of importance and support. But, given the secrecy of her father's affairs, Carmen began to feel increasingly guilty about her own secret relationship. She wanted to be able to tell her parents about the relationship, but her withdrawal from the family made her feel helpless to do so. She did not know how to reconnect with them. The problem area was identified as that of interpersonal deficits because it appeared that her inability to communicate to her parents was resulting in feelings of isolation and guilt that were contributing to her depression.

Middle Sessions (5–8)

The strategies used to ameliorate her interpersonal deficits included role playing, clarification of feelings, techniques of initiating and deepening relationships, and techniques of interpersonal problem solving. The focus of the middle sessions was to help Carmen label her feelings and find the words to express those feelings. The therapist and Carmen explored what made it difficult for her to start conversations, what she was worried her mother or friends might think if she told them how she felt, and how she would feel if she expressed her feelings more. The therapist provided psychoeducation about ways in which people typically negotiate within a relationship.

In the beginning, Carmen had difficulty even relating to the therapist what had occurred since the previous session and how she had felt about the events. Using their own conversation in the sessions, the therapist demonstrated to Carmen how revealing information about herself could help others like the therapist and her family better understand and respond to her needs, thereby making her feel better about herself. Carmen role-played with the therapist conversations that she would like to have with her mother regarding her desire to date. She discussed how she would handle various reactions her mother might have. She also discussed her feelings about the conflict in her parents' relationship and its effect on her ability to communicate with them. She was afraid that if she wasn't the perfect daughter, she would exacerbate her parents' marital stress. To try to maintain this image, she withdrew from talking about herself. By relating events to feelings, the therapist helped Carmen to see that the withdrawal was creating more problems in her relationships with her parents and making her feel worse about herself. Between sessions, Carmen experimented by talking more to her mother about her feelings. Over the course of several conversations, her mother was able to successfully discuss the issue of boyfriends, and Carmen negotiated a reasonable compromise, which further encouraged Carmen to continue expressing her feelings to others. Her improvement was noticeable in her increased openness with the therapist, as well.

Termination Sessions (9–12)

As Carmen continued to practice communication, she and the therapist discussed her increased sense of closeness and support within her relationships and the decrease in her depressed mood. She was engaging in more social activities with friends and was talking more to both her mother and father about the everyday events in her life. Her parents, as a result of Carmen's treatment and the discussion about contributing factors, made a commitment to work on their relationship with their daughter. The mother reported that she and the father were trying to increase their communication with each other in the same way that Carmen was improving her communication with them. The therapist recommended that the parents seek marital counseling, but they refused. Carmen said that her parents appeared to be getting along better; there was a decrease in fighting, and her father had not spent any nights out of the home.

During the final sessions, Carmen appeared less critical of herself and was finding people very accepting of her in social interactions. She was enjoying a new social self-confidence. At termination, she denied any sad mood, sleep difficulties, fatigue, or suicidal ideation, and reported decreased guilt and self-blame as well as increased self-esteem.

CHAPTER 14

Termination Phase

A termination date is set with the patient and family at the beginning of treatment. The adolescent is reminded about the specific termination date at least 2–4 weeks prior to its occurrence. Twelve weeks is the time frame chosen for the clinical trial assessing the efficacy of IPT-A. It is a reasonable duration for adolescents, who are reluctant to stay in treatment for any significant length of time. It not only gives the patient time to make some changes but also provides a finite time within which to try to achieve them. Of course, the time period can be modified in either direction. The important issue is to retain its time-limited nature by setting the initial treatment contract for the number of weeks that seem most appropriate for that adolescent. The therapist then must work within this time frame while maintaining the balance of time between the different phases of the treatment. Following the acute treatment, we recommend continuation and maintenance treatment. While we do not yet have empirical data on the efficacy of continuation and maintenance treatment for adolescents, research with adults suggests that attending less frequent sessions for 1 year or more following the acute treatment can help prevent relapse and recurrence (Frank, Kupfer, Wagner, McEachran, & Cornes, 1991). Studies following adolescents 2 years after acute cognitive-behavioral therapy showed that they experienced significant relapse and recurrence, suggesting the need for continuation and maintenance treatment (Birmaher, Brent, & Kolko, 2000). A time-limited and brief treatment can provide hope that the symptoms will go away and that the patients can return to a normal life quickly, and continuation or maintenance treatment may help ensure that these improvements last.

TERMINATION WITH THE ADOLESCENT

The termination phase of treatment should include a review of the course of treatment (i.e., the strategies learned and the changes that have occurred as well as unfinished business), preparation for handling interpersonal stresses after the conclusion, and assessment of the adolescent's need for further treatment. While the therapist begins to raise the issues of termination several weeks prior to termination, discussion of the identified problem area should continue.

Tasks of Termination

There are several tasks that the therapist should engage in during the final phase of treatment while still continuing to facilitate work on the identified problem area. The main tasks include the following:

1. Elicit feelings about ending treatment.
2. Review warning symptoms of depression.
3. Recognize interpersonal competencies.
4. Review interpersonal problems that can be stressful.
5. Review specific interpersonal strategies that have been helpful.
6. Brainstorm about the application of these strategies to future situations.
7. Evaluate need for further treatment.

Elicit Feelings about Ending Treatment

One of the most difficult issues facing the patient is the loss of the relationship with the therapist. Particularly with adolescents, the therapist often has become a role model of interpersonal functioning, in addition to becoming a source of guidance and support that previously may have been missing from the adolescent's life. Several weeks prior to termination, the therapist should remind the adolescent that their work together will be coming to a close and ask the adolescent how he feels when he thinks about no longer attending treatment sessions. The therapist must address the adolescent's concern about how he will do without this support and identify other sources of support; otherwise, the likelihood of a recurrence of the depressive symptoms will increase.

The therapist should discuss the end of treatment as a time of potential grieving and warn the patient of the possibility that his depressive feelings may reoccur. It is sometimes difficult for adolescents to admit that they really had needed the help, that they may have grown to depend on the sessions, and that they have enjoyed the weekly meetings. They tend to be reluctant to outwardly discuss their feelings when initially asked. It is helpful if the therapist begins by mentioning some possible feelings that the adolescent may be experiencing and allows the adolescent to acknowledge which ones ring true. Other adolescents have felt more comfortable expressing these feelings in writing and have brought in poems at the end of treatment that they have written about the therapy as well as their relationship with the therapist. These poems depict the rich emotional attachment that the adolescents have made even in the brief treatment. Adolescents may be hesitant to admit attachment to the therapist or the value of the therapy, particularly if they had been against the treatment initially. Alternatively, some adolescents may feel sadness at the end of therapy, which they may interpret as a return of their depression. They may either be upset by the return of the sadness and/or hope that it will allow them to continue their relationship with the therapist a little longer. The therapist needs to educate the adolescent about the difference between depression and sadness about ending the relationship. The therapist might say to the adolescent:

> Feeling sad, worried, or even angry that we are stopping our work together are common feelings at this time. It is normal to feel these things. We have gotten to know each other, and you have told me very personal and important things about yourself. These feelings are not the same feelings that you had when we started working together, and they do not mean you are becoming depressed again. They are probably more temporary feelings of sadness about leaving something that has become comfortable and a source of support. I will miss working with you, but I know it is important for you to be on your own and to use what you have learned here in your other relationships.

The therapist should make every reasonable attempt to link feelings about termination with the specified problem area. For example, feelings of termination may resemble the feelings that the adolescent experienced before the role transition or may be related to feelings experienced during a grief reaction.

The therapist attempts to help the adolescent use his newly developed skills in the discussion of termination:

THERAPIST: I was wondering how you are feeling about ending your visits to the clinic for therapy?

PATIENT: I feel fine. I am not really thinking about it much.

THERAPIST: Really? You aren't wondering what it will feel like when you might have another argument with your mother and we won't be meeting to dissect it together, looking for another approach to the problem?

PATIENT: Well, I guess I am a little worried about that.

THERAPIST: Ending therapy can be a time of mixed emotions. It might be helpful to think about some of the strategies we have discussed and how they might help you in our discussion about ending therapy. Can you tell me any strategies that might help us prepare for the end of treatment?

PATIENT: I don't know.

THERAPIST: Right now, I am not sure if I know your concerns because you aren't discussing your feelings directly with me. You might leave here and feel badly that you didn't get to say some of the things that you are feeling or that I didn't understand what you were feeling. Isn't that what happened with you and your mom—that she couldn't tell what you were feeling? What could you do to keep that from happening in our relationship?

PATIENT: I guess I could tell you more, but that is hard.

THERAPIST: Why don't you give it a try? Remember there is no wrong answer; it is simply a matter of letting me know what this therapy experience has been like for you, how it feels to be ending, and what else you might like to discuss before we stop meeting.

PATIENT: Well, I am sort of scared about forgetting to use the skills that we've worked on after treatment ends, but really happy also about not having to come here anymore. I also am sad that we won't be talking any more because it is still hard to talk to people in my family the way that I talk to you.

THERAPIST: That was great. You now have made it clear to me the types of mixed feelings that you are having about ending treatment, which are very common at this time. Now you and I can talk about them and decide how best to handle them.

Through this exchange the therapist is able to elicit the feelings of the adolescent as well as demonstrate how these interpersonal strategies can generalize from the identified problem area to a multitude of situations. The adolescent then gets added practice using the skills and experiencing the interpersonal rewards that result from their use.

Sometimes adolescents have difficulty seeing how the strategies can generalize between relationships and situations. For example:

THERAPIST: So, we've talked about the need to tell people what you are feeling when they have done something that makes you sad or angry rather than assume that the person knows how you are feeling. We practiced this with your parents. Is there anyone else with whom this might also be helpful?

PATIENT: I don't know.

THERAPIST: Well, let's think. Who else do you feel doesn't understand you a lot?

PATIENT: Well, sometimes my teacher but that's different.

THERAPIST: How is that different?

PATIENT: Well, she just thinks I don't care about my schoolwork sometimes.

THERAPIST: And what do you want her to know about your schoolwork?

PATIENT: I want her to know that when I feel sad I just can't make myself do my schoolwork but I really do care about it, and, now that I am feeling better, I have been doing a lot more of it. I wish she would say something about my improvement.

THERAPIST: That's good. Now what about the strategy of telling people how you feel when they say or do certain things? Do you think you could use that strategy with your teacher to help her to better understand you and help you feel better about school?

The therapist is demonstrating for the adolescent how to take apart a situation and then figure out what might be helpful to do and say in the situation to make it better. By outlining the process first for the adolescent, the therapist may facilitate the adolescent's ability to do it himself with other examples.

Review Warning Symptoms of Depression

It is important to review the list of positive depression symptoms obtained during the initial clinical interview as well as areas of interpersonal conflict described during the interpersonal inventory and treatment. The therapist might say to the adolescent:

> Do you remember how you felt when you first began treatment? How did you know that you were depressed? What were your symptoms? Let's review them. Your symptoms of depression included sad mood, trouble falling asleep, a change in your appetite, not wanting to be with your friends, and crying a lot. Are you still having any symptoms

of depression similar to those you had when you began treatment?
Are they bothering you less or the same or more? What kinds of prob-
lems were you having with your family or friends when we started
treatment? Do you remember the problem area we identified after re-
viewing your important relationships? Has the problem improved?

The therapist and adolescent will put these symptoms and conflicts into
several categories: depression symptoms, areas of conflict between parent and adolescent that are part of a normal developmental process (e.g.,
hanging out with friends before all the homework is completed), and the
identified problem area that was the focus of treatment. Each category
should be reviewed with respect to progress made during the course of
treatment. Adolescents who suffer from depression often appear to have
personality-style disturbances. However, we find that when the depression remits, many of these personality traits are no longer evident.

Recognize Interpersonal Competencies

Throughout the termination phase, the therapist should help the adolescent recognize his competence by discussing accomplishments in the
treatment. The therapist should focus on the goals of treatment initially
laid down, the progress made, and the strategies learned with a view toward independent application by the adolescent in the future. The therapist should ask the adolescent:

What is the identified problem that we have been focusing on? What
changes have been made in this area during treatment? What were our
goals? What strategies did we discuss and use to achieve these goals?
Are there any goals that we did not meet? What are they? How might
you continue to work on them after therapy is completed?

These goals are very specific to each patient and will have been achieved
to varying degrees during the course of the therapy. Each problem area
will be discussed in the context of the initial goals and their final
achievement. Typically a major goal of therapy has been to improve the
adolescent's self-esteem by helping him to be more effective in resolving
the identified problem area and experiencing more positive interpersonal
interactions. In reviewing the accomplishments of the treatment, the adolescent should be helped to see that the improvements were not solely
the work of the therapist but the result of hard work and changes by the
adolescent. The therapist might say:

How do you think you are going to feel when you and I stop meeting?
What might be difficult for you when you stop treatment? What will

you miss? What will you worry about? Who else might provide you with support and guidance? You have worked really hard in these sessions, and I think you have learned a lot. I hope that you continue to work hard to use these strategies after therapy ends. You did a good job of using them in situations between sessions. They will become more second-nature for you the more you use them.

The therapist's role is to stress that the adolescent has acquired a mastery of and/or competence in interpersonal skills that will be maintained beyond the end of treatment. This can be accomplished by reviewing the adolescent's successful "work at home" experiences.

Review Specific Interpersonal Strategies

During the final phase of treatment, it is important to highlight the interpersonal strategies that were discussed and used successfully to address the adolescent's identified problem area. It is often easier for the adolescent to hold on to these strategies when they have been highlighted in some way during the middle phase of treatment. One way the therapist does this is by labeling the strategies, such as using "I statements" to express your feelings to another person. During termination, the therapist should explicitly ask the adolescent to identify and explain what strategies he has used during the treatment. The therapist might say:

You know that we have been focusing these past few weeks on learning different ways to communicate, to set up communications, and to negotiate within your significant relationships. We have discussed specific strategies that have worked for you. Can you tell me the strategies that we have been practicing together? Which ones do you think have worked best for you or felt the most comfortable?

By engaging in this discussion, the therapist is continuing to foster the notion of social competence in the adolescent and increase the adolescent's comfort and familiarity with the strategies. This discussion naturally lends itself to continued discussion of the identified problem area:

THERAPIST: That is great that you could identify the strategies that we have been discussing. Can you tell me how you have continued to use these strategies to work on the problems in your relationship with [name]? Has there been a time in the past week when you have used any of these strategies or a time when you think you should have used the strategies?

PATIENT: Let me think. Yes, I guess I did use one with my sister.

THERAPIST: Tell me what happened.

PATIENT: Well, my sister was really annoying me, and I felt like I was about to explode, but then I thought of you and our discussions. So I took a deep breath and calmed myself down, and then I said to her, "I really feel irritated when you keep teasing me that way. It makes me feel badly about myself. Can you stop doing that?"

THERAPIST: Then what happened?

PATIENT: My sister looked at me and said, "What happened to you?" because I usually explode. But then she stopped teasing me.

THERAPIST: That's great. You were able to stop yourself from saying something in anger that might have made you feel worse and were able to then say how you felt about what she was saying to you. And then you ended up feeling better rather than worse.

The therapist is trying to help make these strategies a natural part of the adolescent's interpersonal repertoire. The therapist encourages him to slow down and examine interpersonal events and how the strategies were used or should have been used in the situations. This process will hopefully demonstrate the use of these skills in everyday life and may help to prevent interpersonal problems that could precipitate recurrence of depressed mood.

Brainstorm about the Application of These Strategies to Future Situations

In fostering the adolescent's internalization as well as generalization of these skills, the therapist should encourage the adolescent to identify specific future situations that may be stressful and to review the use of the new skills in these other situations. The therapist may ask:

> What situations are coming up that you anticipate might be difficult for you to negotiate or may be stressful? What strategies have you learned in treatment that might be helpful in this situation? What are some of the steps that you might take to handle this situation?

This type of review can help to increase the adolescent's self-esteem and help him feel equipped to handle future interpersonal situations. The therapist should help the adolescent identify people in his life who might help remind him of the identified strategies and support him in their use. Still, there are times when the adolescent has difficulty making the connection between a strategy discussed in a past session and a future situation in which it may be helpful. For example:

THERAPIST: So, you have mentioned that you will be moving to a different neighborhood at the end of the year. Transitions can sometimes be difficult, especially when you have to start new somewhere. What kinds of strategies have you learned in therapy that might help with the transition?

PATIENT: I don't know.

THERAPIST: Let's think back on the difficulties that we have worked on together over the past few months. We identified that your depression was related to arguments you were having with your parents about your involvement in activities at school and your desire to be with your friends more than your family. What did we talk about doing to help solve those arguments and prevent others from happening?

PATIENT: I don't see how any of that will help with switching schools.

THERAPIST: What did help you deal with the problems with your parents?

PATIENT: Learning to tell them how I felt and trying to understand their point of view.

THERAPIST: How do you think those two strategies could help in the upcoming move situation? What might happen to you when you move?

PATIENT: Lots of things but not like arguing with my parents.

THERAPIST: Sometimes, in transitions, two people can get into disagreements about a variety of things such as specific decisions about how to plan the move, how the move will affect your routine schedule of activities and time with friends. How can those strategies you mentioned help you in this situation?

PATIENT: I have no idea.

THERAPIST: Well, I will give you a start. Telling your parents how the move might be stressful and that you want to speak to them about seeing your old friends after you move—would that help you to feel to feel better during the move?

In cases where the adolescent is having difficulty making the connection between strategies and future events, the therapist can help by generating some of the connections when the patient is unable. Hopefully, a few suggestions might be enough to get the patient to generate his own connections.

Throughout the treatment and termination, the therapist must continue to emphasize that the work that has been done surrounding the identified problem area frequently leads to more successful relationships for the adolescent outside of treatment. The therapist should identify the changes that she observes in the adolescent: the efforts made to improve communication and see another person's point of view, attempts made to negotiate a dispute, improved insight into his own feelings about a relationship, successful mourning of the loss and the establishment of new relationships. The therapist and patient together highlight how specific strategies have enabled him to make improvements within his identified problem area. A frequent secondary gain of the work on the identified problem area is increased satisfaction across many of his significant relationships and the development of new relationships. The therapist should help the adolescent see the connection between the improvements in interpersonal functioning and the improvements in mood. Specific strategies employed by the adolescents should be identified so that they may be applied to other similar situations. The therapist emphasizes that the strategies are good basic communication and interpersonal problem-solving skills that will be useful in multiple aspects of the patient's life, both in the identified problem area currently as well as in the future with family and friends, in school, and on the job.

Case Example

Allison is a 14-year-old who presented with a major depression that appears to have been precipitated by a dispute with her mother about curfews and dating. The treatment focused on increasing her communication skills, enabling her to better negotiate with her mother. Specifically, the therapist helped Allison to discuss her feelings more clearly with her mother, clarifying her own expectations for curfew and dating as well as clarifying and trying to understand her mother's point of view and expectations. For example, Allison explained to her mother that she wanted to spend more time with her friends. Her mother explained to her that it was all right to spend time with friends as long as she was assured that Allison would be supervised and doing safe activities. They were able to agree that Allison could stay out later if she was at a friend's house and her mother had confirmed that the parents were home and were responsible supervisors. Once she was able to gather all of this information, the therapist helped Allison learn how to negotiate a compromise that would make both her and her mother feel better. This ability to negotiate a compromise replaced Allison's earlier approach of all-or-nothing thinking in the disputes that had led them to an impasse in their relationship, and to Allison's depressed mood.

While showing improvement in her "work at home" negotiating about her curfew and evening activities with friends, Allison was still tentative when she tried to independently generate ideas about what strategies to use. She was increasingly competent in implementing these; therefore, the therapist's goal during termination was to increase Allison's confidence in her ability to select the right approach to a dispute with less need for guidance from the therapist. In addition, Allison and the therapist discussed other people to whom she might turn for guidance after treatment has ended. They were able to identify her sister and her current boyfriend as sources of support. They also discussed how continued sessions at decreased frequency (i.e., continuation or maintenance sessions) might enable her to continue to feel good and give her the opportunity for continued therapeutic support to feel more comfortable with her new interpersonal skills. By emphasizing the adolescent's competence, the therapist will facilitate the adolescent's ability to work through her problems independently following termination.

TERMINATION WITH THE FAMILY

Terminating treatment with an adolescent also means terminating work with the family. Ideally the therapist will conduct a final termination session with the adolescent alone and then have another joint termination session for the adolescent and family. The therapist also may see the family alone if necessary or if the adolescent prefers it that way. Prior to meeting with the family, the therapist explores with the adolescent what he would like to share with his parents and what he doesn't want to share with them, thus protecting the adolescent's confidentiality. The goals of the final session for the family are similar to those for the adolescent. They include a review of the patient's presenting symptoms, initial goals for the therapy, achievement of these goals, and discussion of the changes in the family interactions and functioning as a result of the therapy. It is important to discuss with the family the possible recurrence of mild symptoms shortly after termination. The need for further treatment, if it is indicated, and management of future recurrent episodes of depression also should be discussed.

Structure of the Family Termination

The structure of the termination process with the family varies by adolescent. Ideally, the therapist has already conducted an individual termination session with the adolescent alone and conducts this final session with the adolescent and family members together. This is beneficial when the therapist has the sense that the family will provide support for the adolescent's accomplishments and will further encourage the adolescent's sense of competence. If the therapist perceives that the family will not be supportive when with the adolescent, it is better to conduct the majority of the session with the family alone, bringing them together briefly at the end of the session to discuss possible future treatment needs and issues to continue to address in their relationship.

Family and Adolescent Together

Many of the identified problems with which the adolescent presented initially for treatment have involved the family and their relationships. They may involve transitions, disputes, grief over the loss of a relationship, or a feeling of isolation within the family. To assess the impact of treatment on the family, the therapist might ask the family members the following:

> How do you feel the family may have changed as a result of [adolescent's name]'s treatment? What things are you doing differently? How do you feel differently about each other? What has improved? What do you feel helped bring about these changes? What still remains a problem?

Hopefully, the therapy will have made significant changes in the adolescent's way of relating to the family and will have affected the family's way of relating to the adolescent. Also, as the depressive symptoms improved during the course of treatment, some interpersonal problems of the family may have been alleviated. These positive changes in the family interactions will be reviewed and supported by the therapist.

Of course, not all adolescents recover from their depression in the course of treatment. In such cases, the termination phase is the time when the therapist reviews the progress that was made and the problems that still persist and would benefit from further treatment. Most likely, the adolescent has made some progress or else the therapist would have reviewed the lack of progress with the parent earlier in the course of treatment and already made some changes either by switching the type of therapy or recommending adjunctive medication. Most likely, then, these are adolescents who are experiencing partial but not complete remission of symptoms. The therapist should review the nature of depression and that some adolescents benefit from a little more treatment or other forms of treatment such as medication or long-term psychotherapy. The therapist, together with the family, should then make an appropriate disposition plan in light of the current status of the adolescent's symptomatology and impairment in functioning.

Family Alone

In some cases, an adolescent's depression has improved and the adolescent has enjoyed the treatment experience, despite having a less supportive family. In these instances, it may be better to meet with the family alone for the majority of the session. The therapist's goal for this meeting is to again emphasize the adolescent's accomplishments in treatment and the areas of the relationship that need further work. The therapist should listen to the family's concerns about treatment and/or the adolescent and respond with supportive recommendations that may include continued treatment for the adolescent and/or treatment for another family member. It is helpful to acknowledge the chronic stressors that make it difficult to recognize and support the adolescent's strengths. For example, the therapist might say:

> I know that during the course of Bill's treatment you have been under a lot of stress at home. As we have discussed in earlier sessions, this has sometimes made it difficult for you to emphasize the positive things that Bill has done as much as you would like to. I have seen a lot of improvement in Bill. Have you? Still there are areas in which he is continuing to have difficulty, such as his relationship with his father. To help Bill continue to feel better, there are several things I think might help. I think both you and Bill would feel better if you had a place of your own to get support for all the stress your family is experiencing. If you feel more support from people outside your family, most likely you will feel better in your interactions with your family. Bill also might benefit from continuing in therapy so he can keep working on improving his relationship with his father and practice his new skills. How does this sound to you?

The goal of this communication is to acknowledge the continuing family stress and its effect on all members of the family and to emphasize the importance of recognizing the adolescent's accomplishments while recommending further treatment so the improvements can continue. The therapist might even coach the parent on how to acknowledge these accomplishments to the adolescent when he joins them for the final few minutes of the session to wrap up treatment.

THE NEED FOR FURTHER TREATMENT

It is a different experience to end treatment when the adolescent has not improved as much as the therapist and adolescent would have hoped. In such cases, usually the adolescent has been making some improvement or else the treatment approach would have been reevaluated earlier on. Still, there are adolescents for whom there has been some improvement, but they are still moderately symptomatic at the conclusion of treatment. It is important for the therapist to openly discuss this issue with the adolescent and his parents. The therapist should initially review how the adolescent was feeling at the beginning of treatment and the depression symptoms that remain at termination. The identified problem areas should be discussed, along with the improvements that have occurred and those changes that have been discussed but have not yet occurred. A discussion should follow in which the parents, therapist, and adolescent discuss whether or not these symptoms warrant further treatment, whether they feel that they might continue to improve on their own after treatment, and the pros and cons to pursuing further treatment. Some adolescents may feel the need to take a break from therapy and choose to address other problems at a later date. This is a decision that needs to be made together with parent, therapist, and patient after listening to the therapist's appraisal of the adolescent's depression and recommendations regarding further treatment.

Continuation Treatment

According to the American Academy of Child and Adolescent Psychiatry Practice Parameters (AACAP, 1998) for the treatment of depression, clinicians should offer all patients continuation treatment for at least 6 months after complete symptom remission to consolidate the response and prevent relapse. This is felt to be true whether it is psychopharmacological or psychosocial treatment. The efficacy of continuation treatment has not yet been adequately studied in children and adolescents; however, the recommendation is based on the efficacy demonstrated in the adult research literature. In the adult studies, patients remain on the same dose of antidepressant used to achieve remission as long as there are no significant side effects. The same phenomenon has been examined in children and adolescents in naturalistic follow-up studies, which show that continued medication and/or psychotherapy can decrease relapse rates (Birmaher et al., 1996b; Emslie et al., 1998). There have been no clinical trials studying the efficacy of continuation treatment with IPT-A. Controlled studies examining the efficacy of continuation treatment for children and adolescents are needed. As a result of our clinical experiences, we concur with the practice parameters and recommend approximately 3 months of continued IPT-A therapy biweekly in order to help consolidate the adolescent's improvements and prevent quick relapse. When shifting from the acute to continuation phase of treatment, the therapist should make the shift explicit and renegotiate the treatment contract with new goals and a new time frame.

Maintenance Treatment

Another treatment option, after completing the acute and continuation treatment for adolescents in complete remission, is to shift to maintenance treatment with IPT-A. The practice parameters also recommend maintenance treatment for patients who are in full remission from their depression (American Academy of Child and Adolescent Psychiatry, 1998). In this case, adolescents would continue with once-a-month sessions of IPT-A for approximately 1 year. There is data for the efficacy of maintenance treatment in preventing recurrence of depression in depressed adults (Frank et al., 1991).

Maintenance sessions may serve a similar purpose for adolescents as they do with adults, that is, to provide enough support for continued use of effective interpersonal strategies to decrease the rate of recurrent episodes. Although psychotherapy is a widely used treatment for depressed adolescents, there have been no published controlled clinical trials assessing the efficacy of a follow-up maintenance psychotherapy treatment for depressed adolescents who have recovered from an acute episode of major depression. There have been several studies that followed adolescents naturalistically after completion of treatment for initial episode, and these suggest a significant risk for recurrence of a depressive episode either as an adolescent or young adult (Lewinsohn, Clarke, Seeley, & Rhode, 1994a; Macaulay et al., 1993).

There is a history of using IPT as a maintenance treatment with adults (IPT-M). A primary reason for considering IPT as a long-term maintenance treatment for adults was the evidence that, even in the face of complete symptomatic remission, patients with a history of recurrent depression continue to show marked impairment in social adjustment (Frank et al., 1990; Klerman et al., 1974). This persistent impairment in social functioning also is confirmed in the studies with depressed adolescents (Puig-Antich et al., 1985b, 1993; Weissman et al., 1999a, 1999b). Psychosocial impairments may contribute in a significant way to a patient's vulnerability to depression and may take longer to improve than the symptoms themselves. If an adolescent is still unable to negotiate his interpersonal environment when no longer depressed, the lack of interpersonal success may precipitate a recurrence or may act as a predisposing vulnerability for a recurrence of depression. Continued treatment, focusing on interpersonal conflict and stress and successful coping strategies within the interpersonal problem area framework, may result in a longer time to recurrence by providing further opportunities to discuss the interpersonal issues and apply the coping strategies to more and varied situations. Maintenance IPT (IPT-M) for adults was designed to maintain recovery and reduce recurrence by continuing to focus on the interpersonal aspects of the patients' initial depressive episode and addressing new issues as they arise. The therapist reinforces the effective strategies learned in the acute phase and fosters acquisition of new ones, thereby hopefully averting the build-up of frustration and anger that could lead to another episode (Frank et al., 1991).

Based upon the evidence for the morbidity of adolescent depression, the persistent social impairments, and the high rate of recurrence, we felt it was important to gather further information on the feasibility of developing and conducting maintenance treatment for depressed adolescents. The therapist may be able to help the adolescent at key points in his development, thereby reducing the developmental social lag that can be caused by depression.

Four adolescents who received IPT-A as part of an acute randomized controlled clinical trial and who met recovery criteria on the Beck Depression Inventory (BDI) and Hamilton Rating Scale for Depression (HRSD) (BDI ≤ 6; HRSD ≤ 9) participated in a pilot study of IPT-AM. The patients were seen once a month for 12 months by the same therapist who treated their acute episode. The therapists conducted the IPT-AM according to a maintenance IPT-A treatment manual outline (Mufson, unpublished manuscript). All sessions were videotaped, and the therapists received regular supervision by an IPT-A expert. The four patients attended their monthly sessions regularly for a year. There was no excessive use of the telephone in between sessions to suggest distress with the decreased frequency of the sessions. The patients continued to report their maintenance sessions as helpful. Their behavior suggests acceptability and feasibility of conducting maintenance sessions with adolescents. However, a large controlled clinical trial is needed to assess its efficacy. The following is a hypothetical case that demonstrates the use of IPT-AM.

Case Example

Joanna was referred to the acute IPT-A clinical trial study by her school guidance counselor because she appeared depressed, was failing in school, and was socially isolated. Joanna lived with her father, mother, and older sister. The family had immigrated to the

United States from South America 2 years prior to Joanna's referral. Joanna had been depressed for 2 years and exhibited symptoms including pervasive sadness most of the time, frequent passive suicidal ideation, early and middle insomnia, mild anhedonia, loss of energy and fatigue, mild hopelessness, and poor concentration. Joanna also reported extreme social discomfort and reluctance to make oral presentations at school. She rarely volunteered answers to teachers' questions in class. Although she reported having friends, she was close to no one and had no confidante. Joanna's depressive symptoms and social discomfort resulted in frequent school absences. Joanna was diagnosed with major depression, moderate severity, and social phobia and was seen for 12 interpersonal psychotherapy sessions with the focus on role transitions. When Joanna's family immigrated to the United States, she was faced with three role transitions: (1) the move into adolescence, (2) her family's increased dependence on her as their primary translator, and (3) the move to a new country. Shortly after the family's move, her older sister developed a severe depression, and the family's reliance on Joanna increased.

During the acute treatment, Joanna focused on developing new communication skills that she practiced in session using role playing, as well as at school with her friends and teachers. She learned how to better negotiate arguments with her parents and to assert herself appropriately with her parents and peers. Her new comfort level was apparent in her behavior with the therapist and by her report in other settings. By the end of treatment, Joanna had several close friends, was able to attend school regularly, negotiated successfully to make up missed schoolwork, and was able to be more open about her feelings with family and friends.

Maintenance sessions were held once a month for 12 months following termination of the acute treatment. In the maintenance phase, Joanna continued to integrate her new communication and negotiation skills into various settings in her life. In session 4, Joanna brought up a difficult family situation with which she was struggling. Her sister's depression had worsened, making Joanna feel pressured to succeed where her sister could not, and making school feel more threatening and negative. The therapist helped Joanna link these symptoms to her feelings about the effect her sister's problems were having on her role in the family and her relationship to school. Joanna was able to identify the need to let her family know how her sister's illness was affecting her emotionally as well as affecting her performance and attendance in school. She again practiced in session how to let her parents know of her discomfort with the situation at home. She then took the skills learned in the role plays home to try with her parents. Her parents were able to respond appropriately and provide her with more support. In month 6 of IPT-AM, Joanna reported that she was doing well emotionally and academically. For the rest of the year of IPT-AM monthly therapy, Joanna reported no depressive symptoms, had a full social life, excelled academically while working part-time, and reported reduced conflict within her family relationships.

Reemergence of Depression Symptoms

Many patients have difficulty with ending treatment; therefore, the decision to recommend further treatment should not be based on the recent emerging discomfort but on a broader view of the patient's clinical history and the course of his treatment. Family members need to be alerted to the possibility of a regression at the conclusion of treatment. The distinction between a regression that will resolve in a few weeks and a recurrence of symptoms should be made. For adolescents who appear to be experiencing mild discomfort as a result of concerns about termination, the therapist might tell them:

> It is very common for patients to feel nervous about ending treatment, particularly if they feel that it has been helpful to them. It is our experience that this discomfort usually goes away several weeks after termination as you begin to recognize your ability to function successfully in the absence of treatment. That is why we usually suggest a 4-week waiting period before making a referral for additional treatment. How do you feel about trying the waiting period? What are your concerns? If possible, let's try the waiting period and see how you feel in a few weeks. If during that time, you feel you need help, you can always call me and more treatment will be arranged.

The family should support the adolescent during this transition. This waiting period is feasible for people who are experiencing mild discomfort, but it is not recommended for adolescents who continue to present with significant symptomatology and/or impaired functioning.

Parents should be informed that depressive episodes might reoccur at some point in the future, particularly during times of stress or change for the adolescent. Early warning signs and symptoms (i.e., general for depression and specific to the adolescent) are reviewed, and appropriate management including referral for a different treatment is outlined. If the adolescent's symptoms do not resolve in several weeks, the therapist should be contacted to determine whether further treatment is necessary. Otherwise, if it is clear at termination that the adolescent needs further treatment, this is the time to arrange for an appropriate referral. If a referral is needed, it should include a psychiatric evaluation to determine the need for medication and/or a course of another type of psychotherapy that may include a different individual psychotherapy or family therapy.

THERAPIST FEELINGS ABOUT TERMINATION

Terminating treatment with the adolescent can be difficult for the therapist as well as for the adolescent. Despite working with the adolescent for a relatively brief period of time, a lot of intense therapeutic work has occurred within the context of a strong patient–therapist alliance. The therapist feels sad about not being able to witness the adolescent's continued growth. The process of saying good-bye to the patient allows the therapist to demonstrate how good relationships can end simply because it is time to move on, rather than a relationship coming to an end only when something has gone wrong in the relationship. It is acceptable for the therapist to express to the adolescent how much she has enjoyed working with him and that she will miss their meetings, but it is important also to convey her happiness that he is well and ready to move on. The therapist can say:

> *It is sometimes hard to believe that we have been working together for almost 3 months and that we are getting ready to say good-bye. I just want you to know that I have really enjoyed working with you and being able to help you feel better. I will miss our meetings. You really worked hard and accomplished a lot of changes that you should feel good about. I feel good that you will be able to continue this work after we stop meeting.*

The therapist is able to express her genuine feelings toward the adolescent, but, at the same time, does not make him feel badly about ending the treatment and leaving the therapist. Instead, she continues to foster a sense of self-confidence, letting him know that this was a positive relationship for both of them. It is possible (outside of a research protocol) to decide that booster sessions (i.e., continuation and/or maintenance) would be helpful to the adolescent, but this decision should be based upon the adolescent's situation, not the therapist's reluctance to end their relationship.

THE NEED FOR LONG-TERM TREATMENT

Even though a patient's major depressive symptoms may have resolved during the course of treatment, additional problems may require that he

seek longer-term treatment. Some patients may need continued supportive psychotherapy when there is still a paucity of social support outside
the therapeutic relationship. Additional psychotherapy is typically recommended for those adolescents who are experiencing such other difficulties as mild eating disorders, adjustments to learning disabilities,
problems coping with a past history of sexual or physical abuse, coping
with a chaotic family, or impaired personality traits that are not addressed in IPT-A. It is generally acknowledged that there is a strong likelihood that depressed adolescents will experience another episode of depression at some point in their life. Many adolescents experience
numerous transient episodes of depressive symptomatology and impaired functioning. For those adolescents who present with numerous
such episodes, long-term treatment might prove useful in stabilizing their
functioning. IPT-A can help stabilize a patient, help treat the acute disorder, and help the adolescent feel prepared for more intensive exploration
of other psychiatric issues that impair the adolescent's functioning in
other domains.

Case Example

Karen, age 17 years old, presented with a major depression associated with a dispute with her parents, particularly her mother.
Following completion of 12 sessions of IPT-A, the majority of her
depressive symptoms had remitted. She had gained a better perspective about her mother's concerns regarding her relationship with her
boyfriend and had been able to negotiate an agreement with her
mother regarding her involvement in activities with him. Since she
was feeling less depressed and was having less conflict with her
mother, she raised the subject of a resurgence of feelings about a car
accident that she had been in several years ago in which she had
been injured. She had spent several weeks in the hospital and still
worried whenever she had to go on a long car trip anywhere. At the
conclusion of IPT-A, Karen, the therapist, and her parents discussed
how much the car anxiety was interfering with her functioning.
Both Karen and her parents expressed concern that it might become
more impairing next year when she would be ready to get her
driver's license. They all decided that Karen would benefit from further treatment focused on her anxiety and avoidance of riding in
cars since her accident.

    In this case example, IPT-A was able to effectively treat her de-
pression symptoms and then enabled her to face the other difficulties she was having and to address the specific phobia with another
type of treatment. Options for other treatment include referral to
another clinic or another therapist, a different therapeutic orientation, medication, or development of a new and different contract

with the same therapist focusing on different issues. This decision should be made jointly with the therapist, adolescent, and responsible parent.

CONCLUSION

The therapist's goals in the termination phase are to balance the tasks of the termination phase with concluding work on the identified problem area. It is crucial to devote a major portion of the termination phase to reviewing interpersonal strategies used in the identified problem area and applying the strategies to ongoing and future situations. The more practice the adolescent gets using the strategies, the more second nature they will become for him. The result will be a greater sense of interpersonal confidence and a reduction in interpersonal conflict or disappointment that could lead to a return of depressive symptoms. Good experiences during this phase of treatment are invaluable to helping the adolescent to feel better about himself and to be able to negotiate successful endings of other relationships at future points in his life. Future treatment may be necessary under certain circumstances when the symptoms may not have fully remitted or when there are other more chronic problems contributing to the adolescent's impairment. The termination phase enables both the adolescent and parent to participate in the review of accomplishments and the identification of areas that still would benefit from further treatment and to make further treatment decisions accordingly.

PART III

Special Issues
in Treating Adolescents

CHAPTER 15

Clinical Issues in the Therapist–Patient Relationship

U p to this point, we have described the typical course of treatment using the IPT-A model. Although we have periodically touched on some of the problems that may arise at various points in treatment, there are several other issues that may impact treatment. These issues may not be specific to IPT-A, but they are handled in a particular way within the IPT-A framework. These can be grouped in the general categories of patient-related, family-related, and depression-related issues.

PATIENT-RELATED ISSUES

Throughout the description of IPT-A in this book, examples are provided of the type of patient–therapist relationship that characterizes IPT-A treatment. In working with depressed adolescents, however, there are several potential issues that may arise within the therapeutic relationship.

Patient Confidentiality

Confidentiality between the patient and therapist is a cornerstone to the therapeutic relationship. Adolescents under the age of 18 are still legally considered minors, and parents legally have the right to know what their adolescents are doing. However, when working with adolescents and their families, the therapist should emphasize to the family that the therapy would be more effective if the adolescent can feel that the conversations are confidential. Both the adolescent and family are instructed that information from the sessions will be kept confidential unless life-threatening. Specifically, confidentiality is maintained unless the therapist feels that the adolescent is at risk of harm to himself or may harm someone else. If the therapist feels the need to share some information from the session with the parents, the therapist first should discuss this with the adolescent, allow the adolescent to express his concerns, explain the reasons for discussing it with the parents, and plan the best way to inform the parents. Clearly communicating with the adolescent and family in this way provides an excellent model for them, showing the value of effective communication even in stressful situations.

The parents should be informed that any information they wish to provide to the therapist is welcome and may be beneficial. However, all phone calls and information from the parents will be shared with the adolescent. The therapist cannot maintain confidentiality with the parents because it would jeopardize the therapist's alliance with the adolescent. Knowing the sessions are confidential and that the therapist will share with the adolescent her conversations with the parent(s) will help the adolescent feel that the therapy session is a safe and secure place to talk.

Substitution of the Therapist for Family or Friend

For many depressed adolescents who feel alienated from family and friends and who are in need of support, the therapist can become a substitute for these missing relationships. In IPT-A, this is acceptable only in certain situations and within certain limits. Often the therapist does take on a role with the adolescent that might have been performed by a family member in order to serve as a bridge while the adolescent tries to reestablish family connections or find outside support. For example, when an adolescent does not have a parent who is able to act as an advocate, the therapist often acts on behalf of the adolescent with the school. Doing so provides the adolescent with alternative role models for effective adult support and communication.

The goals of IPT-A include helping the adolescent to develop his own coping resources and supports outside of the therapeutic setting that can be maintained after the conclusion of therapy. Therefore, it sometimes becomes necessary to clarify with the adolescent the limits of the therapeutic relationship and how it differs from a friendship. The therapist should encourage the adolescent to find appropriate sources of support and/or role models outside the therapeutic relationship. The therapist should explain that she could help the adolescent practice the skills needed to establish these relationships, but that this is practice for the real relationship building needed outside of treatment. It is important during these discussions to continue to encourage the adolescent's expression of affect so that his feelings can be identified and related to what is occurring in his interpersonal world.

The Excessively Dependent Patient

Similar to the situation described above, depressed adolescents frequently experience a level of fatigue or malaise so severe that they feel unable to act upon any initiative and unable to make any decisions on their own. They may ask for specific advice about how to resolve a problem or may try to have the therapist do some of the negotiating with their parents, teachers, or peers instead of doing it themselves. The therapist must be wary of intervening too directly because the therapist does not want to deprive the adolescent of developing his own coping and negotiation skills to use in the future. Still, adolescents often need the added support and authority of the therapist when trying to negotiate and/or communicate with their parents. In these cases, the therapist can help the adolescent develop a series of steps toward specific interpersonal objectives. These steps should involve a progressively decreased role for the therapist and increased demand on the adolescent to function more independently of the therapist. If the work that the adolescent needs to do is with a parent or teacher, it can be helpful to schedule a meeting with any such third parties to help them understand what the adolescent is expected to work on and to help them determine ways that they can be a support and assistance to the adolescent's work outside of the therapy sessions.

Case Example

Maria is a 16-year-old female who is experiencing a role dispute with her mother. They argue about almost everything, including when to do homework, cleaning her room, spending time with her friends, and how to dress. The arguing has become so severe that Maria and her mother were avoiding speaking to each other at all times except for emergencies. The therapist was trying to help Maria learn to better express what she wanted regarding one or two of these issues and to practice in the session how to speak to her mother about them. While reluctant to role-play in the session, Maria would eventually practice ways to have conversations. However, in between sessions she was unable to apply the skills to situations with her mother. Instead, she would call the therapist on the phone and ask the therapist to talk to her mother. To facilitate a discussion between Maria and her mother, the therapist invited her mother to participate in a therapy session with Maria. The therapist hoped that she could coach Maria to express herself in the session to her mother. Instead, Maria refused to speak and wanted the therapist to express her feelings and opinions as they had been rehearsing them in earlier role plays.

Maria was being overly reliant on the therapist to explain and negotiate her position on the areas in dispute. While the therapist tried to model appropriate discussion during the initial part of the session, she did not continue to do so. If she had continued, Maria would have lost an opportunity to develop her own communication and negotiation skills. The therapist explained to the mother that they had been working on Maria's developing more effective communication skills so that she could better let her mother know how she is feeling and what she needs. Maria's mother agreed that this was an important issue for Maria. The therapist then turned to Maria and told her that she would not "speak for her" any more in the session but was willing to help her explain her point of view to her mother. Turning to the mother, the therapist discussed with her ways in which she could engage Maria in a conversation. The therapist educated both Maria and her mother on the importance of learning to negotiate with each other rather than having to have the therapist do it for them.

If the adolescent's demands on the therapist are inappropriate, such as phoning her during the middle of an argument so the therapist can negotiate for him or wanting to go places together outside of treatment, the therapist must explore the reasons for these needs and explain to the adolescent the appropriate boundaries for the relationship. The therapist might say:

> It is not unusual for patients to feel closeness to their therapists, but it is important to remember that there is a difference between your friendships and your relationship with me. I am here to support you, to help you learn new ways of coping with conflicts and situations outside the therapy. But my goal is to enable you to find fulfilling relationships outside of therapy and to develop your own positive coping strategies. Maybe we should talk about how you can establish friendships with other people who could engage in these activities with you or focus on how to enter into negotiations when you are in a dispute.

When a Patient Wants to Share a Therapist

Sometimes an adolescent may bring along a family member or friend to therapy and would like the therapist to treat the other person. It is not the role of the IPT-A therapist to explore the underlying motivations. The therapist should explain to the adolescent that she is that adolescent's therapist and is there to help the adolescent. Consequently, the therapist is interested in the other people in the adolescent's life, but the therapist must refer the other person for an evaluation for treatment by another therapist. Treating both the patient and the patient's friend could lead to problems for the therapist if each adolescent shares information with the therapist that they do not want the other adolescent to know. Such situations would compromise the therapist's ability to maintain confidentiality and create conflicts of interest that would make it impossible for the therapist to act professionally toward both as patients. Thus, it is best to refer the patient's friend to another clinician.

PATIENT-INITIATED DISRUPTIONS TO TREATMENT

Cancellation and Lateness to Sessions

When working with adolescents in IPT-A, the therapist takes a different stance on missed appointments or lateness than when working with adults. The therapist allows greater flexibility of scheduling sessions and does not interpret missed sessions as resistance—at least not initially— until proven otherwise. The therapist, though, should examine whether the adolescent is not attending the session because he feels worse and is unable to get out of the house, whether practical problems in his life (e.g., transportation, financial issues, or household responsibilities such as babysitting for a younger sibling) are impeding his attendance, or whether the adolescent is feeling better and has returned to involvement in activities with peers and/or family members that hinder attendance. The therapist is similarly nonjudgmental about lateness. The therapist might say:

> *These past few weeks I have noticed that you have been missing sessions or late, and I was wondering how you are feeling about coming for therapy? Have you been feeling better? Worse? How so? What do you think keeps you from getting here or causes you to be late?*

If there is no worsening of depressive symptoms associated with the lateness, the therapist should stress that the more time they have together, the more they can accomplish. If the adolescent continues to miss consecutive sessions, then the therapist again needs to explore what may be preventing the adolescent from getting to treatment. It is possible that the patient currently is not interested in treatment. In this case, the possibility of ending treatment early should be broached with the adolescent since treatment cannot be very effective if the adolescent does not attend sessions. This decision needs to be made on a case-by-case basis after the therapist ascertains the reasons for the missed sessions. If someone or something is impeding the adolescent's attendance, then perhaps the therapist can help the adolescent resolve the problem and enable the adolescent to complete his course of treatment.

In treating the adolescent, the therapist often relies on the telephone as a means of staying in contact with the adolescent either between initial sessions or when sessions are missed. In the beginning, telephone contact is believed to enhance the development of the therapeutic alliance. If the adolescent has failed to attend a session, the therapist can hold a brief session over the telephone to maintain continuity until the adolescent comes in for a session. However, therapy should not regularly occur on the telephone. If such a pattern begins to develop, it is necessary to have the adolescent attend a session to discuss these therapeutic difficulties.

Resistance to Treatment

Treatment resistance can present in a number of different ways, including not attending treatment, physically attending treatment but not participating in the session, and failing to follow through on plans and recommendations developed in treatment sessions. First and foremost, the therapist must consider whether or not IPT-A is the appropriate treatment for the adolescent and whether the problem is that another treatment might be optimal and IPT-A is not helping the patient. The therapist should discuss this possibility with the adolescent and his family, and if they agree, the therapist should refer them for another type of treatment.

There are some adolescents who attend the session, are passively compliant during the session, but do not truly participate in the process of treatment. In these cases, we recommend that therapists first highlight this pattern of response to treatment for the adolescent, reminding him of the reasons treatment was sought and the necessary role he must play in the process for it to be effective. It is also important to give the adolescent the opportunity to talk about any concerns he may have about the treatment and how the therapist might help him to be more proactive in the sessions. If this does not help to alleviate the resistance, the therapist must evaluate whether IPT-A is an appropriate treatment for him at this time, given its short-term nature and demands for active involvement by the adolescent.

Noncompliance with "Work at Home"

Partially related to treatment resistance is noncompliance with assignments to complete "work at home," that is, to practice new interpersonal skills in between sessions. The success of a short-term treatment such as IPT-A depends on generalization of the skills taught or modeled to situations outside of the therapeutic setting. Therefore, work at home or in school or in other settings in which the adolescent practices interpersonal skills is important to the effectiveness of the treatment. That being said, when an adolescent is not compliant with such assignments, the therapist must consider a number of issues. First, it is crucial for the therapist to give the adolescent the message that this work is important by regularly inquiring about assignments given during the preceding session. Early in treatment, the therapist must take care not to engender treatment resistance by giving the adolescent the message that he has failed or disappointed the therapist by not doing this work. When work at home is not completed, the therapist should inquire as to what got in the way of doing the work and any specific obstacles. These might be life events, behaviors of significant others in his life, or the result of emotions such as fear or depression that keep the adolescent from trying something new. It is actually most helpful to anticipate and discuss these possible obstacles during the session when the assignment is given, to help the adolescent predict the obstacles and discuss ways to proactively manage them.

The therapist also must determine if the assignment was too difficult or if they did not practice the necessary skills adequately for the adolescent to be successful in completing the work. It is helpful for the therapist to accept at least partial responsibility for work not being completed, particularly early in treatment, so that the adolescent is not too discouraged to try again. This tends to make it more likely that the adolescent will be willing to try an assignment in the future and more likely that he will honestly let the therapist know if he feels the assignment is too difficult. The following clinical example illustrates how this can be used to better facilitate the therapeutic process and the subsequent completion of assignments for outside the session.

Case Example

Brian is a 14-year-old boy who is no longer interested in playing football. According to Brian, his father takes great pride in Brian's proficiency at the sport and would be very upset to learn that his son no longer wants to play. Brian reports feeling extremely anxious about talking to his father. The therapist role-played this discussion with Brian a few times in the preceding session and encouraged him to go home and have the conversation with his father. Brian reluctantly agreed, but when he returned the following week he stated that he tried but was not able to have the conversation.

THERAPIST: That is OK. Let's talk about what happened. You said that you tried. What did you do?

PATIENT: Well, one day when he got home from work I went into the living room where he was watching TV, and I said that I had something I wanted to talk to him about.

THERAPIST: What exactly did you say?

PATIENT: "Dad can I talk to you about something?"

THERAPIST: How did your dad respond?

PATIENT: At first he didn't say anything. I think he didn't really hear me, or it didn't register, but then I said it again, and he responded kind of irritated and just said, "What?"

THERAPIST: And what did you do then?

PATIENT: Well, I tried to talk, but I was nervous because he seemed already mad, so I just ended up saying "never mind."

THERAPIST: Did you ever get another chance to try?

PATIENT: I forgot to try again.

THERAPIST: OK. Well, we actually can learn a lot from what you did try. Actually, I think I realized where I might have made a mistake. Although we practiced this several times, we really didn't talk enough about how to set up the conversation and how to pick a time to have it. We should have practiced that part. We also should have thought more about the different reactions your dad could have to you trying to have this conversation and worked out how to handle those different ways. So, let's back up and work on some of this. Let's start with the issue of when to try to talk to your dad. Do you have some thoughts as to when are good times and when are not so good times to have an important conversation with your dad?

PATIENT: Not when he is in a bad mood—I guess not after work. He really needs a chance to unwind. He is kind of expecting problems and complaints from people, and all he really wants to do is relax. Maybe on the weekend is better.

THERAPIST: That sounds like a good idea. Some people find it works best when you are doing something with him that you both enjoy. Can you think of anything like that?

PATIENT: Well, if we are working on a project around the house or if we were out for a burger.

THERAPIST: It sounds like those might be good times to have this kind of discussion with your dad. Now that we have a better idea as to when you would have the discussion, let's talk a bit more about how you could go about starting the conversation to ensure that he is really listening to you and realizes how important this is to you.

The therapist would continue in this vein, attempting to work out more of the details of the interaction and uncover more of the potential obstacles. The more prepared the adolescent feels to handle the details and process of the assignment, the more likely he is to follow through with it the next time.

Early Termination

Adolescents will, at times, seek to terminate a course of treatment early. Sometimes the adolescent expresses this desire directly and sometimes more passively by not attending treatment sessions or arriving late to sessions. Before reacting to an adolescent's desire to terminate early, the therapist must investigate the reasons the patient wants to do so. It is important to discern whether the adolescent is terminating because he feels better, because the treatment has not satisfactorily met his therapeutic needs, or because the parents want termination. Adolescents often have what appear to be transient episodes of depression that may remit quickly and/or spontaneously. In such a case, the therapist would be wrong to force the adolescent into continuing the treatment and perpetuating the sick role. The therapist should support the adolescent's feelings of well-being, review the changes that may have occurred in the time that the adolescent did receive treatment, and inform the adolescent that he may return for treatment at a later date if the feeling of well-being does not last and he would like more treatment.

The therapist cannot force the adolescent to remain in treatment, however, it is important to reeducate the adolescent about the possibility that his depression will recur. The therapist should explain that, even though he is feeling better now, it could still be helpful to practice skills a little longer with the hope of preventing a relapse in the future. This is particularly important if specific impending stressors can be identified or if the flight to health is largely in response to a recent positive life event, the effects of which could subside quickly. A common example of the latter is the improvement that many adolescents experience when summer arrives and school is no longer in session. During the summer, there are many fewer demands placed on most adolescents. For these adolescents, however, the return to school several months later can be considerably stressful and trigger a relapse. In such cases, continuing treatment through the transition can be helpful to preventing such a relapse. As part of this process, the therapist should help the adolescent identify what he can do to protect himself against future depressive episodes and specifically how the adolescent can manage particular stressors. This should include a discussion of the warning signs of the adolescent's depression and the steps to follow if he begins to experience these signs.

If the adolescent wishes to terminate due to dissatisfaction with the treatment, the therapist must examine the therapeutic contract in light of the adolescent's expressed needs and either renegotiate the contract, if possible, or refer the adolescent for treatment that may be more congruent with his needs.

FAMILY-RELATED ISSUES

Family Encouragement of Early Termination

If the parents want the adolescent to terminate the therapy, a meeting should be set up between the parents and the therapist. If the parents refuse to attend, the problem should be discussed over the telephone with the goal of arranging a face-to-face meeting. Parents may wish to terminate their child's treatment for several reasons, which may include feeling threatened by the therapist and worrying that their role is being usurped; thinking that because their child is in therapy, they are bad parents; worrying that a "family secret" such as incest or alcohol abuse may be revealed; or feeling threatened by the changes the adolescent is making in the treatment, even if these are beneficial changes (e.g., increased independence). The therapist must try to determine which of these reasons are contributing to the parents' desire to have their child leave treatment.

Depending upon the particular reason, the therapist will need to respond with clarification and reassurance that the parents' involvement is welcomed and, perhaps, provide a referral for family or individual treatment for other family members. Another useful strategy in cases where the adolescent wants to continue but the parents are resistant is to work with the adolescent on using effective communication to tell the parents that he wants to continue in treatment and how it is helpful to him. The therapist can work in the sessions on how the adolescent can negotiate a compromise with his parents, such as continuing for several more sessions but not necessarily the entire course of treatment.

If the parents persist in their request to end the treatment, the therapist is obliged to do so unless there are clear indications that termination of therapy constitutes neglect. Actionable indications may include severe depressive symptoms such as suicidal ideation or indications of sexual or physical abuse in the household. Referral to another therapist and/or notification of a child protective service agency are mandatory in such cases.

Patient Feeling the Blame for Family Problems

Another problem can occur in the therapy when patients take the blame for problems within the family due to the patient's style of internalizing responsibility for issues that are largely external to him. It also can occur when the patient has become the scapegoat of the family's problems, although the problem really involves the family as a whole or specific other family members. Often the assumption of blame arises from a combination of these factors. The therapist should recognize when this is occurring and identify the reason for it by determining whether this reflects a pattern of internalizing responsibility or whether family members are doing or saying things that are creating this situation. Once the origins of the problem have been identified, the therapist can use a combination of education and interpersonal communication and negotiation techniques to address this issue.

This is a time when more directive techniques are often necessary. It may be important to meet with the patient's parent(s) or guardian(s) to help clarify the issues and intervene on behalf of the patient. In cases where the adolescent is internalizing responsibility for a family problem, the parents can hopefully join as allies with the therapist in clearly identifying for the adolescent those things that are out of his control and not related to him. In cases where family members are labeling the family problems as being the adolescent's problem, the therapist can work with the family to see how this is not the case and how detrimental it is to the adolescent to place this burden on him. The therapist must be careful not to enter into family therapy, but rather to clarify the issue on behalf of the adolescent and then possibly assist him in accessing therapeutic help from a different provider to address the issues. Consultation and intervention with the family, of course, should only be done after the therapist has talked to the patient about involving the family members.

DEPRESSION-RELATED ISSUES

Problems Due to Hopelessness and Helplessness of Depression

Two of the symptoms commonly associated with depression are hopelessness and helplessness. Both of these pose challenges to treatment of any kind. The adolescents may not fully engage in treatment due to the belief that, like all else in their life, nothing can help, nothing can get better, or they can't do anything to help themselves. It is important for the therapist to perceive these reactions as different from treatment resistance and to understand them as a symptom of the adolescent's depression. In accordance with the IPT-A model, therapists should educate the adolescent about these symptoms and the impact they can have on motivation and functioning both in and outside of treatment. The therapist highlights thoughts and actions that reflect these symptoms and emphasizes that these are issues that can be addressed in the treatment. Addressing these symptoms involves helping adolescents to focus on taking very small steps and emphasizing how very small changes can lead to changes in their moods and functioning. It is helpful to use the analogy of the snowball effect, explaining how one small change can lead to another and another to the point that the result is larger and the changes are more significant. It is also important to identify those times when the adolescent does make positive changes or positive things happen for him that he may not recognize. Sometimes the changes or events are small and can be overlooked, especially by a depressed adolescent who is looking at himself and his life through a "gray" lens.

The Dysthymia Dilemma

A final challenge posed by the nature of depression on treatment occurs with the specific disorder of dysthymia. This involves patients with dysthymia alone or what is commonly referred to as double depression, a combination of an acute major depression and longer-standing dysthymia (Brent, Kolko, Birmaher, Baugher, & Bridge, 1999; Goodman et al., 2000). Patients with dysthymia have often experienced a mild to moderate depression for a considerable amount of time. Chronicity of the depression predicts the severity of impairment at presentation for treatment as well as the duration of the impairment (Kovacs et al., 1994). By definition, a diagnosis of dysthymia in children and adolescents requires the duration of at least 1 year. The symptoms of dysthymia are often less severe than those commonly found with major depression and can go undetected or be mislabeled for some time. Patients with dysthymia and/or double depression often have difficulty defining the onset of their symptoms and sometimes do not even recognize their symptoms because they cannot remember experiencing anything different. Diagnosis and tracking of symptom changes can be more difficult with these patients.

Our clinical experience suggests that adolescents with dysthymia may have somewhat more difficulty engaging in treatment. They frequently do not have the motivation of more acute symptoms nor the recognition that they can feel better. As a result, their motivation is lower than is necessary to truly "work" in treatment. Consequently, a treatment course of only 12 weeks at times does not seem long enough for them. These patients need particular help with recognizing their symptoms and becoming motivated to work in therapy to feel better. Some of these patients have come to see their symptoms as being part of their personality and often so have their families and friends. Therapists must educate both the adolescents and their parents about the symptoms of depression and how what appears to be a trait may not be one, once the depression is alleviated. By helping them to distinguish the effects of the depression from enduring aspects of the adolescent's personality, the therapist may be able to enervate them to engage effectively in treatment. Emphasizing the ability to make small changes can improve motivation, but it is possible that some of these adolescents may benefit from a longer course of treatment and/or adjunctive medication.

CHAPTER 16

Special Clinical Situations

Special clinical situations not specifically discussed in the preceding chapter, but which may occur, are described here. They include non-nuclear families, parental depression, the suicidal teenager, the assaultive teenager, school refusal, substance abuse, notification of Special Services for Children in cases of physical and sexual abuse, learning disabilities, sexually active adolescents, and homosexual adolescents. These are issues that apply to some but not all adolescents and can cross all problem areas. Indications for medication will be discussed in a separate chapter.

NON-NUCLEAR FAMILIES

Due to the high divorce rate as well as increases in single-parent families, adolescents often live in non-nuclear families, which include homes of other relatives, foster homes or group homes, and single-parent families. Reasons for these alternative arrangements include death, abandonment, intervention by protective services for children, irreconcilable differences among family members, and illness. Living with other relatives, such as grandparents or aunts and uncles, is a common alternative. Living with a known relative has the advantage of providing a familiar home for the adolescent. Still, the adolescent has become a new member of an existing family structure and needs to make a place for himself. Foster care forces the adolescent to move into a preexisting family unit composed of many unfamiliar nonbiologically related members. Temporary placement causes stress for the adolescent, who does not know how long the living arrangement will last and consequently how attached to become to the family, and whether to make an effort to find a role in the family. In a group home, the adolescent no longer has a primary caretaker but is one of a group. The adolescent must learn to be part of a group and learn the rules of the community without the benefit of a parent. For the therapist, the task with these adolescents is to engage the relative, foster family, or leader of the group home as the parents would be engaged. It is especially important in the group home situation to identify one responsible person who will act as a liaison between therapy and the home and also act as the adolescent's advocate or supporter in the group environment. As with the parents, these people are important in the adolescent's daily life and must be educated about the nature of depression, ways to support the adolescent's recovery, and, if necessary, participate in the treatment to facilitate changes in the home environment that will play a role in the adolescent's recovery. If the therapist determines that the current home is not viable for the adolescent's recovery, alternative arrangements need to be found. The therapist can handle this directly or work with another mental health worker who can facilitate a move.

PARENTAL DEPRESSION

In our clinical experience, we find that a significant percentage of depressed adolescents come from families in which one or both parents are either currently or previously depressed. This is a finding that is well supported by clinical and epidemiological research (Downey & Coyne, 1990; Lieb, Isensee, Hofler, Pfister, & Wittchen, 2002; Monck, Graham, Richman, & Dobbs, 1994a, 1994b). When the therapist is working clinically with the adolescent, the psychiatric condition of the adolescent's parents is revealed through the parents' own reports, descriptions provided by the adolescent, and/or reports of other individuals involved in the treatment such as a school professional, social service agencies, and past treatment providers. Parental depression impacts the interpersonal context of the adolescent's depression and the course of treatment. Awareness and understanding of the mental health status of an adolescent's parent is critical to understanding the adolescent's depression and developing the most effective treatment plan. In cases where the parent is depressed, it is often necessary for the adolescent's therapist to help the adolescent by first helping the parent. This must be done in a way that preserves the integrity of the adolescent's treatment and demonstrates respect for the parent and his or her situation. Often it is best for the therapist to meet separately with the parents to educate them about her role as the adolescent's therapist and to lay the groundwork for providing the parent with a referral for his or her own treatment. It is important to explain this plan to the adolescent in the context of the IPT-A framework—that is, focusing on the impact of depression on the parents' as well as the teen's interpersonal functioning. Any alleviation of parental depression is likely to reduce the stress the adolescent is facing.

Not all parents, unfortunately, are open to intervention for themselves or their child, sometimes in part due to the parents' depression and accompanying feeling of hopelessness and/or sense of being overwhelmed by family demands. Parental resistance to the adolescent's treatment may present as a lack of emotional support for the treatment, failure to attend scheduled sessions or return the therapist's phone calls, or overt opposition to the adolescent's attendance at sessions. In these situations, the therapist with adolescent approval should attempt to intervene with the parent during an in-person meeting or over the phone if the parent is unable to attend a session. The therapist should try to join with the parent and understand what their concerns are about psychotherapy. Often the parents experience feelings of guilt that they have difficulty expressing. They feel responsible for the adolescent's difficulties in light of their own depression. At other times, their denial of their own difficulties causes them to be unable to appreciate the significance of their adolescent's problems. The therapist, using an empathic and nonjudgmental approach, as well as psychoeducation, can alter the parents' perspective and enjoin them to support the treatment. It is important that the parents hear directly the valuable role that they can play in helping the adolescent, as opposed to only focusing on the parents' role in creating the adolescent's difficulties. If the parents continue to be resistant to collaborating with the therapist and attending sessions, the therapist will need to work with the adolescent on a modified treatment plan.

Depressed parents often model a depressive interpersonal style that can range from ineffective communication and conflict negotiation skills to social withdrawal and helplessness. Therefore, when these adolescents try to practice new interpersonal skills, they face an uphill battle. The adolescent may effectively use a new skill, but the family's response may be guided by their own depression and consequently send a message to the adolescent that the approach does not work or that change is unlikely. The therapist must be aware of this possibility and help the adolescent to experience success in his attempt to use new skills. The therapist and adolescent will need to do more in-session practice of interpersonal strategies as well as have the adolescent identify others in his life with whom he can practice these skills. Another option is to invite the family into the session so the therapist can facilitate the skills practice for everyone in the session. Enlisting the parent as "coach" and "collaborator" in the treatment can foster the parent's willingness to support the adolescent's experiments with new skills, both during and outside of the session. The adolescent should have a good sense of the obstacles he may encounter when he goes home to practice these skills. By helping him anticipate all possible family responses, as well as his own responses, he is less likely to feel frustrated by the difficulties when they occur. Having a good grasp of the role of parental depression in the family and its impact on him allows the adolescent and therapist to develop realistic treatment goals and focus on the relationships that can have the greatest impact on increasing his feelings of support and decreasing his depressed mood.

THE SUICIDAL PATIENT

Although completed suicide in adolescence is an infrequent event, there has been a threefold increase in the rate of completed suicides among white males between the ages of 15 and 24 years. Overall, the incidence of suicide increases in each of the teenage years, peaking at age 23. Over the past decade, there has been a decrease in suicide rate for the middle-aged and elderly, while suicide becomes more common in the young. Suicide attempts and suicidal ideation are highly prevalent in adolescents, although recently there has been a decline in adolescent suicide rates (Shaffer, 1988; Shaffer & Greenberg, 2002), which has been attributed to the increased rates of antidepressant prescriptions among adolescents (Shaffer & Greenberg, 2002). Evaluation for suicidality is a critical part of the initial evaluation, and suicidality should be monitored throughout the treatment. The adolescent should be asked about thoughts of death, wanting to die, and suicidal plans. Specific questions the therapist might ask include:

> *Do you ever feel so bad that life isn't worth continuing? Do you think about death a lot? Do you think about your own death? Does death sometimes seem like a welcome relief from life? Do you think of killing yourself?*

If the adolescent answers positively to these questions, the therapist should ask if the adolescent has ever made a suicide attempt and if a current plan is being considered. The therapist should be very specific in questioning the adolescent to obtain specific answers about ideas, plans, and attempts. The therapist wants to assess the intention and lethality of past suicide attempts and future plans; for example:

Have you ever tried to kill or hurt yourself? When? What did you do? What happened? Did you receive medical treatment? Did you tell anybody? What did you think would happen?

Questions pertaining to future attempts would include:

What are you thinking of doing to hurt yourself now? How close have you come to doing it? What has stopped you? Would you be able to tell anyone before you hurt yourself?

Based upon the therapist's assessment of past suicide attempts, current suicidal ideation or plans, and the stability of the home and family, the therapist must determine whether the adolescent is an acute suicide risk. If the therapist is uncertain, a second opinion should be sought. Any adolescent who is an acute suicide risk is not a candidate for IPT-A and will in fact require psychiatric hospitalization. An adolescent with suicidal ideation may or may not be a candidate for IPT-A, depending upon the adolescent's capacity to establish and maintain a therapeutic alliance with the therapist. The cornerstone of this alliance is that the adolescent assures the therapist that no suicide plan will be attempted, but that if the suicidal urge becomes so compelling, the therapist will be notified immediately and, if the therapist is not available, the adolescent will go to an emergency room immediately. The task of the therapist is not only to monitor the adolescent's suicidality but also to address the inappropriate use of suicide as a coping mechanism. The therapist might connect the patient's suicidal feelings with feelings of anger, despair, frustration, and hopelessness. The therapist might say to the adolescent:

It sounds as though you think about hurting yourself when you feel hopeless to change your situation. It also sounds like you feel very angry about the way you are treated. In your anger and hopelessness, you are unable to see alternatives to resolve the situation other than by killing yourself. I believe that there are other ways to handle these feelings and that there are better solutions to your problems. Let's try to work on some other solutions together.

THE ASSAULTIVE PATIENT

There are occasions when adolescents are so upset that they know no other way of venting their frustration than through aggressive and violent behavior. Assessment for thoughts of hurting other people should be done in conjunction with the assessment of suicidal behavior. The therapist might ask:

> *Have you ever had thoughts of hurting another person? If so, whom? Have you ever lost control and hit someone? Do you ever feel life could get so bad that you would consider doing so? Do you have a plan for how you would do it? What is your plan?*

As in the assessment of suicide, it is very important for the therapist to ask highly specific questions about the intent and the feasibility of carrying through with the action. Based upon the assessment, the therapist must determine whether the adolescent is at risk of harming another person. If this is deemed to be so, the therapist, according to the law (per the *Tarasoff* decision [*Tarasoff v. The Regents of the University of California*, 1976]), must hospitalize the patient and has a duty to warn the intended victim of the patient's threats (Southard & Gross, 1982). An adolescent who is at serious risk for homicidal behavior is not a candidate for IPT-A. An adolescent who expresses anger and hostility in vague threats to others may be a candidate for IPT-A if a therapeutic alliance with the therapist can be established, if the adolescent has the capacity to control assaultive behavior, and if the adolescent is capable of making an agreement with the therapist that violence will not be enacted while in treatment. The therapist also should educate the adolescent to more appropriate methods of problem solving and ways to diffuse anger. The therapist might say:

> *When you make those threats (e.g., to hurt your father), it sounds as though you are very angry and would like to get him to change his behavior with you. However, violence is not an acceptable solution to most conflicts and feelings of rage and anger. What other ways do you think you could address your anger with [name]? What conflict precipitated the anger? What other ways could you solve the conflict? What could you do when you get angry to help yourself calm down so you could discuss your feelings more rationally (e.g., listen to music, go for a walk, call a friend).*

SCHOOL REFUSAL

As a result of their feelings of fatigue, poor concentration, and anhedonia, some adolescents who are depressed find themselves unable to get themselves to school each day. Moreover, when they find that they have been out of school for a week or two, they then conclude that they are too behind to catch up, are embarrassed to go back to school after their absence, and consequently remain home from school for an extended period of time. It is important that the therapist question the adolescent and parent about school attendance during the initial evaluation.

The therapist should ask:

> *Are you attending school? Do you go every day? How many days have you missed this month? Are you regularly late to school? When you are at school, do you cut classes? How often? What are your grades? Are they the same or better than those you received before you became depressed?*

After obtaining permission of the parent(s) and adolescent, the therapist should contact the school to confirm the adolescent's report. The therapist's role should be to stress the importance of returning to school and enlisting the assistance of the parent(s) or school in ensuring the adolescent's return. The therapist should explain to the adolescent that although reluctance to return to school and embarrassment are common, the embarrassment will dissipate after the first day, and being productive in school will improve the adolescent's mood. In addition, the adolescent should be told that as the depression resolves, his concentration will improve. Throughout the treatment the therapist should continue to check on the adolescent's school attendance and performance and be in contact with the school as necessary.

THE SUBSTANCE-ABUSING ADOLESCENT

Part of a screening and history should include a complete history of drug and alcohol use and abuse. Other family members should be interviewed about drug use as well, even though family members may be ignorant of such abuse. For example, the therapist might ask:

> *Have you ever used or experimented with any drugs or alcohol? Have you ever tried marijuana? Not even once? What about cocaine or crack? Hallucinogens? When did you first try marijuana? How often did you use it? Does it interfere with your school or family life? Have you ever tried to stop using marijuana? What happened? Has using marijuana ever caused you to do things you might not ordinarily do? Give me an example. Have you ever sought treatment because of your marijuana problem? What happened? Do any of your friends use marijuana? What about your family—does anyone use any drugs or alcohol?*

If necessary, the adolescent should be referred for drug treatment before IPT-A is started. In order to participate in IPT-A, the adolescent must not be abusing or using any substances and must make a commitment to try not to use substances during treatment so that he can see how therapy affects his mood separate from the drugs. The therapist might say:

> *For me to work with you and use IPT-A to treat your depression, it is very important that you not use drugs during the time you are in therapy. If you do, the therapy will not be effective. Sometimes adolescents use drugs, hoping they will make them feel better, but usually they feel worse. It will be difficult to see if therapy is helpful if you still use drugs, even just a little bit. Can you stay drug-free during this time? How do you feel about trying to say no to drugs? If you do use drugs, it is important that you tell me so I can help you most effectively. IPT-A may not be the right therapy for you now. Will you be able to tell me if you use drugs?*

With some adolescent patients, the therapist might suggest a weekly drug screen to monitor possible drug abuse. The therapist could suggest this as a way to alleviate any difficulty the patient might have in telling the therapist about drug use, difficulty that could engender guilt about not having revealed this information to the therapist. The therapist should present this therapeutic maneuver as nonpunitive. If the adolescent does use drugs during the time of IPT-A, that is a clear indication that the therapy is not providing the help the patient needs for this problem, and alternative treatments should be suggested. If the therapist feels that the drug abuse is a primary problem and the depression is secondary to the drug abuse, the adolescent should be referred to a drug treatment center.

Within the IPT-A framework, the therapist can help the adolescent deal with peer pressure and family dynamics that may lead to drug use, and engage a family member as another source of support for the adolescent's abstinence from drugs. The therapist might ask:

> *What happens when you see other kids your age doing drugs? How do you feel when you join them? How would you feel if you didn't join them? How does [the substance] make you feel different about yourself? Is it difficult to say no when someone offers it to you? What makes it difficult? What goes on at home when you get the feeling of needing to find some drugs? Does it make the problems go away? What is another way to deal with these problems? Is there anyone you feel close to who doesn't use drugs who you could talk to when you feel an urge to get high or when you feel upset?*

PROTECTIVE SERVICE AGENCIES

Protective service agencies have the purpose of protecting the welfare of children when their environment is harmful. Each state has its own agency for accepting and dealing with reports and its own laws governing when and how to report a case. A child may already be in the jurisdiction of a protective service agency when therapy begins, or it may be the duty of the therapist to report the child to a protective service agency if information about possible harm to the child is raised in the course of treatment. Contacting a protective service agency can disrupt the therapeutic alliance with the child or parent. The therapist must be alert to this possibility and work with the adolescent and parent to help them understand the reasoning behind the actions. Parent and adolescent should be told that the report is being made to alleviate a stressful situation for both of them and to provide help. The therapist should emphasize that the protective service agency is a means to provide them with increased social support so that the family can function better.

SEXUAL ABUSE

The therapist should carefully evaluate the adolescent for any past history of sexual abuse or current abuse. The therapist should ask:

> Has anyone ever made you uncomfortable to be alone with him or her? How so? What happens when you are alone with [him or her]? Has [name] ever touched you in a way that made you uncomfortable? What did [he or she] do? When does or did it happen? How many times? Is it still going on now? When did it stop? Does anyone else know about it?

Frequent symptoms that might indicate a past history of abuse include depression, suicide attempt, sexual promiscuity, and conduct problems. Evaluating for sexual abuse requires sensitivity and time. The adolescent may not reveal the abuse during the initial visit but instead may reveal it during the course of treatment, as the patient begins to trust the therapist. If the abuse is currently ongoing, the therapist is required by law to contact the protective service agency for children to intervene with the family and to provide the appropriate social services to the family and the adolescent. If the abuse is current, the adolescent may not be appropriate for treatment with IPT-A because IPT-A is not designed to deal with the acute or long-term consequences of sexual abuse. In this case, the patient should be referred for treatment that is designed to treat the problems associated with sexual abuse. If the abuse is in the past, the therapist still needs a detailed history of the interpersonal context in which the abuse occurred so that an accurate picture of the familial relationships can be created.

LEARNING DISABILITIES

Depression is commonly associated with cognitive impairments that appear most pronounced during the acute stages of depression. A psychosocial history will help the therapist distinguish between long-standing learning disabilities and impairments secondary to the depressive episode. The therapist should ask:

When did you begin to have trouble in school? How were your grades when you were younger? When did you begin to have trouble concentrating in class and/or doing your homework? Does it seem like it has gotten worse since you have been feeling sad or that it is about the same? What is difficult about doing your schoolwork? Concentrating or not understanding the material? Can you give me an example?

The task of differentiating between learning disability and depression is made more difficult when the patient has long-standing depressive symptoms or a personality style that presents as what appear to be cognitive limitations. Psychological or educational testing can be useful in identifying learning disabilities. When learning disabilities are diagnosed, special educational resources are necessary, and the therapist will need to arrange for this in conjunction with the school system. Cognitive impairments secondary to the depression will resolve when the depressive symptoms resolve. The child and parents should be told of the etiology of the child's impairments and revise their expectations accordingly.

THE SEXUALLY ACTIVE ADOLESCENT

Adolescence is a time in which there is an increase in sexual feelings and behavior and often a first intimate sexual encounter. The therapist should question as to whether the adolescent is sexually active and, if so, whether he or she is using birth control and practicing safe sex. The therapist should explore knowledge of sexual issues such as pregnancy and sexually transmitted diseases. For example, the therapist might ask:

Are you currently in a relationship? Do you have a physical relationship with your partner? Do you practice birth control? What type? Are you aware of how sexual diseases are transmitted? Do you take

precautions to prevent this from happening to you? If so, what kind of
precautions? If not, what prevents you from practicing safe sex?

If the sexually active female adolescent appears to lack such knowledge
and has not been using birth control, it is important to make the appropriate referral to a gynecologist or pediatrician. The therapist may also
discuss the importance of birth control with the adolescent—male or female. The therapist should explore the adolescent's feelings about sex,
sexual fantasies, and fantasies about pregnancy. While it is important for
the therapist to impart factual information about the sexual behavior,
the therapist should also connect sexual feelings and/or behavior to the
adolescent's feelings about his or her relationship with his or her parents,
boyfriend, or girlfriend, and to the adolescent's feelings of loneliness and
self-worth. In this manner, the therapist may be able to assist in identifying interpersonal conflicts or feelings of depression that may be contributing to inappropriate or risky sexual behavior.

THE HOMOSEXUAL ADOLESCENT

Adolescence is a time when individuals begin to form intimate relationships usually with partners of the opposite sex and for some adolescents
with partners of the same sex. Exploration of sexual relationships with
different partners is common. Those adolescents who find their sexual
interest is exclusively with partners of the same sex can feel isolated and
alone. It also is possible that the adolescent is comfortable with and has
accepted his sexual orientation. In such a situation, the therapist must be
supportive of the decision. Those adolescents who feel attracted to both
same-sex and opposite-sex partners may feel confused about their sexual
orientation. The role of the therapist is to help the adolescent explore his
or her sexual feelings and concerns about orientation in a nonjudgmental context. In addition, it may be appropriate to identify the association between the adolescent's state of confusion and the depression.

CHAPTER 17

Crisis Management

Crises are not infrequent during the treatment of a depressed adolescent. The crisis can be a direct result of the adolescent's family or social problem and can pose a direct threat to the adolescent's treatment. Crises should be handled swiftly and decisively to protect the adolescent and the treatment. A crisis is a major change in the patient's living situation, interpersonal relationships, family relationships, or emotional well-being that jeopardizes the patient's psychological health and overwhelms the patient's capacity to cope with the situation. The IPT-A therapist's approach to and management of a crisis will be presented here. Specific crisis situations will be discussed.

ASSESSMENT OF THE CRISIS

The first task facing the IPT-A therapist is to determine the nature and origin of the crisis. This should be accomplished by speaking to the adolescent and other parties involved. The initial contact should be in person but can be over the phone. Frequently, the first word of a crisis is communicated by telephone. The IPT-A therapist needs to elucidate the events surrounding the crisis and assess the adolescent's reaction and the family's response to the crisis. It must first be determined whether the crisis is a response to the therapist or to issues being addressed in the therapy. Did the therapist miss early warning signs that such a crisis was likely, or was the patient or family concealing information that would have allowed the therapist to anticipate and prevent the crisis? Alternatively, the event may have been unpredictable and a response to events not under the control of the therapist, patient, and family.

The next step for the therapist is to bring the patient in for an emergency session as soon as possible. In the case of suicidal or homicidal ideation, if an appointment cannot be set up soon enough, the patient should be sent to the nearest emergency room. When meeting in the emergency session, the therapist must determine the need for and level of family involvement. When dealing with an adolescent under 18 years of age, it is mandatory for the therapist to notify the parent if there is a significant risk to the patient and the crisis is verified. The level of involvement will vary with the different types of crises and the nature of the patient's relationship with the family members. The therapist must be careful to elicit the entire story from the adolescent regarding the precipitant and the accompanying emotions. After hearing the whole story, the therapist must again assess whether there is a need for hospitalization due to risk of the patient getting hurt or hurting others. In addition, the therapist must evaluate whether there is a need to involve other agencies or parties, such as medical or legal consultations or protective services for children in evaluating or intervening in the situation.

If the patient is evaluated as being able to remain in outpatient treatment, the IPT-A treatment contract should be reexamined and revised as necessary. Such items in the contract that may change include the frequency of the sessions, involvement of the family, frequency of phone calls between therapist and patient, and the identified problem area that is the focus of the treatment. At times the crisis may suggest that a significant problem area was overlooked, or there may be an interaction between two problem areas, thus requiring a shift in the focus of the sessions. The therapist also may choose to meet more frequently in the weeks following the crisis, until the patient's situation stabilizes.

Management of the individual crises varies by the situation. The most significant decision the therapist must make is whether to hospitalize the patient and/or whether IPT-A must be terminated and another form of treatment begun. If the decision has been made to involve the family, it is important to meet with the family separately as well as conjointly with the patient to see how the problem is understood and how it can best be resolved. The therapist might conduct several sessions with the family to assist in negotiating the resolution of the precipitating conflict and then resume individual treatment with the patient. If the protective service agency is notified, the therapist should work with the agency to rectify the patient's situation so that no further harm can come to the patient.

In this chapter, management of the following specific issues will be presented: runaways, pregnancy, illness in the patient or family, involvement with the law, violence, and premature termination by the patient. The other issues that can require crisis management, such as suicidal behavior and homicidal behavior, are discussed in the chapter on special issues in working with adolescents.

TYPES OF CRISES

Running Away

It is not uncommon for adolescents who are experiencing a significant amount of conflict in the home to threaten to run away. In such a situation, the therapist must do a careful assessment as to the intent of the adolescent and the anticipated consequences. For example, the therapist might ask:

> *Are you thinking of running away? Where would you think of going? Have you ever run away before? If yes, where to and for how long? What was it like for you and for your family? Now, what are you trying to get away from? What do you think will happen back home if you run away? What do you think running away would be like for you? What do you hope would be different for you?*

The therapist needs to obtain a history of previous attempts to run away in order to better assess the likelihood of the patient actually running away. To assist in finding an alternative action, the therapist and patient together should generate a list of options. These options might include writing a list of people (e.g., friends or relatives) the patient could call when distressed, identifying a friend or relative's house the patient could go for a "cooling-off" time, visiting the emergency room to speak with a mental health professional, calling a hotline for runaways (assuming one is available), going for a walk, writing feelings down, or any one of a number of suggestions to help the adolescent either find alternative care or vent feelings rather than act on them in a potentially destructive manner. In addition, the therapist should examine the likelihood of the event occurring in light of the therapeutic relationship. The therapist should ask the patient to tell the therapist if he is running away, where he is going, and to maintain contact if he does run away. If there is a good therapist–patient alliance, the therapist should try to get a commitment from the adolescent that he will not run away in between sessions. With such a commitment, the therapist can then begin to work on understanding the desire and/or need to run as a maladaptive communication style perhaps within the problem area of interpersonal role disputes. If possible, the therapist should try to help the patient to generate alternative solutions to the problem that would not entail running away. Treatment should assist the patient in acquiring more adaptive communication skills and problem-solving techniques.

Pregnancy

Adolescent pregnancy can be a desired event sought by the adolescent. It may also be one thrust upon her by the absence of adequate birth control measures or by a violent sexual act such as rape. The situation can be further complicated by the family's response to the pregnancy and by the quality of the relationship with the boy. Regardless of the type of situation it is, the first question to address is whether the patient is really pregnant. Upon the first suspicion of pregnancy, the patient should be referred for a gynecological exam and pregnancy test. Once the pregnancy has been confirmed, it is the therapist's role to help the patient evaluate her options: to have and keep the baby, to have the baby and give it up for adoption, to have an abortion, or to involve the other biological parent. Given the patient's feelings, the therapist needs to discuss how the pregnancy or abortion would affect the adolescent's life and to explore the feelings associated with the various actions. The therapist also must discuss with the adolescent the realities of taking care of an infant. The therapist might say to the adolescent:

> *What do you imagine it will be like to have a baby at your age? What would you like about it? What would you not like about it? How would you feel around your friends? How do you feel it will change your relationships with your friends? Your family? How do you feel about the father of the baby? What do you expect from your relationship with him?*

The therapist must also discuss whether or not the patient's parents are aware of the pregnancy and, if so, what their attitudes are toward the patient. It is often helpful if a parent is notified early on in the pregnancy, particularly if the patient chooses to carry to term and may be expecting support from the family. The therapist should help facilitate discussion between parent and patient regarding who will take care of the child, expression of each of their concerns about the situation, and alternative solutions. The patient must be educated as to the impact the infant will have on her life. Ultimately it is the patient's choice whether or not to keep the baby. The therapist's role is to make sure it is an educated decision.

Illness in the Patient or Family

When the patient presents with a medical illness, it is important for the therapist to make sure the appropriate medical care is being received. The therapist needs to consult with the treating physician so treatments can be coordinated if necessary. A similar strategy should be undertaken when coping with an illness in a family member. The therapist should consult with the physician to ensure a complete understanding of the situation so he or she can better help the patient cope with the illness and its implications. The treatment will likely focus on coping with the illness and the feelings it elicits in the patient and any subsequent conflicts that may arise with family members.

Involvement with the Law

An antisocial act necessitating legal intervention committed by the adolescent in IPT-A could jeopardize the treatment. Incarceration obviously puts an immediate end to treatment. If the patient is not incarcerated, the therapist should contact the involved law enforcement agents, frequently a probation officer, in an effort to assess all the facts surrounding the incident. The severity and consequences of the act should be taken into consideration by the therapist, who will need to decide if IPT-A can continue or whether another type of treatment, including residential treatment or hospitalization, would better meet the patient's needs. If it is determined that IPT-A can continue, the therapist will need to address the antisocial act with the adolescent and help the patient understand that further antisocial acts may not only disrupt treatment but also have serious legal consequences as well. The therapist might ask the adolescent:

What were you feeling when this occurred? What led up to its happening? What did you feel when it was over? What were you hoping would result from this behavior? Do you feel it might happen again? What else could you do in such a situation if it happened again? How does this relate to the problems we have been talking about in therapy?

The initially agreed-upon problem area should be reassessed at this time, and the new act should be included in the relevant problem area. Treatment will need to focus on acquiring other more adaptive problem-solving and communication skills in addition to focusing on management of emotions.

Violence

Violent acts against persons or objects by the adolescent can occur without legal involvement. Here, too, the IPT-A therapist must thoroughly assess the event by talking to the adolescent, the family, and any other involved parties (i.e., school officials, siblings). Can the patient continue living in the present household, or is another act of violence likely to occur? The adolescent who has gone out-of-control may need hospitalization or placement in a residential treatment facility. The therapist must assess the patient's intent to commit future violence and whether there is a specific target for the violence. If the patient reports specific intent and target, the therapist is obligated to hospitalize the adolescent. If the adolescent, the family, and the therapist feel the patient can control further violent impulses, IPT-A can continue, but there must be a renegotiation of the treatment contract. The violent act will need to be understood by the adolescent and the therapist in the context of one of the defined problem areas. Connections will need to be made between the patient's depressed and angry feelings and the violent behavior. Specifically, a clear plan of action regarding how to handle another violent incident must be elucidated and agreed upon by the patient, therapist, and family. The plan may include termination of IPT-A treatment, referral for residential treatment, or hospitalization following a second incident, depending upon the severity of the behavior. A primary focus of treatment should be increased communication of feelings in a nonviolent manner and acquisition of better problem-solving skills.

Premature Termination by the Parent

There are times when a patient's family will sabotage the treatment by withdrawing the patient from treatment abruptly and unexpectedly. In such cases, if possible, it is important for the therapist to meet with the patient's family to inquire about their treatment concerns and discuss whether termination is believed to be an appropriate disposition at this time. The therapist might say:

> It appears that you have some concerns about your [son/daughter] continuing in treatment. I feel it might be helpful for your and your [son/daughter] if we could talk about some of these concerns. What are you feeling that is causing you to withdraw your [son/daughter] from treatment? What aspects of the treatment are you unhappy with? What aspects of the treatment are you pleased with? What are your plans for your [son/daughter] following removal from treatment? How can we work together to best help [name]?

The discussion and/or meeting allows the therapist the opportunity to correct any misperceptions about the treatment that might be causing the termination. If the therapist is unable to alter the family's decision to terminate and believes that the patient is not at risk for harm to self or others and that it would not constitute medical neglect, the therapist is obligated to abide by the family's decision. If the therapist feels that termination is contraindicated and is a risk to the patient, the therapist must report the case to a protective service agency to try to ensure that the patient is provided with the appropriate treatment either with herself or another mental health provider.

SUMMARY

Crises may arise with adolescents in brief treatment. The therapist's most important decision is whether or not the adolescent can remain in IPT-A or whether the adolescent must receive other types of services either at the same or another facility. Once the decision has been made for the adolescent to remain in IPT-A, the therapist's first step must be to renegotiate the therapeutic contract in order to better address the crisis-related interpersonal problem. With the new contract, the therapist can move forward to address the new information about the patient's interpersonal relationships and the context of the depression.

CHAPTER 18

The Use of Medication in Conjunction with IPT-A

The use of IPT-A in combination with medication has not been studied in a clinical trial; however, it is frequently used this way in our general outpatient pediatric psychiatry clinics with benefits to the adolescent. Most of the clinical trials have included a homogenous sample of adolescents who typically have a depression disorder with a possible anxiety disorder, excluding adolescents with other disorders. In the clinics, the adolescents may present with depression and other comorbid disorders that may require a combination of medication and IPT-A. The most recent study of IPT-A delivered in school-based health clinics attempted to recruit a more heterogeneous sample of depressed adolescents and included adolescents with other comorbidities such as attention-deficit/hyperactivity disorder (ADHD) and substance use (Mufson et al., 2004a). Consequently, we are beginning to gain knowledge about treating adolescent depression in the context of its comorbid disorders. This chapter explores the use of IPT-A in combination with medication for the treatment of depression and for addressing the comorbid disorders of depression.

THE USE OF ANTIDEPRESSANTS IN CONJUNCTION WITH IPT-A

Antidepressant medication is not contraindicated during IPT-A and, in fact, may be a useful adjunct treatment for severely depressed adolescents whose symptoms do not remit during the initial phase of treatment. There is good evidence for the efficacy of selective serotonin reuptake inhibitors (e.g., fluoxetine) for the treatment of adolescent depression (Birmaher & Brent, 2002; Emslie et al., 1997, 2002), and that assessment is included in the Academy of Child and Adolescent Psychiatry's (1998) Practice Parameters for the treatment of adolescent depression. This chapter reviews the guidelines used to decide if antidepressant medication is indicated. The types of antidepressant medication currently in use for depressed adolescents and their administration are recounted. This section is written for the adolescent clinician who may or may not be familiar with the clinical use of antidepressant medication. Readers are referred to Martin, Kaufman, and Charney (2000) and Columbia University College of Physicians and Surgeons' Treatment Guidelines for Adolescent Depression (Shaffer & Finkelson, 2002) for a more in-depth discussion on the use of antidepressants in adolescent depression.

THE DECISION TO TREAT WITH ANTIDEPRESSANT MEDICATION

The main goal of any acute phase of treatment, medication, or psychotherapy is to achieve a timely treatment response, measured by remission of the depressive symptoms. Therefore, if your patient is not responding as well as you would like to your initial psychotherapeutic treatment of choice, it is advisable to consider adding an adjunctive treatment. Our guidelines are to consider antidepressants if there is little or no remission of symptoms after 4 weeks of IPT-A.

Early open clinical trials using tricyclic antidepressants (TCAs) for the treatment of adolescent depression were encouraging. However, later and more well designed randomized control clinical trials were unable to demonstrate the efficacy of TCAs as compared to a placebo (Birmaher & Brent, 2002). The development of the newer generation of antidepressants, selective serotonin reuptake inhibitors (SSRIs), were a vast improvement compared to the TCAs because of their lower side effect profile and low lethality when taken in an overdose. Their availability has resulted in an overall increase in the use of medications for the treatment of depression (Olfson, Marcus, Weissman, & Jensen, 2002), and their use has been suggested as a factor in the reduced rate of completed suicides in this age group (Shaffer, 1988). Evidence from several randomized controlled clinical trials has demonstrated the efficacy of the SSRIs as compared to placebo for treating adolescent depression (Emslie et al., 1997, 2002; Keller et al., 2001; Mandoki, Tapia, Tapia, & Sumner,

1997; Simeon, Dinicola, Ferguson, & Copping, 1990). While there is evidence for the efficacy of paroxetine for treating depressed adolescents (Keller et al., 2001), there are recent concerns about an association between paroxetine and an increase in the number of suicide events in these adolescents. Consequently, there is a ban on using paroxetine and other SSRIs, except fluoxetine, for depressed adolescents in the United Kingdom, and the Food and Drug Administration in the United States is urging caution by suggesting that physicians refrain from prescribing SSRIs other than fluoxetine for depressed adolescents until medical authorities conclude their investigations of this association.

To date there have been no published studies comparing psychotherapy to medication or comparing medication, psychotherapy, and combined treatment, as has been done in adults. The multisite Treatment of Adolescent Depression Study (TADS) is currently under way and will provide important information about the use of cognitive-behavioral therapy with and without medication. The adult data support the clinical use of combined medication and psychotherapy treatment (American Psychiatric Association, 2000b; Keller et al., 2000). Patients who are suicidal and/or severely impaired may require hospitalization; however, with the availability of the SSRIs, suicidality is no longer a mandate for hospitalization. Adolescents who have depressive symptoms meeting DSM-IV criteria for major depression should be considered for a trial of medication and/or psychotherapy. Based upon our outpatient clinical experience, we find that a substantial percentage of adolescents who initially present for treatment with signs and symptoms of major depression improve during the course of several weeks with nonspecific psychotherapeutic intervention alone. Therefore, most adolescents who can be treated on an outpatient basis are monitored closely for several weeks before starting antidepressant medication.

Adolescents who are receiving IPT-A are monitored clinically by the treating therapist and through self-report scales (e.g., the Beck Depression Inventory [BDI]) and clinician-rated scales (e.g., the Hamilton Rating Scale for Depression [HRSD]) on a regular basis. This information is systematically reviewed every 4 weeks and sooner if the treating clinician thinks it is necessary to do so. If after 4–6 weeks of IPT-A treatment, the adolescent is still significantly depressed based on clinical impression and substantiated by a HRSD 25 (scores range from 0 to 40 on the 24-item HRSD), and if the adolescent remains significantly impaired in the areas of school and relationships, antidepressant medication is recommended as an adjunctive treatment to IPT-A. More recent experience treating adolescents experiencing more chronic depression (either dysthymia or chronic major depression) suggests that medication might be beneficial from the outset of treatment to help alleviate the hopelessness and listlessness that often characterize these adolescents and thereby enable them to more actively engage in psychotherapy. The clinician should discuss with the adolescent and his parents the reasons for considering medication. They should be told that the adolescent is still showing significant signs of depression or signs of significant anhedonia and lethargy, and that in such instances medication can often be beneficial. If the primary clinician is not a child psychiatrist, a referral should be made to a child psychiatrist.

INTEGRATING PHARMACOLOGICAL TREATMENT WITH IPT-A

It is important for the pharmacological therapy and the IPT-A to be coordinated. Currently, it is common practice for child and adolescent psychiatrists to provide the psychopharmacological treatment and refer to a non-MD clinician for the psychosocial treatment. If the adolescent is receiving IPT-A from a non-MD clinician, communication between the therapist and psychiatrist is a requirement for optimal patient compliance and care. The therapist will be conducting the therapy in which the adolescent discusses feelings, thoughts, and solutions to problems. The psychiatrist prescribes medication and monitors efficacy and side effects. All problems with the medication should be reported to the psychiatrist. Similarly, the psychiatrist should inform the therapist of any psychological or social issues the adolescent has revealed. The adolescent should be told that the therapist and psychiatrist will be communicating with each other regularly. The adolescent and parent should be informed what role each therapist plays in the treatment.

Appointments should be made so as to enhance the adolescent's participation in the treatment and maximize his or her return to a full and active life. Appointments should be coordinated between the treating clinicians so that the adolescent is not faced with the same appointment time for each clinician. Appointments scheduled for the same day in succession may be best for this purpose, except in instances where a clinical decision is made to provide multiple visits in a given week. This is done when an adolescent is severely depressed and minimally functioning in school.

The child psychiatrist should inform the clinician about the medication before the clinician's next appointment with the adolescent. The treating clinician should know the dose the adolescent is prescribed, any reported side effects, and the expected timetable for improvement. In turn, the treating clinician should inform the psychiatrist about any information relevant to the adolescent's mental status or the adolescent's taking of medication. Such information should include changes in mood or suicidal ideation, side effects, missing doses or not taking the medication, and stressful life events. Weekly phone contact between the psychiatrist and clinician is usually adequate for communication.

PHARMACOTHERAPY

Pharmacological Agents

The major classes of medications used for the treatment of adolescent depression include selective serotonin reuptake inhibitors (SSRIs), mixed agents, antianxiety agents, and neuroleptics. Psychosis precludes treatment with IPT-A and requires treatment with antipsychotic agents. Antianxiety agents include buspirone (Buspar), lorazepam (Ativan), clonazepam (Klonopin), and alprazolam (Xanax), and may be used in conjunction with antidepressants in the early stages of pharmacological treatment. Indications include nervousness, agitation, anxiety, severe insomnia, and concurrent panic attacks. The SSRIs include paroxetine (Paxil), fluoxetine (Prozac), fluvoxamine (Luvox), sertraline (Zoloft), citalopram (Celexa), and escitalopram (Lexapro). Venlafaxine (Effexor) is a serotonin and norepinephrine reuptake inhibitor. Bupropion (Wellbutrin) is a noradrenergic and dopaminergic reuptake inhibitor. Nefazodone (Serzone) has a mixed serotonin effect. The SSRIs are reviewed in this chapter. The reader is referred elsewhere for a comprehensive treatise on the use of SSRIs and antianxiety and neuroleptic agents (Birmaher & Brent, 2002).

Administration of Antidepressant Medications

If the adolescent has received a medical exam by a pediatrician within the past 3 months, medical clearance can be obtained from the pediatrician prior to starting medication. If there has been no physical exam, then it is at the child psychiatrist's discretion to determine whether routine labs can be performed with the results sent to the psychiatrist or whether the adolescent should be evaluated by a pediatrician.

When the adolescent is medically cleared for a trial of antidepressant medication, the psychiatrist will meet with the adolescent and parents to review the expected benefits, possible side effects, and the proposed course of treatment. Prescriptions are given to the parents or another responsible adult who will be instructed on appropriate administration of the medication. The adolescent patient is not made responsible for his or her medication, but rather the filling of prescriptions and supervision of daily dosing is under the direction of the parent. Depression is associated with significant morbidity and mortality. Even though the current medications are not fatal in overdose attempts, precautions need to be taken to prevent such an occurrence. Therefore, all medications are to be kept in a locked cabinet out of reach of the depressed adolescent and other children in the household.

Side Effects and Complications of Antidepressant Medication

SSRIs and mixed agents have fewer side effects than the older TCAs. However, side effects can occur. The most common include headaches, gastrointestinal disturbance including decreased appetite, central nervous system effects including agitation and disinhibition, sexual dysfunction effects including impotence or anorgasmia. Activation can occur with SSRIs and must be distinguished from the onset of a hypomanic or manic episode because the treatment is significantly different. Activation is treated with a reduction of dose or discontinuation of medication, whereas hypomania will require the use of a mood stabilizer. Many side effects will subside or disappear within a few days to a week, and lower dose or discontinuation of the drug will cause them to remit completely. Serotonin syndrome, although uncommon, is also associated with the use of SSRIs and is characterized by fever, confusion, rapid heart rate, and muscular rigidity (Zajecka, Tracy, & Mitchell, 1997). It requires immediate medical attention and active intervention. Medications can take up to 4–6 weeks before an adequate response is achieved, but the side effects occur early on in the treatment. Sudden discontinuation of the SSRIs can result in discontinuation syndrome (Zajecka et al., 1997). Symptoms include dizziness, anxiety, diarrhea, fatigue, headache, insomnia, irritability, nausea, tremor, and visual disturbance (Black, Shea, Dursun, & Kutcher, 2000). Symptoms will resolve in 1 day to 3 weeks without treatment and will rapidly disappear with a small dose of the discontinued agent. Therefore, if a decision is made to discontinue medication, the medication should be tapered off slowly over a period of at least 2 weeks. This also allows for the psychiatrist and clinician to monitor carefully the resumption of depressive symptoms that would indicate that a longer course of treatment is necessary.

Pharmacological treatment of adolescent depression can become complex if the first agent chosen is not effective. In such instances a change in medication or the use of an adjunctive medication may be necessary. The American Academy of Child and Adolescent Psychiatry (1998) has published guidelines for the use of antidepressants and presents a decision tree for the psychiatrist to follow based on length of treatment and response. Most of the clinical trials examining the use of medication in depressed adolescents have focused on acute treatment;

therefore, the recommendations for continuation and maintenance phar-macotherapy are based largely on clinical experience. Current recom-mendations are that all patients should be offered continuation treat-ment for at least 6 months after complete symptom remission. Those adolescents who had a slower time to remission (i.e., greater than 3 months) or have factors that place them at risk for recurrent or persis-tent depression such as comorbid disorders, early-onset depression, or family history of recurrent depression or family discord should be con-tinued on medication for at least 1 year or longer to prevent relapse of symptoms (American Academy of Child and Adolescent Psychiatry, 1998; Birmaher & Brent, 2002). Typically, the antidepressants are con-tinued at the same dose at which the adolescent attained remission of the acute symptoms based upon the adult studies, as long as there are not significant side effects (American Psychiatric Association, 2000b). Simi-larly, as in the acute treatment, discontinuation from the continuation therapy should occur gradually to avoid withdrawal effects.

A major concern in the administration of antidepressant medica-tions is an overdose. There are no reports of lethal overdoses with any of the SSRIs. Nonetheless, the possibility of an overdose occurring should be minimized by careful and continuous assessment of the patient's suicidality, a strong therapeutic alliance in which the adolescent assures the therapist that no suicidal action will be performed without seeking help first, and by following the guidelines listed in the preceding section on storage and administration of medication. Overdoses require imme-diate medical care. Treatment is administered in an emergency room.

Treatment of Comorbid Disorders

While clinical trials assessing efficacy of treatments have typically in-cluded a homogeneous sample of depressed adolescents with few comor-bidities, research has found that for children and adolescents with a di-agnosis of major depression, it is estimated that 40–70% are comorbid for a second psychiatric disorder and another 20% report the presence of a third psychiatric disorder along with their depression (Birmaher, Ryan, Williamson, Brent, & Kaufman, 1996a). These comorbid disor-ders can affect the course of the depression. The question then is how does a clinician decide which disorder to treat first. The guideline fol-lowed by most clinicians is to identify the primary disorder to target by assessing which disorder is currently causing the most distress and im-pairment. This is not always an easy distinction to make; however, it is easier and better than targeting the primary disorder as the one which started first. It is very difficult for adolescents to tease apart which symp-toms began first, but they usually are able to say which symptoms are causing them the most distress at the time they are presenting for treatment. Regardless, it is necessary to treat the comorbid disorders that frequently co-occur with depression.

Most of the adolescent depression clinical trials of psychotherapy (Brent et al., 1997; Mufson et al., 1999; Rosselló & Bernal, 1999) excluded adolescents with comorbid disorders other than anxiety. Mufson et al. (1999) demonstrated that when the adolescents recovered from depression in treatment with IPT-A, their comorbid anxiety disorder typically remitted as well. Similarly, the same medications found to be effective for depression are also found to be effective for anxiety (Research Units of Pediatric Psychopharmacology Anxiety Group, 2001) so that the use of SSRIs can simultaneously target both disorders. A more recent study of IPT-A included adolescents with other comorbidities such as ADHD, substance use, and disruptive disorders (Mufson et al., 2004a). The number of adolescents with each disorder is too small to do analyses by diagnostic subgroups.

There are medication studies that address the treatment of depression and its comorbid disorders. Depressed adolescents with ADHD are found to respond less well to SSRI treatment (Birmaher & Brent, 2002). It is generally recommended when treating an adolescent with comorbid depression and ADHD to treat the ADHD first with medication and then treat the depression with an SSRI if the symptoms are still present, though this approach is not empirically validated. This approach is most helpful because (1) an adolescent with ADHD is going to have a difficult time focusing in the session if untreated and (2) the school difficulties that result from untreated ADHD are significant and could be contributing to feelings of hopelessness and conflicts with peers and teachers in school and with parents at home, which in turn could be exacerbating the depression. If appropriately medicated, the adolescent will be better able to utilize IPT-A to address the depression symptoms and interpersonal issues that remain.

IPT-A is not the treatment of choice for adolescents with substance-abuse disorders. The situation is less clear about what to do with those adolescents who are occasional users of substances such as marijuana and alcohol. As stated in Chapter 16, it is important to make a contract with the adolescents to refrain from substance use while in IPT-A and to explain the possible role of these substances in self-medicating their depressive symptoms. In our clinical experience, we find that the less frequent users are typically able to stop their substance use during the course of treatment, especially if their peer group is not made up solely of substance users. The success is greatest when the therapist can continually link the adolescent's usage of substances to depressive feelings and demonstrate how it does not actually improve those feelings but in fact can exacerbate them. Teaching interpersonal skills to enhance competence in the identified problem area can contribute to the adolescent's decreased need for substance use.

Disruptive behavior disorders such as oppositional defiant disorder and conduct disorder also are common comorbid disorders. Oppositional defiant disorder symptoms often seem quite connected to the irritability and conflict associated with the depression and often can be targeted in treatment at the same time. Conduct disorder is more complicated in that it is frequently associated with poor compliance with treatment and involvement with other agencies. Conduct disorder can both precede the depression as well as be a complication of a preexisting depressive disorder and can persist even when the adolescent's mood has improved (Kovacs, 1996). Much more data is needed on how IPT-A and other psychosocial and pharmacological treatments address the difficulties of treating depression in light of varying comorbidities. There are studies showing that these comorbid conditions, along with others such as eating disorders and posttraumatic stress disorder, do affect the course of treatment for depression (Birmaher et al., 1996a, 1996b; Hughes et al., 1999). Therefore, the comorbid disorders must be assessed and addressed in order to successfully treat the depression. There is a paucity of research addressing the issue of treating depression and the comorbid disorders, and much more research is needed to provide adequate guidelines for clinicians.

CONCLUSION

The guidelines for the use of IPT-A in conjunction with medication evolved from our clinical experience in using IPT-A to treat depressed adolescents in both university hospital-based and community settings. The use of IPT-A in combination with medication holds promise for addressing the challenges that arise in treating chronic adolescent depression as well as partial treatment responders, and the comorbid conditions. Combined psychotherapy and pharmacotherapy may also be beneficial in preventing recurrence and treating depressed adolescents efficiently and cost-effectively. More research is needed to address these conditions, and we look forward to studying the effectiveness of IPT-A and medication for addressing these treatment issues.

CHAPTER 19

Current and Future Research in IPT-A

The past decade since the publication of the first edition of this book has been a period of active research in the efficacy and effectiveness of IPT-A. There has been increasing recognition of its promise as a treatment intervention for adolescent depression and increasing demand for training in IPT-A all over the world. It is being included in several clinical psychology and psychiatry residency-training programs, and the research base continues to expand. This chapter provides an overview of the past decade of IPT-A research and a look at where we are heading in the future.

EFFICACY RESEARCH

The first author initially conducted both an open clinical trial and a controlled clinical trial of IPT-A. The open trial provided preliminary support for the use of IPT-A. The purpose of the open trial was to gain experience in IPT-A and to determine if the treatment was feasible and acceptable to the adolescent population. The sample consisted of 14 12- to 18-year-olds who were referred to a hospital outpatient clinic due to depressive symptoms or who responded to an advertisement for the treatment of adolescent depression. The results of this study indicated a significant decrease in adolescents' depressive symptomatology and in symptoms of psychological and physical distress. Adolescents also demonstrated significant improvement in their general functioning at home and at school. Finally, none of the adolescents qualified for a DSM-III-R (American Psychiatric Association, 1987) depression diagnosis at the end of treatment (Mufson et al., 1994).

Although these results were promising, their significance was difficult to determine in the absence of randomization and a comparison group. In addition, since the only therapist was the developer of the adaptation, treatment effects could be attributed to the specific therapist's skill rather than the treatment techniques themselves. To test that premise, the author needed to train other therapists and assess treatment efficacy as delivered by other trained therapists.

The next study was a randomized controlled clinical trial comparing IPT-A to clinical monitoring in a sample of clinic-referred depressed adolescents (Mufson et al., 1999). Adolescents were identified using a clinician-rated scale, the Hamilton Rating Scale for Depression (HRSD), and a self-report measure, the Beck Depression Inventory (BDI), as well as two clinical interviews, the Schedule for Affective Disorders and Schizophrenia for School Aged Children (K-SADS; Chambers et al., 1985) and the Diagnostic Interview Schedule for Children Version 2.3 (DISC 2.3; Shaffer, Fisher, Dulcan, & Davies, 1996a). Adolescents with a diagnosis of major depressive disorder who were not currently suicidal or psychotic and were not diagnosed with a chronic medical illness, bipolar I or II, conduct disorder, substance abuse disorder, eating disorder, or obsessive–compulsive disorder were included in the study. Of the 57 adolescents who were determined to be eligible for the study, 48 agreed to be randomized.

Adolescents were randomized to IPT-A or clinical monitoring. Clinical monitoring was originally designed to be the closest approximation to a waitlist condition and was to be considered an "ethical waitlist." Patients were assigned a therapist, had one session a month but could call if they needed another session. If they needed more than one session, it would be seen as a failure to be maintained in the condition, and they would be removed from the study and referred for more treatment. Although funded in this form, the Institutional Review Board (IRB) review required significant modifications to the condition. Adolescents in the clinical monitoring condition would receive once-monthly 30-minute sessions with a therapist with the option for a second session each month. They were also seen bimonthly by the independent evaluator. During the 1 week of the month without a face-to-face meeting, the therapists needed to have a phone contact with the adolescent to assess clinical status and safety. Thus, the adolescents in the clinical monitoring condition received a therapeutic check-in at least 3 out of 4 weeks of the month. Treatment in both conditions was provided for 12 weeks.

Therapists received training in IPT-A consistent with the training program in the National Collaborative Study for the Treatment of Depression (Elkin et al., 1989). Adolescents in IPT-A had weekly 45-minute therapy sessions with additional parent sessions during the initial and termination phase and when needed in the middle phase of treatment. Adolescents enrolled in the study, in either treatment condition, were assessed at weeks 0, 2, 4, 6, 8, 10, and 12. The outcomes assessed included diagnosis and symptoms levels (HRSD, BDI, Clinical Global Impression Form [CGI]) as well as global and social functioning (Children's Global Assessment Scale and Social Adjustment Scale—Self-Report Version, respectively), parent–child relationship (Parental Bonding Instrument), life events, and social problem-solving skills (Social Problem-Solving Inventory—Revised).

The results of this controlled trial were promising with respect to the efficacy of IPT-A in comparison to clinical monitoring. Treatment outcome was assessed in several ways. First, with respect to rates of treatment completion, significantly more IPT-A patients (88%) completed treatment than did the control patients (46%). Given the rates of noncompletion, particularly in the control group, all subsequent analyses were conducted using both a completer sample ($N = 32$ adolescents) and an intent-to-treat sample ($N = 48$ adolescents). In addition, all analyses were conducted on outcome measures at termination while controlling for the baseline assessment of the measures.

For both the completer and the intent-to-treat samples, IPT-A patients reported significantly fewer depressive symptoms. Using standards for recovery set forth by the National Collaborative Study for the Treatment of Depression (Elkin et al., 1989), significantly more IPT-A patients than control patients met the recovery criteria for major depression. The results of this study revealed that treatment with IPT-A also resulted in improved overall social functioning as compared to treatment in the control condition, as well as improved functioning in the domains of peer and dating relationships. While treatment for many teens focused on family issues, there was a nonsignificant trend toward improvement with IPT-A. This may be due to the likelihood of greater difficulty or longer period of time needed to effect changes in the more entrenched relationship patterns with family. The lack of improvement in family relations also may be due to the perceived high rates of depression in the parents of these teens that may have hampered the parents' ability to alter their behavior and communications in response to the adolescents' efforts to change their interactions.

Finally, although these results were somewhat tentative due to some missing data, IPT-A patients demonstrated better skills than control patients in certain areas of social problem-solving skills, including positive problem-solving orientation and rational problem solving. With respect to the latter, IPT-A patients exhibited better performance in the generation of alternatives and solution implementation and verification. Although further research with different comparison groups and across different adolescent populations is needed, the results of this randomized controlled trial suggest that IPT-A is an efficacious treatment for adolescent depression.

A second research group also has been conducting efficacy studies of IPT for depressed Puerto Rican adolescents, using a different modification of the adult manual tailored to the Puerto Rican culture. Rosselló and Bernal (1999) conducted a study of IPT versus cognitive-behavioral therapy (CBT) versus waitlist condition for depressed teens. They found that IPT and CBT resulted in a greater reduction in depressive symptoms than the waitlist condition. Also, IPT was significantly better than the waitlist condition at increasing self-esteem and improving social adaptation. This study provided additional support for the efficacy of the interpersonal approach to depression in adolescents.

EFFECTIVENESS STUDY

We recently have completed an effectiveness study of IPT-A in comparison to treatment as it is usually delivered in school-based health clinics in urban New York City schools. This investigation is guided by a public health model of clinical intervention and intervention research (Lebowitz, 2000). Studies conducted according to a public health model occur in actual-practice settings and face all the realities and complexities of those settings and the people served by them. Such research aims to address some of the potential limitations of more traditional efficacy trials, including a lack of generalizability and practicality. Using a public health model seems particularly important for evaluating treatments to be provided to more impoverished communities and to adolescents in general, as both of these populations are highly likely to receive services outside of hospitals or research clinics.

The school setting was chosen for this study because school-based health clinics have emerged as an important treatment setting for adolescents with mental health problems (Leaf et al., 1996). They provide an alternative and uniquely available community-based setting for providing care to adolescents, particularly in the current health care climate in which services can be difficult to access and are increasingly costly.

Through this study, we hoped to gain further support for the effectiveness, generalizability, feasibility, and cost-effectiveness of IPT-A.

This project was significant in that it was one of the first attempts to implement and assess the efficacy of an evidence-based psychotherapy for the treatment of adolescent depression in a community setting. Even more unique, the therapists trained to deliver IPT-A in this study were those clinicians already employed in the school-based clinics, including social workers and psychologists who were not necessarily experts in the treatment of adolescent depression or in IPT-A. The results demonstrate the efficacy of IPT-A as compared to treatment as usual (TAU) for adolescent depression in reducing depression symptoms and improving global and overall social functioning (Mufson et al., 2004a). The study suggests that IPT-A is a viable and effective treatment model for school-based health clinics. It can be learned and successfully conducted by social workers and psychologists working in the clinics with a feasible amount of ongoing supervision by an expert clinician. Further work is needed to assess the extent to which the results can be generalized to other school-based health clinics and community settings serving other socioeconomic and ethnic populations.

GROUP PSYCHOTHERAPY

Group therapy is often believed to be an effective treatment modality for adolescents. Group therapy puts the adolescent in contact with peers who have similar difficulties, who can provide support for each other, and who can provide each other with opportunities to practice new skills. Specific goals can include (1) enabling group members to perceive the similarity of their needs, (2) generating alternative solutions to particular conflicts, (3) learning more effective social skills, and (4) increasing awareness of others' needs and feelings (Corey, 1981). These goals are consistent with the goals of interpersonal psychotherapy.

There are several studies already demonstrating the efficacy of CBT as a group treatment for depressed adolescents. After a decade of treating depressed teens, we were continually impressed by the challenges the depressed teens faced in practicing new communication strategies and problem-solving techniques outside of the therapy session. One way to overcome this stumbling block was to conduct group treatment that would allow for more varied practice opportunities within the group setting. A group setting allows patients to try new skills or strategies immediately and to obtain feedback from others regarding interpersonal experiments. Group members can role-play different communication skills and obtain validation of their experiences or advice on what to do differently.

Another important factor for adapting IPT-A for group is the cost-effectiveness of treating adolescents in a group and its potential for use in other settings such as school-based health clinics and community clinics. School-based health clinics and mental health clinics in general are understaffed for the patients' needs. Group therapy is one way of meeting the needs of more patients without additional personnel. Consequently, if group IPT-A treatment (IPT-AG) proves to be efficacious and acceptable to depressed adolescents, it will provide an important treatment option to overburdened staff and clinics, particularly in underserved settings.

IPT originally was adapted for group treatment by Wilfley, MacKenzie, Welch, Ayres, and Weissman (2000). Specifically, the adaptation was for the group treatment of adult binge eaters. Group IPT-A is an adaptation using both the original IPT-A Manual (Mufson et al., 1993) and the Adult Group Interpersonal Psychotherapy Manual (Wilfley et al., 2000). IPT-AG has the same primary goals as the individual treatment, with two additional goals: (1) to increase the adolescents' experience with positive social interaction and reduce social isolation, and (2) to increase the positive resolution of interpersonal difficulties in a supportive group setting. The structure of the group consists of two pregroup individual sessions with the parent(s) and the adolescent followed by 12 90-minute group therapy sessions. The work of the initial phase is conducted in the individual format to enable the therapist to obtain sufficient information about the adolescent's depression syndrome and significant relationships.

Middle phase and termination work largely takes place in the group setting. Treatment also includes one additional session midway through the group with the adolescent and parent and similarly an additional session following completion of the group as well to address future treatment needs. As in the individual treatment, the therapists emphasize the development of competence and independence rather than fostering a more dependent relationship on the therapists. Group exercises are designed to have the adolescents help coach each other to use better communication and problem-solving skills. In addition, they report to each other on "work at home" and learn from each other's mistakes and successes. The same problem areas are addressed, although there is less direct work with each adolescent's problem area and more facilitated learning through discussion of other group members' difficulties (Mufson et al., 2004b).

We have conducted five pilot groups of IPT-AG with groups of depressed Latina and African American adolescents seeking treatment at a university hospital. Adolescents are included with the diagnosis of adjustment disorder with depressed mood, major depression, dysthymic disorder, and depression not otherwise specified. Each group has a maximum of eight and a minimum of four adolescents. It appears that—based on adolescent reports, our initial clinical impressions, and limited data—adolescents find IPT-AG interesting and helpful. Also, adolescents reported improvement in depressive symptomatology.

A preliminary randomized clinical trial comparing the group adaptation of IPT-A (IPT-AG) and IPT-A for treating depression in adolescents has recently been completed. While the data has yet to be analyzed, it was apparent during the trial that the adolescents found the treatment acceptable. More work is needed to determine the efficacy of IPT-AG, but it holds the potential for being an important cost-effective treatment option for overburdened staff and clinics. If the treatment is efficacious, we hope to conduct a more extensive clinical trial.

FUTURE WORK

Based upon the promise of IPT-A suggested by the clinical trials that have been cited, the IPT-A research program is expanding. Dr. Jami Young and Dr. Laura Mufson are beginning to examine the potential of IPT-A as a preventive intervention in early adolescents presenting with subsyndromal symptoms of depression. A preventive group IPT-A intervention (IPT-AST) has been developed, and a preliminary study of its acceptability and efficacy will be under way shortly. Dr. Lisa Miller at Columbia University has adapted the group IPT-A manual for use with depressed pregnant adolescents, and Dr. Dan Pilowsky is in the process of developing IPT for the treatment of prepubertal youths.

THERAPIST TRAINING

Research systematically evaluating the efficacy of manual-guided training or the essential components of a good training program has yet to be performed for any type of psychotherapy (Rounsaville, Chevron, Weissman, Prusoff, & Frank, 1988). The type of training program components necessary to train particular types of clinicians in specific settings is largely unknown; however, different programs have been developed for delivery in varied settings. The treatment manual provides the foundation for all the models of training, and the level of specificity and flexibility in the manual influence the training models used in various settings. The goal is to develop a shared language and a specified procedure in an agreed-upon sequence among the therapists participating in the trial (see Appendix C). We will continue to conduct research on implementing and disseminating IPT-A to a myriad of settings such as school-based health clinics and primary care settings as well as develop new training programs to address these issues.

CONCLUSION

Long-term follow-up studies are needed to establish the long-term impact of IPT-A, particularly given the documented patterns of recurrence and persistence of depression in adolescents. An important area of clinical application is the use of IPT-A as a continuation and/or maintenance treatment following treatment for the acute episode of depression. There is increased demand for continuation and maintenance treatments that can be used in conjunction with the acute, brief treatment models. Finally, it will be important to eventually test the efficacy of IPT-A combined with medication for the treatment of adolescent depression.

Our research program over the past decade has provided support for the efficacy of IPT-A in both clinic and community settings. IPT-A adaptations hold promise for addressing treatment problems that accompany adolescent depression such as partial treatment response, comorbidity, the need to prevent recurrence, and the need to treat efficiently and cost-effectively. We look forward to studying the effectiveness of IPT-A and its new adaptations and to facilitating the effective use of IPT-A both in research settings and general clinical practice.

CHAPTER 20

A Comprehensive Description of an IPT-A Case

CASE OVERVIEW

JT is a 16-year-old boy and is in the 11th grade at a public high school. He reluctantly came for an evaluation with his parents after 5 months of a deteriorating relationship with them. JT's chief complaint was intractable conflict with his parents, particularly his father. Although initially he denied depressive symptoms, eventually he acknowledged experiencing sad and irritable mood, poor concentration, initial insomnia, fatigue, and feelings of hopelessness. He denied feeling suicidal, but he admitted that he sometimes wished that he were dead. He added that he often wondered how his parents would respond if one day he was gone.

JT transferred to his current school in the 10th grade (about 1½ years ago) because he and his family moved to a new apartment in another part of the city. He reported that he always experienced conflict with his parents, especially his father, but that the conflict increased when he changed schools and escalated further during the past several months. He reported the onset of some symptoms at approximately 2 years ago but experienced a significant increase in symptoms over the course of the past several months. He associated the increase in his symptoms with mounting pressure from his parents regarding his academic performance as they began to discuss post-high school education options. JT reported being angry with his parents because they wouldn't let him spend more time with his friends, and they were "constantly complaining" about the friends he had chosen. He insisted that he actually spent very little time with his friends due to his parent's restrictiveness and that he had begun to skip school occasionally in order to spend more time with them. He admitted that some of his new friends were different from his friends in his previous school but denied that they were a bad influence. Another source of family tension for JT was that his father, the superintendent of an apartment building, insisted that JT work for him all weekend and several nights a week, whenever he was not doing homework.

JT believed that his depression was related to his relationship with his parents, particularly his father. He had a slightly better relationship with his mother, but he felt that she was "a puppet" to his father and doubted she would ever stand up for him regardless of her own beliefs. When asked about his goal for treatment, he had difficulty identifying something specific but eventually stated that he wished he could have a better relationship with his parents and that they would trust him more to do the right thing and give him space to be a teenager. He stated emphatically that he did not think his parents and their behavior would ever change.

JT's parents reported that he wanted to spend all of his time with friends; he wasn't fulfilling his responsibilities or following rules at home, especially curfew, and he was often truant from school. Reportedly his overall grade-point average had dropped from a B+ to a C+ during the past semester. JT's father claimed that "he has always been a difficult kid" but he had become more so over the course of the past several months. They reported that when JT was at home he often chose to spend his time alone in his room and rarely spent time with them or his two younger brothers (ages 13 and 10). Their goal for treatment was for JT to accept his responsibilities and "behave like a member of the family." JT's mother added that she wanted her son to feel better and "feel good about himself." In such cases where the parents' and adolescents' goals don't obviously match, the therapist should try to find the common ground between the goals. In this instance, the therapist could relate JT's wish to have a better relationship with his parents to being more of a member of the family. His desire for more trust could also play a role in his mother's goal for him to feel good about himself. Relating the family members through their goals provides a common ground from which to begin the treatment.

INITIAL-PHASE SESSIONS (1–4)

In accordance with the IPT-A model, the overall treatment goals for JT were to decrease his depressive symptoms and improve his interpersonal functioning. To this end, the goals for the initial phase were (1) to further identify JT's depressive symptoms and educate JT and his parents about depression; (2) to educate JT and his parents about IPT-A treatment, including their roles in the treatment; (3) to relate JT's depression to the interpersonal context in which it occurs; (4) to review current and past interpersonal relationships as they relate to current depressive symptoms by conducting an interpersonal inventory; and (5) to identify JT's interpersonal problem area and establish a treatment contract. For JT, the initial phase occurred over the course of five sessions including one joint session with JT and both of his parents in between his first and second individual sessions.

Depression Diagnosis and Education

JT was initially reluctant to acknowledge depressive symptoms during the pretreatment evaluation. As the initial phase of treatment began, he became more open about the extent and severity of his symptoms. JT acknowledged that the symptoms discussed above occurred with considerable frequency and were distressing to him. He also acknowledged additional symptoms, including feelings of worthlessness and several somatic symptoms including stomachaches and headaches with no known medical origin. He confided that his poor concentration was having an impact on his functioning in school. JT was diagnosed with a major depression, moderate severity. The therapist helped JT understand how his emotional and physical experiences were part of his depression:

> JT, your sad and angry feelings as well as the other things you are reporting such as having difficulty sleeping, feeling tired, feeling down on yourself, and thinking that things will never get better are all symptoms of what is called depression. Similarly, the conflict you are having with your parents and the decline in your school performance are symptoms of your depression. The conflict may have played a role in the cause of your depression and is made worse by your depression. Depression can affect your life in many ways, and it is very important to get help for it as soon as possible. At the same time, it is important for you to know that depression is not uncommon.

JT appeared relieved to have his symptoms explained to him as being part of a clinical depression. As the therapist explained to him that depression is something experienced by other teens and that it is likely that treatment will help him to feel and function better, he seemed more at ease. As part of the explanation of the medical model of depression, JT was assigned the limited sick role. The therapist explained:

*JT, you and your parents have noted that you don't seem to be func-
tioning as well in school during these past months. When people experience depression they often have difficulty at school and/or work as
well as sometimes in activities in which they are typically very good.
They also may have less interest in things that previously interested
them. This is part of the depression. It seems like this is happening to
you. I am going to ask you and your parents to accept the fact that for
some time you may not function as well as usual due to your depression. This means that, despite trying hard, for a short time your grades
may not be what they were before becoming depressed. This, however, does not mean that you should give up or pull away from school
or other activities. Actually it is very important that you continue to
attend both school and activities and that you work as hard as you
can. Eventually, as your symptoms improve, you will find yourself
functioning better again.*

The therapist went on to describe IPT-A treatment, including the focus of the treatment and JT's role in the treatment. Finally, they discussed his parents' potential involvement in the treatment. The therapist
met with JT and his parents later that week. Half of this session was
conducted with the parents alone and half with JT. The focus was on educating the parents about JT's depression and the impact of his depression on his functioning. In addition, the therapist explained the IPT-A
model and the parents' roles in the treatment. The therapist informed the
parents that the majority of the treatment would be conducted alone
with JT and that they might be asked to participate in the middle part of
treatment to work on specific communication and problem-solving skills
if it appeared likely to be helpful. Although they agreed to JT's and their
own participation in the treatment, JT's father stated that he did not really believe that JT's problems were about depression. He saw it more as
laziness and oppositional behavior. He agreed, however, to give the
treatment time and to keep an open mind.

During this session, the therapist bore witness to some of the interaction patterns between JT's parents. His father clearly dominated the conversation and left little room for his mother to speak. She spoke meekly
and hesitantly, rarely stating anything that was not supporting her husband, although she did say that she believed JT was depressed and felt
strongly that he needed help. She hinted that she too had struggled with depression in the past and that she understood how hard it could be.

Interpersonal Inventory

The main focus of the following two individual sessions was on completing the interpersonal inventory. This process began with the creation of a

closeness circle as a schematic representation of JT's most significant relationships and the extent to which he felt close to each of the identified
people. For the circle, JT identified his parents, his two brothers, Robert
(age 13) and Charlie (age 10), his cousin Gary, his Aunt Laurie, and his
three friends Brad, Karl, and Ian as being those with whom he had the
most significant relationships. Figure 20.1 is a replication of his closeness circle.

As depicted, JT identified his brother Charlie and his friends Brad
and Karl as being the people to whom he felt closest, although he did not
feel he could tell them everything. He identified Ian and his aunt Laurie
as being in the next circle, stating that he could talk to them about some
personal issues and felt pretty close to them. He stated that his mother
and his cousin Gary were people he could only talk to about specific
problems. Finally, he placed his brother Robert and his father in the
outer ring, stating that he did not feel close to them at all.

Following the completion of the closeness circle, the therapist began

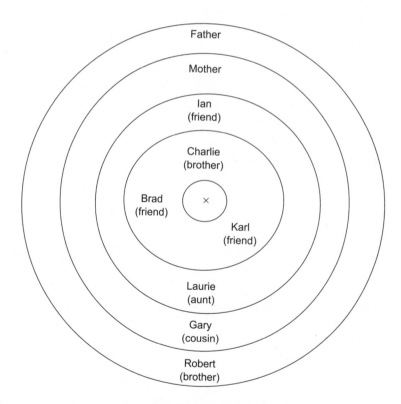

FIGURE 20.1. JT's closeness circle.

the interpersonal inventory with JT. They systematically went through each of the relationships, exploring the positive and negative aspects of the relationships, desired changes in the relationships, expectations for one another in the relationships, interaction patterns in the relationships, and the impact of JT's depression on the relationships. This process was initially difficult for JT, as he had a tendency to respond with generalities and global statements. He had difficulty seeing the gray areas in his relationships, tending to see them as all good or all bad. For example, in discussing his relationship with his father, JT and the therapist had the following exchange:

JT: My father is just a jerk. I shouldn't have even put him in the circle—its not like he would ever change, anyway.

THERAPIST: Well, let's talk about your relationship with your father more specifically. What are some of the negative aspects of your relationship with your father? [The therapist chose to begin with the negative issues, as this was clearly JT's focus and would likely be somewhat easier for him to discuss.]

JT: Too many to count—we really don't have a relationship.

THERAPIST: Sometime when things have been really bad for a while, it can seem hard to make sense of what is specifically wrong in the relationship, but this is important for us to do here. Just take your time and think specifically about the things that are bothering you about the relationship.

JT: My father never listens to anyone else—not me, not my mother—he is always in a bad mood and tired. He is always yelling at me and thinks I can't do anything right.

THERAPIST: You sound angry and frustrated right now as you talk about this. Can you give me a specific example of something that you and your father might argue about and how that conversation might go?

JT: Well, spending time after school or on Saturdays with my friends. My dad just thinks I should always be working.

THERAPIST: Can you think of a time in the last week when you had an argument about this? [The therapist tries to get an example from the previous week. The "here-and-now" focus on IPT begins even in the interpersonal inventory.]

JT: Yeah, 2 days ago.

THERAPIST: Can you tell me specifically what happened?

JT: I came home from school and asked if I could go to the park for a couple of hours with my friends. My father just glared at me and then said, "I am sure you have better things to do with your time. If you don't have any work to do I could use your help in an apartment."

THERAPIST: And how did you feel?

JT: I was mad—and he knew it.

THERAPIST: And what did you say or do?

JT: I just went into my room and turned on my music.

THERAPIST: Did you ever talk to your dad about how you felt?

JT: There is no use. It's not like he cares or anything. Besides, he knows how I feel. [At this point in the treatment, the therapist is trying to gather specific information in order to make a diagnosis of the interpersonal issues related to JT's depression. This is not the time for intervention into a specific interaction pattern. Such an intervention comes in the middle phase of the treatment once all necessary information to make an accurate assessment has been gathered.]

THERAPIST: Can you remember a time with your dad when it did not feel this way?

JT: No, not really. Well, it used to be that sometimes we would have fun together, but that was a long time ago, and he was still a jerk a lot of the time.

THERAPIST: What is it that you and your father used to enjoy together? [The therapist tries to get detailed information about what was enjoyable in the father–son relationship. This may prove helpful during the middle phase, when the therapist will try to remind JT and his father that they did enjoy some activities together.]

JT: We both used to like baseball a lot. He used to come to my games, and we would watch on TV, but that all changed when I decided to stop playing when we moved. Then he just got on my case more about my school work, and he always expected me to do his job for him in my free time, making me work so hard for him on weekends!

The therapist needed to help guide JT into giving examples of interactions that they could examine in detail. The specifics are necessary to help the therapist identify the interaction patterns that typify this relationship and to identify the specific issues that may be the focus of treatment. The therapist completed the interpersonal inventory over the course of the second and third individual sessions. Some of the information that was gathered is presented in the following paragraphs.

Within his immediate family JT had a number of conflictual relationships. The most conflictual of these was with his father. Although he
outwardly insisted that this relationship did not matter to him, based on
the extent of his symptoms and the association between conflicts with
his father and the exacerbation of his symptoms, this clearly was not the
case. JT and his father had considerable difficulty communicating with
each other. His father had difficulty listening to others' opinions and
presented as dogmatic and closed-minded. JT experienced a great deal of
anger in his interactions with his father but rarely communicated this directly. Instead, he engaged in more passive–aggressive behaviors such as
being truant from school or withdrawing from any contact. He had considerable difficulty communicating assertively with his father. His conflict with his father increased substantially during JT's transition to the
new school. Several things occurred at that time. JT, who was a standout
player on his baseball team at his old school, chose to not try out for the
baseball team at his new school because he believed he would not make
it. JT's father saw this decision as JT giving up and being more concerned with his social life than his future. As the therapist and JT talked
about this decision and his father's reaction, JT shared that his father
had aspired to be a professional baseball player but had to leave school
early in order to work and help support his younger siblings. JT also acknowledged that he was angry at his father for the fact that they had to
move. He explained that he had felt settled and established in his previous school and that his father announced the move to his family very
suddenly. Reportedly, they moved to be closer to the apartment building
in which his father had recently become the superintendent. JT explained that his father had not given anyone in the family a say in the
move and that in part his decision not to play baseball was his way of
getting back at his father for forcing the move.

As the therapist progressed through the inventory, it became apparent that JT evidenced difficulty with effective communication in many of
his relationships. This was not unlike his mother's pattern of interacting,
for which JT expressed considerable disrespect and frustration. He saw
his mother as a doormat and acknowledged feeling "hurt" that she did
not stand up for him more. JT denied outward conflict with his mother
but explained that they had less and less contact with each other. They
used to talk about things in his life, and he had always liked how interested she seemed. Since he began to feel depressed he had withdrawn
from her. Her attempts to talk to him and get him to open up, he said,
"drive me crazy, and so I often yell at her and walk away." When asked
how his mother responds, JT said she just walks away and doesn't talk
to him. He thinks she probably feels hurt. JT and the therapist more
briefly reviewed the other relationships in the circle that appeared to be

less central to his depression. JT picked several that represented his relationships in general and illustrated certain communication or interaction patterns.

Therapist Decision: Selecting a Problem Area

Several interpersonal issues appear associated with JT's depression. JT clearly had considerable disputes in his relationship with his father. The two were not communicating well, particularly about their feelings, and had very different expectations of each other and their relationship. JT also had clearly experienced an increase in symptoms that had never abated and only worsened, beginning with his transition to a new school. JT had clear interpersonal deficits, particularly in his ability to communicate his feelings effectively and assertively. The therapist saw JT's conflicts with his father as being the primary issue related to his depression, while the transition issues and skills deficits were important but secondary. They seemed to impact JT most significantly through their effects on his conflicts with his father. Therefore, the selected problem area was *interpersonal role disputes,* specifically, disputes related to his father's unilateral decision to move and the impact of the transition on JT.

Setting the Treatment Contract

During the final session of the initial phase, the treatment contract was set. This involved several different tasks: (1) the therapist reviewed with JT her perspective on the association between his interpersonal problems and his depression and depicted this association with a depression circle; (2) the therapist identified the interpersonal problem area and sought feedback from JT regarding this interpersonal diagnosis; and (3) the therapist reviewed the structure and parameters of the next component of treatment, including JT's role in the treatment.

The therapist began this process with the following dialogue:

> *JT, over the course of the past few weeks we have talked about your relationships and your depression in considerable detail. You have helped me to understand what is and isn't working in your relationships and the likely association between your relationships and the depression you are currently experiencing. Based on this discussion, it appears to me that mild signs of depression began a year and a half ago—around the time that you moved and changed schools—but your depression worsened about 5 months ago at the end of the summer or the beginning of this school year. The increase in your symp-*

toms seemed most closely related to the increased conflicts with your father and the impact of his decision to move on your friendships and your academic performance. Sometimes when people do not communicate their feelings and make their wishes known to others, they get depressed. It seems hard for you talk about your feelings with certain people, such as your father and some of your new friends. The two of you have been unable to talk about the move and how his expectations for you of late make you feel. Your anger at your father about the move also has complicated your adjustment to your new school. As a result of being depressed, you have withdrawn from people, particularly family members, and feel more hopeless that things at home and in school will improve. Your concentration has decreased, and you have become tired, both of which have contributed to problems with your grades. The worse you do in school, the worse you feel about yourself and the more your parents are on your case. Can you see how the things happening in your relationships and your depression interact in this loop? Based on what you have told me, I think you are having trouble finding your way out of this cycle of conflict. Here is a picture of how I see these things fitting together [Figure 20.2].

Therefore, it seems to me that we should focus the treatment primarily on your arguments with your father. If we can help you and your father to communicate better, understand each other, and negotiate better, this is likely to help you feel better and function better in a number of areas. How does this sound to you? Is this the way you see it, or do you have different ideas? It is really important that you let me know and share any questions or disagreements you may have with my understanding of this.

To ensure that JT understood the framework of the problem area, the therapist asked him to explain the ideas in his own words. Although JT agreed with the therapist's conceptualization of the problem, he expressed considerable pessimism about the therapist's ability to help him in his relationship with his father. The therapist responded by acknowledging JT's hesitation and explaining concretely how they would proceed.

It is not uncommon for adolescents to feel that there is no way of fixing the problem. The truth is there is no guarantee here, but we have a number of options as to how we can proceed, and I believe that we may be able to improve things. The steps may be small and they may take some time, but I hope that you can give it a chance. I will work with you on one or two specific issues or disputes with your father, and we will work on how to better communicate with him. We also

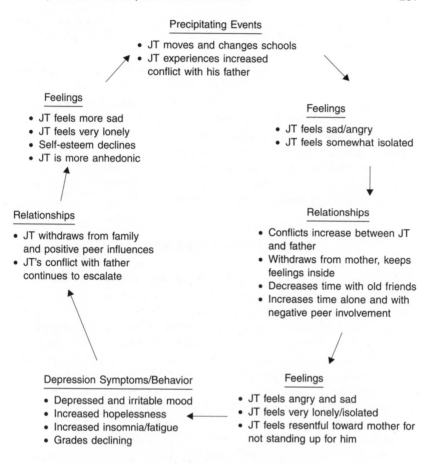

FIGURE 20.2. JT's depression circle.

can meet with your father and maybe your mother so that I can help you to work out these issues with them. As you know, this treatment lasts for 12 weeks and we are beginning our second month, but there is plenty of time to work through some of these issues. I want you to work hard in these sessions. Your job will be to bring in specific examples of interactions with your father and to practice, in session and outside of session, different ways to communicate and negotiate with him. As part of this process we also may address issues in some of your other relationships—relationships that are going well and those in which you are having some difficulty. Our primary focus, though, will be on your relationship with your father and specific sources of con-

flict in that relationship such as your friendships, academic work, and
required work with your father. Does this sound OK to you?

JT did agree to the treatment contract. Although he was nervous
about trying to work things out, he did hope that things would get
better. The therapist further reviewed the parameters of treatment and
expectations for JT. She reexplained the limited sick role and asked JT
for a commitment to attend school and to refrain from smoking marijuana or using any substances during the treatment. It was important to
be able to track his symptoms unaffected by substances. Some of his
marijuana use was likely a way of self-medicating his depression since he
most often smoked after an argument with his father.

MIDDLE-PHASE SESSIONS (5–8)

The primary focus of the middle phase of treatment was on JT's role dispute with his father. This phase consisted of individual sessions 5–8 as
well as one joint session with JT and his parents, although the work continued into the termination phase as well. Preliminary assessment of the
dispute between JT and his father suggested that they were in the renegotiation stage, trying to work out their differences but ending up in arguments each time. Therefore, the goal was to define and resolve the dispute by first clarifying expectations and then modifying communications
and expectations (see Chapter 11). Early middle-phase sessions were
used to further clarify the stage of dispute and the goals. The therapist
was unsure about the ability of both JT and his father to make the necessary changes to bring about full resolution to the dispute but was opti-
mistic that small steps could be made to decrease the frequency of the
conflicts. The general strategies used in the treatment were (1) exploration of the dispute, (2) identification of dispute patterns, (3) conducting
a decision analysis to determine resolution of the dispute, (4) modifying
expectations where necessary, and (5) improving communication and negotiation skills.

Discussion of the role dispute between JT and his father had begun
during the interpersonal inventory; however, more details were gathered
during the middle phase. One of the first challenges the therapist faced
was to narrow the focus of the sessions to one or two specific conflicts
between JT and his father. This is a common problem when an adolescent has a highly conflictual relationship with someone, particularly a
family member. JT had a tendency to make many global negative statements about his relationship with his father. The therapist had to be
tuned in to this tendency and remind JT that, although focusing on a

specific issue could feel trivial given all that he felt was wrong in the relationship, it was the best way to begin to bring about change. Other issues were likely to fall into place or be easier to address once some gains had been made in a specific area.

Therapist Decision: Selecting a Specific Issue to Address

THERAPIST: JT, although I know that you have some very negative feelings about your father and your relationship, and you say that there are many things wrong in this relationship, we need to select a starting point. It is best for us to focus on one primary issue to start. I usually like to start with something small and not the most difficult problem. Do you have a specific conflict or issue that you think we should start out addressing?

JT: I want my father to trust me more and give me the chance to be a teenager and get off my back about school and work.

THERAPIST: I do understand all that, but you just named a lot of different issues. I see that they are all very important, but can we think of one issue to start with?

JT: I guess, trust. I want him just to trust me. It's not like I am getting into trouble all the time.

THERAPIST: OK, that's great. We are starting to narrow this down, but trust is still a really big issue. Could you tell me what kinds of things he does that make you feel that he doesn't trust you?

JT: He won't let me go out with my friends. Well, at least rarely during the day and almost never at night. If I get to go out, I have to be in by 10, even on the weekend and that is only every few weeks or so.

THERAPIST: So you want to get to spend more time with your friends? Is that correct?

JT: Yeah, basically.

THERAPIST: OK, let's work with that issue. Can you explain your perspective and your father's perspective on this conflict?

JT: I want to be able to spend time with my friends and relax, and my father just wants me to work. He thinks I am only getting into trouble or being lazy if I am with my friends. It's like he was never a teenager.

The therapist's task here was to narrow the focus of treatment and interventions to a specific issue in order to increase the probability that treatment can proceed in a productive direction. There were many issues that could have been selected. The issue that is chosen is less important than ensuring that the issue or conflict is defined as specifically as possible and has potential for successful resolution, to give hope to the adolescent that the situation can improve.

Therefore, treatment initially focused on JT's anger at his dad for abruptly moving the family, his subsequent desire to spend more time with his friends, and his father's resistance to this. The first two sessions of the middle phase focused on understanding the feelings about the move and friends that were fueling the dispute on both sides, as well as the specific patterns of communication between them. This particular topic of conflict posed an additional challenge to the therapist. It was clear that JT's father's resistance to his spending time with friends had increased since he changed schools. This was possibly due to his withdrawal from his involvement in baseball and the decline in his academic performance, possibly due to different expectations of teenage behavior, and possibly due to the choice of friends that JT had made. The father's resistance was likely due in part to his legitimate concerns about JT's new friends and poor grades, and his disappointment at JT's withdrawal from baseball. The therapist also had some concerns regarding the decisions and choices that JT was making regarding his friendships and some of his activities, and needed to address them as part of the exploration of the dispute.

THERAPIST: It is important that we have a clear understanding of what you feel your father's opposition is to your spending time with friends. Did he oppose this as much prior to your move to this new school?

JT: Not as much. He has always been tough on me to work really hard, but he never really had a big problem with me spending time with my baseball buddies or my cousin. I also didn't want to go out as much then. It was different.

THERAPIST: Well, you are older now, so of course you are looking for more freedom. You said before that your dad doesn't let you go out because he thinks you are lazy and he doesn't want you to relax and have a good time.

JT: Yeah, well, that's part of it. I mean he has always had this thing about working hard, especially as the oldest in the family.

THERAPIST: Kind of like he had to?

JT: Yeah, that is part of it, I think. It's like he wants things to be better for me than it was for him, but then he wants me to have to work as hard as he did. Sometimes I don't even believe him that he always had to work and never had fun. Maybe it's true but . . .

THERAPIST: Do you really believe that this is the reason? What might have made your father feel differently about your spending so much time on baseball rather than these new friends?

JT: I don't know.

THERAPIST: It is hard to know. You are right that it is OK for you to want to be a teenager. I am curious though about this change in your dad's attitude about your being with friends since you changed schools. What do you think caused this shift?

JT: He doesn't like my new friends. He thinks they are all bad. He never even gave them a chance. Besides, it was his decision to move. It's not my fault that these were the guys I met when we moved.

THERAPIST: I hear that you are angry at your dad about the move, and I want to get back to that, but first I wonder if you think he is a bit concerned about your safety with your new friends?

JT: Maybe a little—probably more concerned about me throwing my future away—but he should know that it's not like I won't do my own thing when it counts. It's not like I don't make my own decisions.

THERAPIST: Well, let me ask you a question. Do you think that your current friends, or at least some of them, are a bad influence or that some of the activities put your safety or future at risk?

JT: Again, it's not like I don't make my own decisions.

THERAPIST: Yes, at times, but it has sounded to me like sometimes it is hard to figure out how to step away from the crowd and do what you know is right.

JT: Sometimes. Yeah, I guess some of his concerns make some sense . . . but some of the guys are really good guys and . . .

JT initially was defensive regarding his current friendships but eventually was able to acknowledge his own ambivalence regarding these relationships and to see some of his father's perspective. This was extremely important for preparing JT to negotiate with his father in the future.

Identifying the patterns of communication between JT and his father required JT's bringing in specific examples of interactions related to the dispute that occurred in the days just prior to the sessions. The therapist, using communication analysis, encouraged JT to provide very specific descriptions of his interactions with his father that included not only what was said and done but also the feelings that were generated by the interactions and how those interactions were related to JT's depressive symptoms. An example of how this technique was employed with JT follows:

THERAPIST: OK, JT, so at the start of the session when we were reviewing your symptoms you reported that you had been feeling somewhat better. Your mood was brighter, you were more hopeful, and your concentration was better until 2 days ago when you had an argument with your father about going out with your friends on Saturday night. Can you recall the details of that conversation with your father, including not only what was said but also how you and your dad were feeling?

JT: I guess so. Maybe not everything.

THERAPIST: Let's try to remember as much detail as you can. I will help you along. How did the interaction start?

JT: I came home from school and was talking to my mother about how some of the guys were going to see Wrestlemania at Madison Square Garden on Saturday night, and I really wanted to go. Then my father walked in right in the middle of the conversation and asked what we were talking about, so I told him—not like I didn't know what he was going to say.

THERAPIST: So, how exactly did you tell your father?

JT: I said that some of the guys were going to Wrestlemania and had invited me and I wanted to go.

THERAPIST: And how did your father respond?

JT: He said, "You're not going. I don't want you in the city getting into whatever trouble with those hoodlums. You don't even watch wrestling. Besides, we have a lot of work to do this weekend in the basement apartment, and you have SATs coming up in 2 weeks."

THERAPIST: How did that make you feel?

JT: Pissed off. I mean he always is passing judgment. The guys who are going aren't the ones who get into trouble—and how does he know I don't like wrestling? Like we ever talk anymore. It's like I am his slave.

THERAPIST: Were you feeling anything else?

JT: Mad at him, of course, that he never trusts me.

THERAPIST: You must have been feeling frustrated and hurt. How do you think your dad was feeling?

JT: I don't know what he was feeling. He seemed mad.

THERAPIST: Could he have been worried about you?

JT: I don't know. Maybe. Who cares?

THERAPIST: Well, even when you don't care, it really spoils your mood. You were feeling better before this argument. What did you say to your dad?

JT: I told him he was a jerk and just left the kitchen and went to my room. I didn't talk to him again until the next day.

THERAPIST: So you didn't tell your father how you were feeling?

JT: He knew.

THERAPIST: I will admit that he probably knew you were angry. That was clear. But sometimes we assume that people really understand our feelings because of our behavior and the truth is they don't. You never told him all the things that you were able to just tell me, such as your feeling that he doesn't trust you. Your dad has no way of knowing how the things he says make you feel if you don't communicate it to him. What could you have said to your father?

JT: I don't know.

THERAPIST: Just try to imagine having a different conversation.

JT: I could have told him that he made me angry when he just said no like that and how I wished he would trust me and how he doesn't even know what guys are going.

THERAPIST: That sounds like a start. Let's think also about your dad's point of view for a minute. You don't have to accept his point of view, but just figure it out so you can find a more effective way to communicate and negotiate with him. What might have been on your father's mind or what might he have been feeling when he responded that way, besides your initial guess that he just didn't trust you?

JT: Well, I know he is stressed about the apartment, so that was part of it. He probably thought I had forgotten that I told him I would help. It's not like I can't help him at other points during the weekend.

THERAPIST: That's a good point. But how would he know you would help him at another time or that you've been studying?

JT: Yeah, I have been studying a lot. He has been working so much he doesn't even know how hard I have been working. Also my grades are up since I started coming here, and he knows that, but he doesn't focus on that when things are going badly.

THERAPIST: I want to get back to that and how it makes you feel, but I just want to finish with what might have been leading your father to respond the way he did. We also have discussed how some of your father's concerns about the guys you have been hanging out with are a little valid. I know you told me you were spending less time with some of them. I wonder if he knows that. We have identified a number of things that might have been on your father's mind when he responded to you. How do you think you could have found out his specific concerns and alleviated some of them by telling him more about your activities and plans?

The therapist went on to explore how and when JT could have addressed these issues in a way that would increase the likelihood that his father would respond in a more positive manner. While exploring several similar interactions with JT in ensuing sessions, the therapist continually highlighted the interaction pattern that had become evident. JT would express his desire to do something with his friends without first addressing some of his father's concerns, causing his father to respond quickly and negatively. JT would get angry and upset and withdraw to his room without ever addressing his father's concerns or expressing his feelings. Over time, JT would feel more depressed and frustrated. Over the course of treatment, JT began to more actively identify alternative ways of interacting and communicating. He became more adept at seeing his father's perspective.

In preparation for a joint session, the therapist began role playing with JT in the session. The therapist and JT alternated playing the roles of JT and his father and practiced interactions related to the dispute. JT wanted to attend a school dance that was coming up, but had not yet broached this topic with his parents. This became the focus of many role plays. An example of one of the role plays follows:

THERAPIST: JT, I know that you really want to go to the school dance. You have said that you do not believe that your father will let you go because he won't trust you and you think he will want you to stay home and study. So, let's think about how you could try to talk to your father about this. Let's start with deciding when is a good time to talk to him. When do you think is the best time to talk to your dad about something that is important to you? When is he most likely to be able to listen?

JT: When he is not stressed out—but he is always stressed out.

THERAPIST: When is your father the least stressed out?

JT: On Sundays or weeknights, after he has had supper and is relaxing, as long as he is not watching a game or something.

THERAPIST: OK, so let's practice having a conversation with your father. Let's pretend it's a weeknight after supper and he is just sitting, relaxing in the living room. How could you start the conversation?

JT: I don't know.

THERAPIST: I would recommend you do two things. First, you want to let him know that you have something you really would like to talk to him about, let him know this is important to you. Second, ask him if this is a good time to talk. If he agrees, then you can proceed to talk to him. Let's try this, would you like play yourself or your father?

JT: I guess my father.

THERAPIST: OK, I will be you. Dad, I have something important that I would like to talk to you about. Is this a good time?

JT: What is it?

THERAPIST: Well, we have a dance coming up at school in 2 weeks on Saturday night. I would really like to go. I know that I would have to work extra hard during the days and get all my work done. I will do that.

JT: Why do you have to go to some dance? How do I know that you won't be off doing something else and getting into trouble?

THERAPIST: Because I am telling you that you can trust me. I would be going with Chad and Kyle, two of my newer friends who are good guys. They work hard at school, and they don't get into trouble. I want to go to the dance. It is over at 11:00 and I will come home right after if that is what you want.

JT: I don't know.

THERAPIST: Could you at least think about it? I really do want to go, and I guarantee I will get all my work done.

The role play stops.

THERAPIST: JT, you played your father very well. You gave me a hard time when I tried to be you. How did you feel with the way I played you?

JT: I guess some of what you said was OK.

THERAPIST: What didn't feel OK?

JT: The part that I will be home right at 11:00 P.M.

THERAPIST: What time seems reasonable to you?

JT: I think 11:30, at least.

THERAPIST: Could you ask your father for an 11:30 curfew?

At points in the session, the role play focused most directly on letting JT's father know how JT felt about his lack of trust and negotiating to build back this trust. JT learned the basic negotiation skills quickly but struggled more with expressing his feelings. The therapist tried to help JT see how helpful it would be to JT's relationship with his father if he learned to speak more directly about his feelings.

Therapist Decision: Role Play versus Work at Home

Both role play and "work at home" are common techniques used with role disputes in order to encourage practice of effective communication and negotiation strategies. The therapist in this case opted to use only role play during the first few sessions of the middle phase as she felt that JT and his father initially would need assistance to negotiate their interactions. Therefore, she chose to keep the practice in-session and then schedule a joint session for JT and his parents in which JT could practice his communication and negotiation skills with the therapist's assistance and mediation if necessary.

In preparation for the joint session the therapist called JT's parents and spoke with both of them about attending, explaining the purpose of the session. JT's father agreed to come in but was somewhat negative on the telephone. His mother was more encouraging, indicating that she thought JT seemed a little better and that he had been a bit more open with her and less reclusive.

Given JT's father's response on the telephone, the therapist decided that it would be best to meet with JT's parents alone, first, to prepare them to support JT's efforts. The therapist spoke with JT and explained that, although they had several sessions to get ready for this meeting, his parents did not, and it might help things go better if the therapist prepared them for the meeting. JT agreed to this, and the therapist met with the parents for about 30 minutes prior to the joint session. In talking to JT's parents, the therapist said:

> JT has been working very hard in his therapy sessions on learning new ways to directly tell you what he is feeling and thinking about the

things that are important to him. He has done a really great job, but what is most important is that he learns to use these skills outside of the therapy sessions in his real life. I know that you all have been through some difficult times together, so I wanted to bring you all in here so that he could try to use these new skills with you. Just like anything that is new, it can be hard for him, especially if he feels nervous or stressed. So, I wanted us to talk together first and figure out the best ways that we can help him. What I really need is for you both to be JT's coaches and supports as he tries to communicate. He has something that he wants to talk to you about, an event at school that he would like to attend, and he selected this as the topic for today. This doesn't mean that we can't talk about anything else, but we will start with this if that is acceptable to you. He has been practicing being more direct and clear when he talks about his feelings, and so when you notice him doing this it would be great if you could let him know. The more positive feedback he gets from the two of you, the more likely he is to continue to try to speak more openly. Is this something that sounds OK to you? Do you have any concerns or questions?

It was very important to give JT's parents a chance to voice any concerns or questions they had and for the therapist to get a sense of whether they were going to be able to be supportive and not sabotage the intervention. JT's mother was very agreeable to this. His father agreed but expressed his concern that they deal with the big issues, for example, his schoolwork. The therapist recognized the importance of this issue and asked them if they had noted any change in this area. Both parents agreed that it had gotten slightly better. They discussed how important it was to them that JT agree to continue to work hard at school and talked about how this could be incorporated into the discussion during the joint session in a way that was likely to be productive.

The focus of the joint session was on negotiating around JT's request to attend the school dance and communicating about the feelings each of the family members was having regarding this request. With the help of the parent preparation meeting, JT's parents were quite responsive and supportive during the joint session. His father stated his concerns strongly and did not back down on certain issues such as school performance, but he was willing to make compromises and responded quite positively to JT's attempts to share some of his feelings with his parents. He was able to verbally acknowledge JT's feelings about school and to state that he was willing to listen to possible solutions. JT's mother was quick to note some of the positive changes that JT had made. JT, with some reminders from the therapist, let his mother and, at times, his father know when they said things that made him feel better.

The therapist did have to work hard to keep them, especially JT's father, focused on the specific issue at hand. By the end of the session, they had come to an agreement that JT could attend the dance if he spent a certain part of each day studying at home and if he committed to helping his father with apartment maintenance on two Sundays of the month. The therapist reminded them that there were other issues that needed to be addressed at another time, but they had done well in achieving this one goal and hopefully had learned effective strategies in doing so that could be used by all of the family members to address their feelings and conflicts that may arise in the future.

The remainder of the middle phase of treatment was spent identifying other issues that JT could address with his family and similar difficulties he had with friends. The therapist helped JT to generalize the skills he had used to resolve the school dance issue to these different situations and relationships. For example, they worked briefly on addressing problems in JT's relationship with his cousin, specifically on how to communicate honestly and directly about his feelings regarding his cousin's breaking his confidence. These strategies were used to encourage him to speak openly with his cousin instead of shutting him out. JT continued to struggle with his initial impulse to shut down and walk away, but he became much quicker at recognizing when he was about to do this and to see the connection between this pattern and his depression.

TERMINATION-PHASE SESSIONS (9–12)

The final four individual sessions with JT focused primarily on issues related to termination, although much middle-phase work continued, especially in session 9. The main focus of sessions 9 and 10 was on continued work regarding the generalization of JT's gains in treatment to other situations and relationships. The first task was to specifically identify JT's treatment gains.

JT needed some help and coaching on this task. He recognized a clear improvement in his symptoms. He reported improved mood, improved sleep, decreased fatigue, and improved self-esteem. In addition, he reported considerably fewer thoughts related to death and increased hopefulness about the future. He continued to feel periodically frustrated with his father and with his difficulty resolving all issues with him, but when reviewing the past several weeks he was able to acknowledge that the conflicts with his father were fewer and less substantial. He reported that his expectations for his relationship with his father had shifted. He no longer felt as responsible for the conflicts nor as responsible for his father's moods. JT agreed with the therapist that he had learned to communicate about his feelings and negotiate topics of conflict in a much more effective way. He still, at times, withdrew and shut down, particularly during discussions with his father, but this was much less frequent. He was expressing his feelings and communicating much more effectively with other people in his life, particularly his mother and some of his friends. The therapist encouraged him to continue working on these issues with other people in his life, particularly his brother and his cousin. He worked with the therapist on identifying ways to use his skills to address other issues in these relationships. A combination of role play and work at home was used to reinforce these discussions.

JT was able to identify potential conflicts and issues that may arise in the future with his father as well as other important people in his life. He discussed how he would use the skills he had learned to manage these situations. JT was particularly concerned about the process of making decisions regarding college and managing his father's reactions to which colleges JT would like to apply. JT also was leaning more to wanting to break away from his relationship with Brad or at least to break away from some of the activities with which he was not comfortable. He expressed considerable anxiety about changing this relationship and concern about how he would manage to do it. JT also was struggling with not wanting his father to think that he was "just giving in to his opinions."

During the final sessions, the focus was on identifying JT's warning symptoms, reviewing his need for further treatment now or in the future, and discussing his feelings about ending treatment. JT initially reported that he felt good about treatment ending. He stated that he felt as if he had made significant gains and was much more confident in his ability to handle problems if and when they occurred in the future. With some discussion, however, he acknowledged feeling anxious about treatment ending and insecure about his ability to handle upcoming challenges. Although he was able to identify his warning symptoms, he felt concerned that if he started to feel sad he would retreat into his old patterns and pull away from people instead of seeking help. The therapist highlighted for JT that one of the most important steps in not falling into old patterns is recognizing those patterns, something that JT now readily did. With some encouragement, JT also was able to acknowledge sadness at the ending of the therapeutic relationship, indicating that it was one of the first times in his life that he had felt really helped by an adult. The therapist acknowledged her feelings about JT, as well:

JT, it has been really nice to work with you. You have worked very hard and made many gains over the course of your treatment. I have looked forward to our meetings and will miss them now that they are ending. At the same time, I feel good about the work that you did and confident that you have learned some new and very valuable skills. You have been willing to take important steps toward working things out in your relationship with your father, and, although that relationship is not exactly as you would like it, it seems much improved. I also am glad to hear that you have had a positive experience in treatment. As we discussed, it is possible that you may feel depressed again someday in the future. I hope that, having had this positive experience, you will be willing to get back into treatment before your symptoms become more severe and affect your school work or other aspects of your life too significantly.

The therapist and JT agreed that, although he was not feeling confident in his ability to sustain his gains once therapy ended, it was important to try. JT acknowledged that in his life he often questioned his abilities and then surprised himself by being able to manage situations. He felt that he wanted to conclude the treatment now but agreed to contact the therapist if he needed a referral for further treatment in the future. The therapist recommended the option of continuation treatment in which he could continue to come but less frequently in order to help him maintain his gains and prevent relapse. This option appealed to JT, and they agreed to meet once a month for the next six months and then reassess his symptoms and functioning before deciding to end treatment completely.

This case highlights many of the key components of IPT-A treatment. It calls attention to some of the places where the therapist must decide in which direction to focus the treatment and the issues involved in making these decisions. Therapists commonly ask us to describe the differences between an IPT-A approach and a cognitive-behavioral approach to treating adolescent depression, as these are the two treatments with the most efficacy data for this population. What follows now is a discussion of the differences and similarities between how an IPT-A therapist and a cognitive-behavioral (CBT) therapist might address the issues presented by JT and his family. We acknowledge that there is more than one treatment approach stemming from CBT, as discussed in Chapter 2, and that these approaches cannot be easily simplified here. At this time, we are not attempting to present a comprehensive view or understanding of either of these perspectives, nor do we purport to be experts on these treatments. Rather, this discussion is meant simply to highlight some of the key similarities and differences between the CBT approach and IPT-A.

A COMPARISON OF COGNITIVE-BEHAVIORAL
AND IPT-A APPROACHES TO THE TREATMENT OF JT

The treatment of JT illustrates both similarities and differences between the CBT and IPT-A approaches to the treatment of adolescent depression. The CBT approach being used is based upon both Beck's (1967) focus on the negative cognitive triads as well as Lewinsohn's (1980) theory of the role of positive reinforcement and pleasurable activities in alleviating depression. Both IPT-A and CBT therapists are active participants in the therapy sessions to focus the treatment on the identified problem and to work collaboratively with the adolescent to solve the problems associated with the depression. They similarly use a method of both open-ended and specific questioning to help the adolescent look at his problem from a different perspective and to generate solutions with some coaching and guidance from the therapist. IPT-A and CBT are alike in their emphasis on the "here and now" and on teaching problem-solving skills. IPT-A, however, is more focused on interpersonal problem solving, specifically about relationship problems as compared to CBT, which is focused on problem solving in general. Nonetheless, in treating adolescents, a CBT therapist also may spend a significant amount of time on interpersonal problem-solving issues.

In the case of JT, the CBT therapist might begin by explaining the cognitive model of depression to JT in an age-appropriate way. That is, she would explain that thoughts, behaviors, and feelings are all linked together so that if you can make changes in one component of the system, the rest will change too. Since feelings are hard to change (i.e., it's hard to become "undepressed"), the therapist tries to treat the depression by changing the other two—behavior and thoughts. The therapist would elicit examples of JT's behavior and thinking when he is and is not feeling depressed.

The next step would be to identify therapeutic goals with JT and his parents. The therapist and parents would have met in a prior joint session in which the therapist provided psychoeducation about depression and solicited their collaboration with the treatment. Once the goals were established, the therapist would teach JT to monitor his mood. She would use simple mood scales and diagrams to show JT the relationship between mood and events and would assign homework based on mood monitoring during the initial sessions. Structured homework using charting and diaries would continue to reinforce the skills being learned throughout the treatment.

Using the information collected during mood monitoring, the therapist would illustrate for JT how positive mood tends to go together with activities that give pleasure or mastery and negative mood with unpleasant, negative activities. The therapist would point out the importance of increasing pleasant activities, a technique called behavioral activation, as a way to influence JT's mood through behavior changes. To do this, the therapist would work with JT to generate a list of fun and confidence-building activities, emphasizing activities that are legal, inexpensive, and feasible. Since JT was not particularly anhedonic, behavioral activation would be brief and would emphasize mastery activities to combat the sense of failure he had due to his academic problems.

Since JT was experiencing substantial difficulties with his father in trying to get permission to spend time with his friends, a large part of treatment would focus on teaching JT problem-solving skills. Specifically, he would be taught how to define the problem, generate options for obtaining his parents' permission, choose the most feasible option, and act on it. If necessary, the therapist would work with the parents to help them understand both behavioral activation as well as approaches to problem solving.

Following that phase of treatment, the therapist would turn the focus to helping JT to feel better by changing his maladaptive cognitions. She would help him identify automatic thoughts and would point out the relationship between pessimistic, self-blaming, catastrophizing types of thoughts and depression. She would coach JT to "talk back" to these maladaptive thoughts and replace them with more accurate and useful ones. For example, instead of thinking "My dad yelled that I can't go out. He doesn't trust me at all, and he thinks I will just get into trouble," JT would think, "My dad is in a bad mood because of the apartment problems, and he feels anxious that I will get into trouble." The homework for the bulk of the remaining session would highlight for JT that, by changing his maladaptive cognitions, his mood was improving.

The above discussion is just a snapshot of how a CBT therapist might have approached the treatment of JT. There are a number of variations of cognitive-behavioral therapy, each with different emphases. Based upon the Beck and Lewinsohn models, commonly used techniques with adolescents would include (1) mood monitoring, (2) behavioral activation, (3) teaching problem-solving skills, (4) changing maladaptive cognitions, and (5) affect regulation. Similar to an IPT-A therapist, a CBT therapist would use role-play techniques to engender change.

As illustrated in the case of JT, the unique characteristics of IPT-A are (1) its conceptualization of depression as a medical illness, (2) the accompanying assignment of the limited sick role, (3) the interpersonal diagnostic assessment, or interpersonal inventory, and (4) the focus on the linkage between affect, interpersonal events, and depression. The main IPT-A techniques utilized in the middle phase of JT's treatment included clarifying feelings as well as expectations for relationships, management and encouragement of affect, behavior change techniques such as role playing, and communication analysis of problematic interactions. In contrast to CBT's assigned homework using charts and diaries, IPT-A's "work at home" typically arises spontaneously from the content of sessions rather than from a predetermined list of good therapeutic homework tasks and tends to focus on promoting a different interpersonal interaction than mood and dysfunctional thought monitoring.

One of the most significant differences in the treatment approaches is that the CBT therapist targets thoughts to change mood and behavior, while the IPT-A therapist targets affect to change mood and behavior. In addition, IPT-A identifies one of four problem areas' frameworks (e.g., grief, role disputes, role transitions, interpersonal deficits) from which to approach the depression interpersonally, a framework not used in CBT. Although CBT and IPT-A approach depression from these different perspectives, they are two time-limited treatments that share similarities as well as some fundamental differences, as described above. This discussion provides a snapshot of a CBT therapist's approach to the treatment of depression and an initial framework in which to begin to think about which patients might benefit from which treatment approach. More research is needed to answer this question.

CLOSENESS CIRCLE

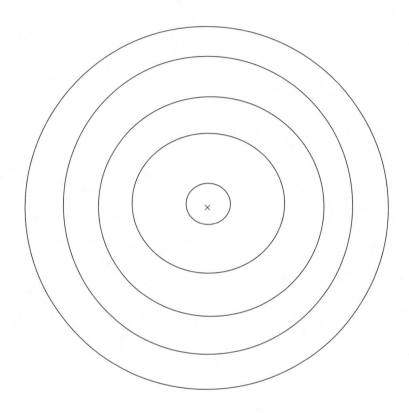

INTERPERSONAL INVENTORY

How to Query about Relationships

GENERAL INTRODUCTORY QUESTIONS

1. I would like to take some time now to talk to you about the important people in your life, people like your mother and father, sisters and brothers, best friend, girlfriend or boyfriend, other close relatives and friends.
2. Let's first make a list of who these people are.
3. Has your depression affected your relationship with the people closest to you? How?
4. We are now going to talk specifically about your relationships with each of these people and how your depression has been affected by or has affected this relationship.

The following are guidelines for the types of questions therapists can use in conducting an Interpersonal Inventory. Keep in mind that the key is to collect very specific details about relationships and interactions that occur in those relationships. Most adolescents will tend to make global, general statements. It is the therapist's job to elicit the details.

INITIAL QUESTIONS ABOUT SPECIFIC RELATIONSHIPS

What do you like about _____?
What don't you like about _____?
Have you ever told _____ how you feel?
What stops you?
What do you think would happen?
How would that make you feel?
Are there any times that you and _____ are together and it is OK?
Can you give me an example?
What are the positive aspects of your relationship?
Are there things in your relationship that you would like to change?

How would you feel if those things were different?
What things would you like to remain the same?
What do you like about those aspects of the relationship?
How does it make you feel when you are with the person?

QUESTIONS RELATED TO INTERPERSONAL ROLE DISPUTES

Are there any things that you and another significant person in your life cannot
    agree on?
What are those things?
What happens between the two of you when you try to talk about it?
How do you feel then? What do you do?
How do you get along with _____?
What does _____ say or do that makes you so angry?
What do you get into conflict about? How often?
What happens? What do you do?
How do you feel when it happens?
Can you tell _____ how you feel?
What stops you from telling _____ how you feel?
What helps you tell _____ how you feel?
Do you think _____ would understand?

QUESTIONS RELATED TO INTERPERSONAL DEFICITS

Do you have difficulty making friends? In what way?
Do you pick your friends or do they pick you?
How do you feel about meeting new people?
What is difficult about meeting new people?
What is OK about meeting and talking to new people?
How do you feel in new social situations?
Can you confide in anyone? Who?
How do you feel after you talk about your personal stuff with _____?
Do you often feel uncomfortable in your relationships? In what way?
Do you have a girlfriend/boyfriend?
What would you like to change about the relationship?
How do you feel about dating?

QUESTIONS RELATED TO GRIEF

Do you know anyone who has died recently?
How close to _____ were you?

How was that for you?
What was difficult about it for you?
Was there anyone who helped you feel better?
How do you think it affects your feelings now?
Is there anyone you talk to about these feelings? Now or in the past?

QUESTIONS RELATED TO ROLE TRANSITIONS

Have there been any changes in your family recently?
Have you had to adapt to anything new yourself, like a new school or new
    neighborhood?
What have they been?
What has it been like for you? Positive? Negative? In what way?
How has the change made you feel about yourself? Your family?
How has the change affected the way you get along with people in the family?
Have there been changes in other areas of your life?
What has been difficult about the change(s)?

Table B.1 illustrates how to use these questions in conducting the interpersonal inventory.

TABLE B.1. Interpersonal Inventory Flow Chart

1. Who are the significant people in your life?
   • Review each relationship—one at a time.
2. Three types of questions to ask:
   • Questions about facts or opinions
   • Questions about events that relate to these opinions
   • Questions about feelings associated with different aspects of the relationship

Example: Relationship with mother

Questions about facts/opinions	Questions about events	Questions about feelings
What do you like about your mom?		
What don't you like about your mom?		
How do you get along? →	What does she say or do that makes you angry? →	Have you ever told her how you feel?
	What do you get into conflict about? How often? What happened? What do you do? Can you give me an example? →	How do you feel when that happens? What helps you tell Mom how you feel?
What are the positive aspects of your relationship? →	What kinds of activities do you enjoy doing together? →	How do you feel when you are doing these things with Mom?
Do you think Mom would understand how you feel in these different situations? →	Can you give me an example of a situation in which you felt Mom showed you she understood? →	How did that make you feel?
Are there things in your relationship you would like to change? →	Can you give me an example of how a situation could be different? →	How would you feel if those things were different?
What things would you like to have remain the same?	→	How do those things make you feel better?

SESSION CHECKLISTS FOR INTERPERSONAL PSYCHOTHERAPY FOR DEPRESSED ADOLESCENTS

INITIAL PHASE

Week 1

- Review treatment plan and introduction to IPT-A.
- Review depression symptoms and confirm diagnosis.
- Review associated psychosocial history.
- Psychoeducation about depression: explain syndrome and treatment options.
- Assign limited sick role.
- Meet with parent(s) and provide psychoeducation about depression and treatment.
- Review session and plan for next session.

Week 2

- Review current depression symptoms for past week.
- Use mood rating.
- Complete closeness circle.
- Relate depression to current problems in adolescent's life.
- Begin interpersonal inventory.
- Evaluate impact of each relationship on mood and mood on relationship.
- Review session and plan for next session.

Week 3

- Review current depression symptoms for past week.
- Use mood rating.
- Continue interpersonal inventory.
  - Review positive and negative aspects of significant relationships.
- Review session and plan for next session.

Week 4

- Review current depression symptoms for past week.

- Use mood rating.
- Complete interpersonal inventory.
- Describe and identify specific problem area.
- Make explicit patient–therapist contract.
  - Agree on identified problem area.
  - Specify adolescent's role in sessions.
  - Specify therapist's role in sessions.
  - State policy on missed or cancelled sessions or late attendance, frequency of sessions.
  - Specify role of parents or other significant people in treatment.
- Review session and plan for next session.

GENERAL MIDDLE-PHASE SESSION STRUCTURE

Sessions 5–8

- Review current depression symptoms (use mood rating).
- Focus on identified problem area.
- Ask about any interpersonal problems in past week.
- Discuss in detail interpersonal events related to depression/irritable mood.

General IPT-A Techniques

- Encourage expression of affect.
- Directive techniques (education, advice giving, limit setting, modeling).
- Link affect to interpersonal events.
- Explore possible changes that could be made.
- Identify dysfunctional communications.
- Practice new communication strategies (communication analysis).
- Practice generating alternative solutions to problems.
- Practice decision-making process (decision analysis).
- Role-play alternative interpersonal interactions.
- Use patient–therapist relationship to provide interpersonal feedback.
- Involve significant others in sessions.

Grief

- Precipitants
  - Death of a loved one resulting in abnormal grief or normal grief.
- Presenting problems
  - Chronic, delayed, or distorted grief reaction.
  - Symptoms of excessive feelings of worthlessness, psychomotor retardation, and/or functional impairment.

- Reliving death vividly as if in present.
- Significant withdrawal or acting out.
- Goals
  - Facilitate the mourning process.
- Strategies
  - Encourage the adolescent to think about the loss in detail.
  - Review relationship with deceased in detail.
  - Connect current behaviors to feelings surrounding death.
  - Improve communication skills.
  - Develop supportive relationships.
  - Reintegrate into social milieu.

Interpersonal Role Disputes

- Precipitants
  - Conflict in a significant relationship.
  - Nonreciprocal expectations (i.e., conflict with parents over rules about dating, curfew, money, values, or responsibilities).
  - Difficulty playing different roles in various facets of their lives (i.e., child in school vs. parentified child at home).
- Presenting problems
  - Verbal arguments with parents and/or friends.
  - Avoidance of interaction.
  - Engaging in forbidden activities in secrecy.
  - Increasing anger and distrust in relationships.
- Goals
  - Define and resolve the dispute (Renegotiation and Impasse Stage).
  - Mourn the loss of the relationship (Dissolution Stage).
- Strategies
  - Explore dispute.
  - Identify dispute patterns.
  - Conduct decision analysis regarding how to proceed with relationship and dispute.
  - Improve communication and negotiation skills.

Role Transitions

- Precipitants
  - Expected or unexpected life transitions.
  - Examples include:
    - Change in family structure due to divorce, separation, illness, or death in the family.
    - Moving to a new school, including moving from middle to high school.

- First experience with dating relationships.
- Attempting to seek autonomy or independence from family.
- Adolescent pregnancy.
- Presenting problems
  - Teen takes on inappropriate responsibilities in family.
  - Poor communication in family system.
  - Lack of clarity in roles and expectations.
  - Teen loses support of impaired or absent parent.
  - Remaining parent less available for parenting.
  - Teen begins acting out or withdrawal from tasks associated with new role.
- Goals
  - Relinquish old role and accept new role.
  - Develop a sense of mastery over new role.
- Strategies
  - Education about the transition.
  - Review old and new roles: feelings and expectations.
  - Social skills assessment and development.
  - Develop social support network.

Interpersonal Deficits

- Precipitants
  - Depression leads to interpersonal skill lags or social withdrawal.
  - Presence of minor or circumscribed deficits exacerbated by depression or life events.
- Presenting problems
  - Social or communication skill deficits.
  - Examples include:
    - Inability to initiate relationships.
    - Inability to maintain relationship.
    - Difficulty expressing oneself verbally or effectively.
    - Difficulty eliciting information from others to establish communication.
- Goals
  - Reduce social isolation.
  - Improve and increase relationships by improving skills and increasing social self-confidence.
- Strategies
  - Review current and past relationships.
  - Explore interactions with the therapist.
  - Identify repetitive patterns and problems in relationships.
  - Highlight skills and strengths.
  - Build interpersonal skills.

TERMINATION: WEEKS 9–12

- Review depression symptoms for past week (use mood rating).
- Review warning symptoms of depression.
- Review identified problem area.
- Review identified strategies used in treatment.
- Review interpersonal successes and efforts to change.
- Discuss generalization of strategies to future situations.
- Discuss feelings about ending therapy.
- Discuss possibilities of recurrence and/or need for future/further treatment.
- Practice/model positive ending to a relationship.
- Meet with parents to review progress of treatment and plans for the future.

References

Alessi, N. E., & Robbins, D. R. (1984). Symptoms and subtypes of depression among adolescents distinguished by the dexamethasone suppression test: A preliminary report. *Psychiatry Research, 11,* 177–184.

Alessi, N. E., Robbins, D. R., & Dilsaver, S. C. (1987). Panic and depressive disorders among psychiatrically hospitalized adolescents. *Psychiatry Research, 20,* 275–283.

Altmann, E. O., & Gotlib, I. H. (1988). The social behavior of depressed children: An observational study. *Journal of Abnormal Child Psychology, 16,* 29–44.

Amato, P. R., & Keith, B. (1991). Parental divorce and the well-being of children: A meta-analysis. *Psychological Bulletin, 110,* 26–46.

American Academy of Child and Adolescent Psychiatry. (1998). Practice parameters for the assessment and treatment of children and adolescents with depressive disorders. *Journal of the American Academy of Child and Adolescent Psychiatry, 37*(Suppl. 10), 63S–83S.

American Psychiatric Association. (1987). *Diagnostic and statistical manual of mental disorders* (3rd ed., rev.). Washington, DC: Author.

American Psychiatric Association. (2000a). *Diagnostic and statistical manual of mental disorders* (4th ed., text rev.). Washington, DC: Author.

American Psychiatric Association. (2000b). Practice guideline for the treatment of patients with major depressive disorder (rev.). *American Journal of Psychiatry, 157*(Suppl. 4), 1–45.

Angold, A. (1988). Childhood and adolescent depression: II. Research in clinical populations. *British Journal of Psychiatry, 153,* 476–492.

Angold, A., Costello, E. J., & Erkanli, A. (1999). Comorbidity. *Journal of Child Psychology and Psychiatry, 40,* 57–87.

Angold, A., Weissman, M. M., John, K., Merikangas, K. R., Prusoff, B. A., Wickramaratne, P., et al. (1987). Parent and child reports of depressive symptoms in children at low and high risk of depression. *Journal of Child Psychology and Psychiatry, 28*(6), 901–915.

Angst, J., Merikangas, K., Scheidegger, P., & Wicki, W. (1990). Recurrent brief depression: A new subtype of affective disorder. *Journal of Affective Disorders, 19,* 87–98.

Baker, V. E., & Sedney, M. A. (1996). How bereaved children cope with loss: An overview. In C. A. Corr & D. M. Coor (Eds.), *Handbook of childhood, death and bereavement* (pp. 109–129). New York: Springer.

Balk, D. E., & Corr, C. A. (2001) Bereavement during adolescence: A review of research. In H. Stroebe & S. Stroebe (Eds.), *Handbook of bereavement research* (pp. 199–218). Washington DC: American Psychological Association.

Balk, D. E., & Vesta, L. (1998). Psychological development during four years of bereavement: A longitudinal case study. *Death Studies, 22,* 23–41.

Beardslee, W. R., Bemporad, J., Keller, M. B., Klerman, G. L., Dorer, D. J., & Samuelson, H. (1983). Children of parents with major affective disorder: A review. *American Journal of Psychiatry, 140,* 825–832.

Beck, A. T. (1967). *Depression: Clinical, experimental, and theoretical aspects.* New York: Harper & Row.

Beck, A. T., Rush, A. J., Shaw, B. F., & Emery, G. (1979). *Cognitive therapy of depression.* New York: Guilford Press.

Bemporad, J. (1988). Psychodynamic treatment of depressed adolescent. *Journal of Clinical Psychiatry, 49*(Suppl. 9), 26–31.

Bemporad, J., & Lee, K. W. (1988). Affective disorders. In C. Kestenbaum & D. Williams (Eds.), *Handbook of clinical assessment of children and adolescents* (Vol. II, pp. 626–650). New York: New York University Press.

Bernstein, G. A., & Garfinkel, B. D. (1986). School phobia: The overlap of affective and anxiety disorders. *Journal of the American Academy of Child and Adolescent Psychiatry, 25,* 235–241.

Biederman, J., Munir, K., Knee, D., Armentano, M., Autor, S., Waternaux, C., et al. (1987). High rate of affective disorder in probands with attention deficit disorder and in their relatives: A controlled family study. *American Journal of Psychiatry, 144,* 330–333.

Birmaher, B., & Brent, D. A. (2002). Pharmacotherapy for depression in children and adolescents. In D. Shaffer & B. D. Waslick (Eds.), *The many faces of depression in children and adolescents* (pp. 73–103). Washington, DC: American Psychiatric Publishing.

Birmaher, B., Brent, D. A., & Kolko, D. (2000). Clinical outcome after short-term psychotherapy for adolescents with major depressive disorder. *Archives of General Psychiatry, 57,* 29–36.

Birmaher, B., Ryan, N. D., Williamson, D. E., Brent, D. A., & Kaufman, J. (1996a). Childhood and adolescent depression: A review of the past 10 years. Part I. *Journal of the American Academy of Child and Adolescent Psychiatry, 35,* 1427–1439.

Birmaher B., Ryan, N. D., Williamson, D. E., Brent, D. A., & Kaufman, J. (1996b). Childhood and adolescent depression: A review of the past 10 years. Part II. *Journal of the American Academy of Child and Adolescent Psychiatry, 35,* 1575–1583.

Black, K., Shea, C., Dursun, S., & Kutcher, S. (2000). Selective serotonin reuptake inhibitor discontinuation syndrome: Proposed diagnostic criteria. *Journal of Psychiatry and Neuroscience, 25*(3), 255–261.

Blos, P. (1961). *On adolescence.* New York: Free Press of Glencoe.

Boszormenyi-Nagy, I., & Krasner, B. R. (1986). *Between give and take: A clinical guide to contextual therapy.* New York: Brunner/Mazel.

Bowlby, J. (1978). Attachment theory and its therapeutic implications. *Adolescent Psychiatry, 6,* 5–33.

Brent, D. A., Holder, D., Kolko, D., Birmaher, B., Baugher, M., Roth, C., et al. (1997). A clinical psychotherapy trial for adolescent depression comparing cognitive, family, and supportive therapy. *Archives of General Psychiatry, 54*(9), 877–885.

Brent, D. A., Kolko, D. J., Birmaher, B., Baugher, M., & Bridge, J. (1999). A clinical trial of adolescent depression: Predictors of additional treatment in the acute and follow-up phases of the trial. *Journal of the American Academy of Child and Adolescent Psychiatry, 38,* 263–270.

Brent, D. A., Perper, J. A., Montz, G., Liotus, L., Schweers, J., Roth, C., et al. (1993). Psychiatric impact of the loss of an adolescent sibling to suicide. *Journal of Affective Disorders, 28,* 249–256.

Brody, G., & Forehand, R. (1990). Interparental conflict, relationship with the noncustodial father, and adolescent post-divorce adjustment. *Journal of Applied Developmental Psychology, 11,* 139–147.

Brown, D., Winsberg, B. G., Bialer, I., & Press, M. (1973). Imipramine therapy and seizures: Three children treated for hyperactive behavior disorders. *American Journal of Psychiatry, 130,* 210–212.

Brown, G. W., & Harris, T. (1978). *The social origins of depression: A study of psychiatric disorders in women.* New York: Free Press.

Brown, G. W., Harris, T., & Copeland, J. R. (1977). Depression and loss. *British Journal of Psychiatry, 130,* 1–18.

Burns, B. J. (1991). Mental health service use by adolescents in the 1970s and 1980s. *Journal of the American Academy of Child and Adolescent Psychiatry, 30*(1), 144–150.

Carlson, G., & Cantwell, D. (1980). Unmasking masked depression in children and adolescents. *American Journal of Psychiatry, 137,* 445–449.

Carlson, G., & Strober, M. (1979). Affective disorders in adolescence. *Psychiatric Clinics of North America, 2,* 511–526.

Chambers, W. J., Puig-Antich, J., Hirsch, M., Paez, P., Ambrosini, P. J., Tabrizi, M. A., & Davies, M. (1985). The assessment of affective disorders in children and adolescents by semistructured interview: Test–retest reliability of the schedule for affective disorders and schizophrenia for school-age children, present episode version. *Archives of General Psychiatry, 42,* 696–702.

Cherlin, A. J., & Furstenberg, F. F. (1994). Stepfamilies in the United States: A reconsideration. *Annual Review of Sociology, 20,* 359–381.

Christie, K. A., Burke, J. D., Reiger, D. A., Rae, D. S., Boyd, J. H., & Locke, B. Z. (1989). Epidemiologic evidence for early onset of mental disorders and higher risk of drug abuse in young adults. *American Journal of Psychiatry, 145,* 971–975.

Clark, D., Pynoos, R. & Goebel, A. (1994). Mechanisms and processes of adolescent bereavement. In R. Haggerty (Ed.), *Stress, risk, and resilience in children
and adolescents: Processes, mechanisms, and interventions* (pp. 100–145).
Cambridge, UK: Cambridge University Press.

Clarke, G. N., Hawkins, W., Murphy, M., & Sheeber, L. B. (1995). Targeted prevention of unipolar depressive disorder in an at-risk sample of high school adolescents: A randomized trial of group cognitive intervention. *Journal of the
American Academy of Child and Adolescent Psychiatry, 34,* 312–321.

Clarke, G. N., Hops, H., Lewinsohn, P. M., & Andrews, J. (1992). Cognitive-
behavioral group treatment of adolescent depression: Prediction of outcome.
Behavior Therapy, 23, 341–354.

Clarke, G. N., Rohde, P., Lewinsohn, P. M., Hops, H., & Seeley, J. R. (1999). Cognitive-behavioral treatment of adolescent depression: Efficacy of acute group
treatment and booster sessions. *Journal of the American Academy of Child
and Adolescent Psychiatry, 38,* 272–279.

Corey, G. (1981). *Theory and practice of group counseling* (2nd ed.). Monterey,
CA: Brooks/Cole.

Costello, E. J., Angold, A., Burns, B. J., Stangl, D. K., Tweed, D. L., Erkanli, A., et
al. (1996). The Great Smoky Mountains Study of Youth: Goals, design, methods, and the prevalence of DSM-III-R disorders. *Archives of General Psychiatry, 53,* 1129–1136.

Costello, E. J., Erkanli, A., Federman, E., & Angold, A. (1999). Development of
psychiatric comorbidity with substance abuse in adolescents: Effects of timing and sex. *Journal of Clinical Child Psychology, 28*(3), 298–311.

Costello, E. J., Pine, D., Hammen, C., March, J. S., Plotsky, P. M., Weissman, M.
M., et al. (2002). Development and natural history of mood disorders. *Biological Psychiatry, 52,* 529–542.

Coyne, J. (1976). Towards an interactional description of depression. *Psychiatry,
39,* 28.

Cytryn, L., & McKnew, D. H. (1972). Proposed classification of childhood depression. *American Journal of Psychiatry, 129,* 63–69.

Cytryn, L., & McKnew, D. H. (1985). Treatment issues in childhood depression.
Psychiatric Annals, 15, 401–403.

Cytryn, L., McKnew, D. H., Zahn-Waxler, C., & Gershon, E. S. (1986). Developmental issues in risk research: The offspring of affectively ill parents. In M.
Rutter, C. E. Izard, & P. B. Read (Eds.), *Depression in young people: Developmental and clinical perspectives* (pp. 163–189). New York: Guilford Press.

Diamond, G. S., Reis, B. F., Diamond, G. M., Siqueland, L., & Isaacs, L. (2002).
Attachment-based family therapy for depressed adolescents: A treatment de-
velopment study. *Journal of the American Academy of Child and Adolescent
Psychiatry, 41*(10), 1190–1196.

Diamond, G. S., Serrano, A. C., Dickey, M., & Sonis, W. A. (1996). Current status
of family-based outcome and process research. *Journal of the American
Academy of Child and Adolescent Psychiatry, 35*(1), 6–16.

Diamond, G., & Siqueland, L. (1995). Family therapy for the treatment of depressed adolescents. *Psychotherapy: Theory, Research, Practice, Training,
32*(1), 77–90.

DiMascio, A., Weissman, M. M., Prusoff, B. A., New, C., Zwilling, M., & Klerman, G. L. (1979). Differential symptom reduction by drugs and psychotherapy in acute depression. *Archives of General Psychiatry, 36,* 450–456.

Downey, G., & Coyne, J. (1990). Children of depressed parents: An integrated review. *Psychological Bulletin, 108*(1), 50–76.

Edelbrock, C. S., Costello, A. J., Dulcan, M., Kalas, R., & Conover, N. C. (1985). Age differences in the reliability of the psychiatric interview of the child. *Child Development, 56*(1), 265–275.

Eissler, K. R. (1958). Notes on problems of technique in the psychoanalytic treatment of adolescents. *Psychoanalytic Study of the Child, 13,* 223–254.

Elkin, I., Shea, M. T., Watkins, J. T., Imber, S. D., Sotsky, S. M., Collins, J. F., et al. (1989). National Institute of Mental Health Treatment of Depression Collaborative Research Program: General effectiveness of treatment. *Archives of General Psychiatry, 46,* 971–983.

Emery, G., Bedrosian, R., & Garber, J. (1983). Cognitive therapy with depressed children and adolescents. In D. P. Cantwell & G. A. Carlson (Eds.), *Affective disorders in childhood and adolescence: An update* (pp. 445–471). New York: Spectrum.

Emslie, G. J., Heiligenstein, J. H., Wagner, K. D., Hoog, S. L., Ernest, D. E., Brown, E., et al. (2002). Fluoxetine for acute treatment of depression in children and adolescents: A placebo-controlled randomized clinical trial. *Journal of the American Academy of Child and Adolescent Psychiatry, 41*(10), 1205–1214.

Emslie, G. J., Rush, A. J., Weinberg, W. A., Kowatch, R. A., Carmody, T., & Mayes, T. L. (1998). Fluoxetine in child and adolescent depression: acute and maintenance treatment. *Depression and Anxiety, 7,* 32–39.

Emslie, G. J., Rush, A. J., Weinberg, W. A., Kowatch, R. A., Hughes, C. W., Carmody, T., et al. (1997). A double-blind, randomized, placebo-controlled trial of fluoxetine in children and adolescents with depression. *Archives of General Psychiatry, 54*(11), 1031–1037.

Erikson, E. (1968). *Identity, youth and crisis.* New York: Norton.

Fendrich, M., Warner, V., & Weissman, M. M. (1990). Family risk factors, parental depression, and psychopathology in offspring. *Developmental Psychology, 26*(19), 40–50.

Fergusson, D. M., Horwood, L. J. & Lynskey, M. T. (1995). Maternal depressive symptoms and depressive symptoms in adolescents. *Journal of Child Psychology and Psychiatry, 36,* 1161–1178.

Fine, S., Forth, A., Gilbert, M., & Haley, G. (1991). Group therapy for adolescent depressive disorder: A comparison of social skills and therapeutic support. *Journal of the American Academy of Child and Adolescent Psychiatry, 30*(1), 79–85.

Fine, S., Gilbert, M., Schmidt, L., Haley, G., Maxwell, A., & Forth, A. (1989). Short-term group therapy with depressed adolescent outpatients. *Canadian Journal of Psychiatry, 34,* 97–102.

Frank, E., Kupfer, D. J., Perel, J. M., Cornes, C., Jarrett, D. B., Mallinger, A. G., et al. (1990). Three-year outcomes for maintenance therapies in recurrent depression. *Archives of General Psychiatry, 47*(12), 1093–1099.

Frank, E., Kupfer, D. J., Wagner, E. F., McEachran, A. B., & Cornes, C. (1991). Efficacy of interpersonal psychotherapy as a maintenance treatment of recurrent depression: contributing factors. *Archives of General Psychiatry, 48,* 1053–1059.

Freud, A. (1958). Adolescence. *Psychoanalytic Study of the Child, 16,* 225–278.

Fristad, M. A., Gavazzi, S. M., & Soldano, K. W. (1998). Multi-family psychoeducation groups for childhood mood disorders. *Contemporary Family Therapy, 20,* 385–402.

Furman, W., & Buhrmester, D. (1992). Age and sex differences in perceptions of networks of personal relationships. *Child Development, 63,* 103–115.

Garber, J., Kriss, M. R., Koch, M., & Lindholm, L. (1988). Recurrent depression in adolescents: A follow-up study. *Journal of the American Academy of Child and Adolescent Psychiatry, 27*(1), 49–54.

Garfield, S. L. (1986). Research on client variables in psychotherapy. In S. L. Garfield & A. E. Bergin (Eds.), *Handbook of psychotherapy and behavior change* (3rd ed., pp. 213–256). New York: Wiley.

Geis, H., Whittlesey, W., McDonald, N., Smith, K. & Pfefferbaum, B. (1998). Bereavement and loss in childhood. In B. Pfefferbaum (Ed.), *Childhood and adolescent psychiatric clinics of North America: Vol. 7. Stress in children* (pp. 73–85). Philadelphia: Saunders.

Geller, B., Zimmerman, B., Williams, M., Bolhofner. K., & Craney, J. L. (2001). Bipolar disorder at prospective follow-up of adults who had prepubertal major depressive disorder. *American Journal of Psychiatry, 158,* 125–127.

Ghali, S. B. (1977). Culture sensitivity and the Puerto Rican client. *Social Casework, 58,* 459–468.

Goodman, S. H., Schwab-Stone, M., Lahey, B. B., Shaffer, D., & Jensen, P. S. (2000). Major depression and dysthymia in children and adolescents: Discriminant validity and differential consequences in a community sample. *Journal of the American Academy of Child and Adolescent Psychiatry, 39,* 761–770.

Gould, M. S., King, R., Greenwald, S., Fisher, P., Schwab-Stone, M., Kramer, R., et al. (1998). Psychopathology associated with suicidal ideation and attempts among children and adolescents. *Journal of the American Academy of Child and Adolescent Psychiatry, 37,* 915–923.

Gray, R. E. (1987). Adolescent response to the death of a parent. *Journal of Youth and Adolescence, 16*(6), 511–525.

Haley, J. (1976). *Problem-solving therapy: New strategies for effective family therapy.* New York: Jossey-Bass.

Hall, G. S. (1904). *Adolescence: Its psychology and its relations to physiology, anthropology, sociology, sex, crime, religion, and education.* New York: Appleton.

Hammen, C. (1999). The emergence of an interpersonal approach to depression. In T. Joiner & J. C. Coyne (Eds.), *The interactional nature of depression: Advances in interpersonal approaches* (pp. 21–37). Washington DC: American Psychological Association.

Hammen, C., Burge, D., Burney, E., & Adrian, C. (1990). Longitudinal study of diagnoses in children of women with unipolar and bipolar affective disorder. *Archives of General Psychiatry, 47,* 1112–1117.

Hammen, C., Rudolph, K., Weisz, J., Rao, U., & Burge, D. (1999). The context of depression in clinic-referred youth: Neglected areas in treatment. *Journal of the American Academy of Child and Adolescent Psychiatry, 38*(1), 64–71.

Hardy-Fanta, C., & Montana, P., (1982). The Hispanic female adolescent: A group therapy model. *International Journal of Group Psychotherapy. 32,* 351–366.

Harold, G. T., Fincham, F. D., Osborne, L. N., & Conger, R. D. (1997). Mom and Dad are at it again: Adolescent perceptions of marital conflict and adolescent psychological distress. *Developmental Psychology. 33,* 333–350.

Harrington, R. C., Fudge, H., Rutter, M., Pickles, A., & Hill, J. (1990). Adult outcomes of childhood and adolescent depression. *Archives of General Psychiatry, 47,* 465–473.

Harrington, R., Whittaker, J., & Shoebridge, P. (1998). Psychological treatment of depression in children and adolescents: A review of treatment research. *British Journal of Psychiatry, 173,* 291–298.

Hersen, H., & Van Hasselt, V. B. (Eds.). (1987). *Behavior therapy with children and adolescents: A clinical approach.* New York: Wiley.

Hetherington, E. M. (1989). Coping with family transitions: Winners, losers, and survivors. *Child Development, 60,* 1–14.

Hetherington, E. M. (1997). Teenaged childbearing and divorce. In S. S. Luthar, J. A. Burack, D. Cicchetti, & J. Weisz (Eds.), *Developmental psychopathology: Perspectives on adjustment, risk, and disorder* (pp. 350–373). New York: Cambridge University Press.

Hetherington, E. M., Bridges, M., & Insabella, G. M. (1998). What matters? What does not?: Five perspectives on the association between marital transitions and children's adjustment. *American Psychologist, 53,* 167–184.

Hoberman, H. M. (1992). Ethnic minority status and adolescent mental health services utilization. *Journal of Mental Health Administration, 19*(3), 246–267.

Holahan, C. J., Moos R. H., & Bonin, L. A. (1999). Social context and depression: An integrative stress and coping framework. In T. Joiner & J. C. Coyne (Eds.), *The interactional nature of depression: Advances in interpersonal approaches* (pp. 39–65). Washington, DC: American Psychological Association.

Horowitz, L. M. (1996). The study of interpersonal problems: A Leary legacy. *Journal of Personality Assessment, 66*(2), 283–300.

Horowitz, M. (1976). *Stress response syndromes.* New York: Jason Aronson.

Howard, K. I., Kopata, S. M., Krause, M. S., & Orlinsky, D. E. (1986). The dose–effect relationship in psychotherapy. *American Psychologist, 41,* 159–164.

Hughes, C. W., Emslie, G. J., Crismon, M. L., Wagner, K. D., Birmaher, B., Geller, B., et al. (1999). The Texas Children's Medication Algorithm Project: Report of the Texas Consensus Conference Panel on medication treatment of childhood major depressive disorder. *Journal of the American Academy of Child Psychiatry, 38*(11), 1442–1454.

Hussong, A. (2000). Perceived peer context and adolescent adjustment. *Journal of Research on Adolescence, 10,* 391–415.

Kandel, D. B., & Davies, M. (1986). Adult sequelae of adolescent depressive symptoms. *Archives of General Psychiatry, 43,* 255–262.

Kashani, J. H., Burbach, D. J., & Rosenberg, T. K. (1988). Perceptions of family conflict resolution and depressive symptomatology. *Journal of the American Academy of Child and Adolescent Psychiatry, 27*(1), 42–48.

Kashani, J. H., Carlson, G. A., Beck, N. C., Hoeper, E. W., Corcoran, C. M., McAllister, J. A., et al. (1987). Depression, depressive symptoms, and depressed mood among a community sample of adolescents. *American Journal of Psychiatry, 144*(7), 931–941.

Kashani, J. H., Orvaschel, H., Burke, J. P., & Reid, J. C. (1985). Informant variance: The issue of parent–child disagreement. *Journal of the American Academy of Child Psychiatry, 24*(4), 437–441.

Kashani, J. H., Rosenberg, T. K., & Reigh, N. C. (1989). Developmental perspectives in child and adolescent depressive symptoms in a community sample. *American Journal of Psychiatry, 146*, 871–875.

Kaslow, N. J., & Thompson, M. P. (1998). Applying the criteria for empirically supported treatments to studies of psychosocial interventions for child and adolescent depression. *Journal of Clinical Child Psychology, 27*, 146–155.

Kazdin, A. E., French, N. H., Unis, A. S., & Esveldt-Dawson, K. (1983). Assessment of childhood depression. *Journal of the American Academy of Child and Adolescent Psychiatry, 22*, 157–164.

Keller, M. B., Beardslee, W. R., Lavori, P. W., & Wunder, J. (1988). Course of major depression in nonreferred adolescents: A retrospective study. *Journal of Affective Disorders, 15*, 235–243.

Keller, M. B., Lavori, P. W., Beardslee, W. R., Wunder, J., & Ryan, N. (1991). Depression in children and adolescents: New data on the "undertreatment" and a literature review in the efficacy of available treatments. *Journal of Affective Disorders, 21*, 163–171.

Keller, M. B., McCullough, J. P., Klein, D. N., Arnow, B., Dunner, D. L., Gelenberg, A. J., et al. (2000). A comparison of nefazodone, the cognitive behavioral-analysis system of psychotherapy, and their combination for the treatment of chronic depression. *New England Journal of Medicine, 342*(20), 1462–1470.

Keller, M. B., Ryan, N. D., Strober, M., Klein, R. G., Kutcher, S. P., Birmaher, B., et al. (2001). Efficacy of paroxetine in the treatment of adolescent major depression: A randomized, controlled study. *Journal of the American Academy of Child and Adolescent Psychiatry, 40*, 762–772.

Kessler, R. C., & Walters, E. E. (1998). Epidemiology of DSM-III-R major depression and minor depression among adolescents and young adults in the national comorbidity survey. *Depression and Anxiety, 7*, 3–14.

Kestenbaum, C. J., & Kron, L. (1987). Psychoanalytic intervention with children and adolescents with affective disorders: A combined treatment approach. *Journal of the American Academy of Psychoanalysis, 15*(2), 153–174.

Kiesler, D. J. (1979). An interpersonal communication analysis of relationship in psychotherapy. *Psychiatry, 42*, 299–311.

Kiesler, D. J. (1983). The 1982 interpersonal circle: A taxonomy for complementarity in human transactions. *Psychological Review, 90*, 185–214.

King, N. J., & Berstein, G. A. (2001). School refusal in children and adolescents: A review of the past 10 years. *Journal of the American Academy of Child and Adolescent Psychiatry, 40*, 197–205.

Klein, D. N., Lewinsohn, P. M., Seeley, J. R., & Rohde, P. (2001). A family study of major depressive disorder in a community sample of adolescents. *Archives of General Psychiatry, 58,* 13–20.

Klerman, G. L., DiMascio, A., Weissman, M. M., Prusoff, B., & Paykel, E. S. (1974). Treatment of depression by drugs and psychotherapy. *American Journal of Psychiatry, 131*(2), 186–194.

Klerman, G. L., Weissman, M. M., Rounsaville, B. J., & Chevron, E. (1984). *Interpersonal psychotherapy for depression.* New York: Basic Books.

Kovacs, M. (1979). The efficacy of cognitive and behavioral therapies for depression. *American Journal of Psychiatry, 137,* 1495–1501.

Kovacs, M. (1996). Presentation and course of major depressive disorder during childhood and later years of the life span. *Journal of the American Academy of Child and Adolescent Psychiatry, 35*(6), 705–715.

Kovacs, M. (1997). Depressive disorders in childhood: An impressionistic landscape. *Journal of Child Psychology and Psychiatry, 38,* 287–298.

Kovacs, M., Akiskal, H. S., Gatsonis, C., & Parrone, P. L. (1994). Childhood-onset dysthymic disorder: Clinical features and prospective naturalistic outcome. *Archives of General Psychiatry, 51,* 365–374.

Kovacs, M., Devlin, B., Pollack, M., Richards, C., & Mukerji, P. (1997a). A controlled family history study of childhood-onset depressive disorder. *Archives of General Psychiatry, 54,* 613–623.

Kovacs, M., Feinberg, T. L., Crouse-Novak, M. A., Paulauskas, S. L., & Finkelstein, R. (1984). Depressive disorders in childhood I: A longitudinal prospective study of characteristics and recovery. *Archives of General Psychiatry, 41,* 229–237.

Kovacs, M., Gatsonis, C., Paulauskas, S. L., & Richards, C. (1989). Depressive disorders in childhood IV: A longitudinal study of comorbidity with and risk for anxiety disorders. *Archives of General Psychiatry, 46,* 776–782.

Kovacs, M., Obrosky, D. S., Gatsonis, C., & Richard, C. (1997b). First-episode major depressive and dysthymic disorder in childhood: Clinical and sociodemographic factors in recovery. *Journal of the American Academy of Child and Adolescent Psychiatry, 36*(6), 777–784.

Kupfer, D. J., Frank, E., & Perel, J. M. (1989). The advantage of early treatment intervention in recurrent depression. *Archives of General Psychiatry, 46,* 771–775.

Leaf, P. J., Alegria, M., Cohen, P., Goodman, S. H., Horwitz, S. M., Hoven, C. W., et al. (1996). Mental health service use in the community and schools: Results from the four-community MECA study. *Journal of the Academy of Child and Adolescent Psychiatry, 35,* 889–897.

Lebowitz, B. D. (2000). A public health approach to clinical therapeutics in psychiatry: Directions for new research. *Dialogues of Clinical Neuroscience, 2*(3), 309–313.

Leon, G. R., Kendall, P. C., & Garber, J. (1980). Depression in children: Parents, teacher, and child perspectives. *Journal of Abnormal Child Psychology, 8*(2), 221–235.

Levy, J., & Deykin, E. Y. (1989). Suicidality, depression, and substance abuse in adolescence. *American Journal of Psychiatry, 146,* 1462–1467.

Lewinsohn, P. M., Antonuccio, D. O., Steinmetz, J., & Teri, L. (1984). *The coping with depression course: A psychoeducational intervention for unipolar depression.* Eugene, OR: Castalia.

Lewinsohn, P. M., & Clarke, G. N. (1999). Psychosocial treatments for adolescent depression. *Clinical Psychology Review, 19,* 329–342.

Lewinsohn, P. M., Clarke, G. N., Hops, H., & Andrews, J. (1990). Cognitive-behavioral treatment for depressed adolescents. *Behavior Therapy, 21,* 385–401.

Lewinsohn, P. M., Clarke, G. N., Rohde, P, Hops, H., & Seeley, J. R. (1996). A course in coping: A cognitive-behavioral approach to the treatment of adolescent depression. In E. D. Hibbs & P. S. Jensen (Eds.), *Psychosocial treatments for child and adolescent disorders: Empirically based strategies for clinical practice* (pp. 109–135). Washington DC: American Psychiatric Press.

Lewinsohn, P. M., Clarke, G. N., Seeley, J. R., & Rohde, P. (1994a). Major depression in community adolescents: Age at onset, episode duration, and time to recurrence. *Journal of the American Academy of Child and Adolescent Psychiatry, 33*(6), 809–818.

Lewinsohn, P. M., Roberts, R. E., Seeley, J. R., Rohde, P., Gotlib, I. H., & Hops, H. (1994b). Adolescent psychopathology II: Psychosocial risk factors for depression. *Journal of Abnormal Psychology, 103*(2), 302–315.

Lewinsohn, P. M., Rohde, P., Klein, D. N., & Seeley, J. R. (1999). Natural course of adolescent major depressive disorder: I. Continuity into young adulthood. *Journal of the American Academy of Child and Adolescent Psychiatry, 38,* 56–63.

Lewinsohn, P. M., Weinstein, M., & Shaw, D. (1969). Depression: A clinical-research approach. In R. Rubin & C. Frank (Eds.), *Advances in behavior therapy* (pp. 231–240). New York: Academic Press.

Lieb, R., Isensee, B., Hofler, M., Pfister, H., & Wittchen, H. (2002). Parental major depression and the risk of depression and other mental disorders in offspring: A prospective–longitudinal community study. *Archives of General Psychiatry, 59,* 365–374.

Liebowitz, J. H., & Kernberg, P. F. (1988). Psychodynamic psychotherapies. In C. J. Kestenbaum & D. T. Williams (Eds.), *Handbook of clinical assessment of children and adolescents* (Vol. II, pp. 1045–1065). New York: New York University Press.

Lowenstein, A. (1986). Temporary single parenthood: The case of prisoners' families. *Family Relations, 35,* 79–85.

Mandoki, M. W., Tapia, M. R., Tapia, M. A., & Sumner, G. S. (1997). Venlafaxine in the treatment of children and adolescents with major depression. *Psychopharmacology Bulletin, 33*(1), 149–154.

Marriage, K., Fine, S., Moretti, M., & Haley, B. (1986). Relationship between depression and conduct disorder in children and adolescents. *Journal of the American Academy of Child and Adolescent Psychiatry, 25*(5), 687–691.

Martin, A., Kaufman, J., & Charney, D. (2000). Pharmacotherapy of early onset: Update and new directions. *Child and Adolescent Psychiatric Clinics of North America, 9,* 135–137.

Marx, E., & Schulze, C. (1991). Interpersonal problem-solving in depressed students. *Journal of Clinical Psychology, 47,* 361–367.

Marx, E., & Schulze, C. (1991). Interpersonal problem-solving in depressed students. *Journal of Clinical Psychology, 47,* 361–367.

Matson, J. L. (1989). *Treating depression in children and adolescents.* New York: Pergamon Press.

McCauley, E., Myers, K., Mitchell, J., Calderon, R., Schloredt, K., & Treder, R. (1993). Depression in young people: Initial presentation and clinical course. *Journal of the American Academy of Child and Adolescent Psychiatry, 32,* 714–722.

McGoldrick, M., & Walsh, F. (1991). A time to mourn: Death and the family life cycle. In F. Walsh & M. McGoldrick (Eds.), *Living beyond loss: Death in the family.* New York: Norton.

Meyer, A. (1957). *Psychobiology: A science of man.* Springfield, IL: Thomas.

Middleton, W., Moylan, A., Raphael, B., Burnett, P., & Martinek, N. (1993). An international perspective on bereavement-related concepts. *Australian and New Zealand Journal of Psychiatry, 27,* 457–463.

Minuchin, S. (1974). *Families and family therapy.* Cambridge, MA: Harvard University Press.

Mitchell, J., McCauley, E., Burke, P. M., & Moss, S. J. (1988). Phenomenology of depression in children and adolescents. *Journal of the American Academy of Child and Adolescent Psychiatry, 27*(1), 12–20.

Monck, E., Graham, P., Richman, N., & Dobbs, R. (1994a). Adolescent girls: I. Self-reported mood disturbance in a community population. *British Journal of Psychiatry, 165,* 760–769.

Monck, E., Graham, P., Richman, N., & Dobbs, R. (1994b). Adolescent girls: II. Background factors in anxiety and depressive states. *British Journal of Psychiatry, 165,* 770–780.

Moretti, M. M., Fine, S., Haley, G., & Marriage, K. (1985). Childhood and adolescent depression. *Journal of the American Academy of Child and Adolescent Psychiatry, 24,* 298–302.

Mueller, C., & Orvaschel, H. (1997). The failure of "adult" interventions with adolescent depression: What does it mean for theory, research, and practice? *Journal of Affective Disorders, 44,* 203–215.

Mufson, L., Pollack Dorta, K., Wickramaratne, P., Nomura, Y., Olfson, M., & Weissman, M. M. (2004a). A randomized effectiveness trial of interpersonal psychotherapy for depressed adolescents. *Archives of General Psychiatry, 61,* 577–584.

Mufson, L., Gallagher, T., Pollack Dorta, K., & Young, J. F. (2004b). Interpersonal psychotherapy for adolescent depression: Adaptation for group therapy. *American Journal of Psychotherapy, 58*(2), 220–237.

Mufson, L., Moreau, D., Weissman, M. M., & Klerman, G. L. (1993). *Interpersonal psychotherapy for depressed adolescents.* New York: Guilford Press.

Mufson, L., Moreau, D., Weissman, M. M., Wickramaratne, P., Martin, J., & Samoilov, A. (1994). The modification of Interpersonal Psychotherapy with Depressed Adolescents (IPT-A): Phase I and II studies. *Journal of the American Academy of Child and Adolescent Psychiatry, 33*(5), 695–705.

Mufson, L., & Velting, D. M. (2002). Psychotherapy for depression and suicidal behavior in children and adolescents. In D. Shaffer & B. D. Waslick (Eds.), of interpersonal psychotherapy for depressed adolescents. *Archives of General Psychiatry, 56,* 573–579.

Nichols, M. (1984). *Family therapy: Concepts and methods.* New York: Gardner Press.

Nissen, G. (1986). Treatment for depression in children and adolescents. *Psychopathology, 19*(Suppl. 2), 152–161.

Offer, D. (1969). Adolescent turmoil. *The psychological world of the teenager: A study of normal adolescent boys* (pp. 174–193). New York: Basic Books.

Offer, D., Ostrov, E., & Howard, K. (1982). The mental health professional concept of the normal adolescent. In S. Chess & A. Thomas (Eds.), *Annual progress in child psychiatry and development* (pp. 593–601). New York: Brunner/Mazel.

Olfson, M., Marcus, S. C., Weissman, M. M., & Jensen, P. S. (2002). National trends in the use of psychotropic medications by children. *Journal of the American Academy of Child and Adolescent Psychiatry, 41,* 514–521.

Orvaschel, H. (1990). Early onset psychiatric disorder in high risk children and increased familial morbidity. *Journal of the American Academy of Child and Adolescent Psychiatry, 29*(2), 184–188.

Osterweis, M., Solomon, F., & Green, M. (Eds.). (1984). *Bereavement: Reactions, consequences, and care* (pp. 99–145). Washington, DC: National Academy Press.

Parker, G. (1979). Parental characteristics in relation to depressive disorders. *British Journal of Psychiatry, 134,* 138–147.

Pine, D. S., Cohen, P., Gurley, D., Brook, J. S., & Ma, Y. (1998). The risk for early adulthood anxiety and depressive disorders in adolescents with anxiety and depressive disorders. *Archives of General Psychiatry, 55,* 56–64.

Puig-Antich, J. (1982). Major depression and conduct disorder in prepuberty. *Journal of the American Academy of Child and Adolescent Psychiatry, 21*(2), 118–128.

Puig-Antich, J., Goetz, D., Davies, M., Kaplan, T., Davies, S., Ostrow, L., et al. (1989). A controlled family history study of prepubertal major depressive disorder. *Archives of General Psychiatry, 46,* 406–418.

Puig-Antich, J., Kaufman, J., Ryan, N. D., Williamson, D. E., Dahl, R. E., Lukens, E., et al. (1993). The psychosocial functioning and family environment of depressed adolescents. *Journal of the American Academy of Child and Adolescent Psychiatry, 32,* 244–253.

Puig-Antich, J., Lukens, E., Davies, M., Goetz, D., Brennan-Quattrock, J., & Todak, G. (1985a). Psychosocial functioning in prepubertal depressive disorders I. Interpersonal relationships during the depressive episode. *Archives of General Psychiatry, 42,* 500–507.

Puig-Antich, J., Lukens, E., Davies, M., Goetz, D., Brennan-Quattrock, J., & Todak, G. (1985b). Psychosocial functioning in prepubertal depressive disorders II: Interpersonal relationships after sustained recovery from affective episode. *Archives of General Psychiatry, 42,* 511–517.

Raphael, B. (1983). *Anatomy of bereavement* New York: Basic Books.

Raphael, B. (1997). The interaction of trauma and grief. In D. Black, M. Newman, J. H. Hendricks, & G. Mezey (Eds.), *Psychological trauma: A developmental approach* (pp. 31–43). London: Gaskell.

Rao, U., Hammen, C., & Daley, S. (1999). Continuity of depression during the transition to adulthood: A 5-year longitudinal study of young women. *Journal of the American Academy of Child and Adolescent Psychiatry, 38,* 908–915.

Rao, U., Ryan, N. D., Birmaher, B., Dahl, R. E., Williamson, D. E., Kaufman, J., et al. (1995). Unipolar depression in adolescents: Clinical outcome in adulthood. *Journal of the American Academy of Child and Adolescent Psychiatry, 34,* 566–578.

Rao, U., Weissman, M. M., Martin, J. A, & Hammond, R. W. (1993). Childhood depression and risk of suicide: A preliminary report of a longitudinal study. *Journal of the American Academy of Child and Adolescent Psychiatry, 32,* 21–27.

Reinecke, M. A., Ryan, N. E., & DuBois, D. L. (1998). Cognitive-behavioral therapy of depression and depressive symptoms during adolescence: A review and meta-analysis. *Journal of the American Academy of Child and Adolescent Psychiatry, 37*(1), 26–34.

Reinherz, H. Z., Gianconia, R. M., Pakiz, B., Silverman, A. B., Frost, A. K., & Lefkowiatz, E. S. (1993). Psychosocial risks for major depression in late adolescence: A longitudinal community study. *Journal of the American Academy of Child and Adolescent Psychiatry, 32,* 1155–1163.

Reinherz, H. Z., Stewart-Berghauer, G., Pakiz, B., Frost, A. K., Moeykens, B. A., & Holmes, W. M. (1989). The relationship of early risk and current mediators to depressive symptomatology in adolescents. *Journal of the American Academy of Child and Adolescent Psychiatry, 28*(6), 942–947.

Research Units of Pediatric Psychopharmacology Anxiety Group. (2001). Fluvoxamine for anxiety in children. *New England Journal of Medicine, 344,* 1279–1285.

Reynolds, C., & Imber, S. (1988). *Maintenance therapies in late-life depression* (MH #43832). Bethesda, MD: National Institute of Mental Health.

Reynolds, W. M., & Coats, K. I. (1986). A comparison of cognitive-behavioral therapy and relaxation training for the treatment of depression in adolescents. *Journal of Consulting and Clinical Psychology, 44,* 653–660.

Rohde, P., Lewinsohn, P., & Seeley, J. R. (1991). Comorbidity of unipolar depression: II. Comorbidity with other mental disorders in adolescent and adults. *Journal of Abnormal Psychology, 100,* 214–222.

Rosselló, J., & Bernal, G. (1999). The efficacy of cognitive-behavioral and international treatments depression in Puerto Rican adolescents. *Journal of Consulting and Clinical Psychology, 67*(5), 734–745.

Rounsaville, B. J., Chevron, E. S., Weissman, M. M., Prusoff, B. A., & Frank, E. (1986). Training therapists to perform interpersonal psychotherapy in clinical trials. *Comprehensive Psychiatry, 27,* 364–371.

Rutter, M. (1979). *Changing youth in a changing world.* London: Nuffield.

Rutter, M., Graham, P., Chadwick, F. D., & Yule, W. (1976). Adolescent turmoil: Fact or fiction? *Journal of Child Psychology and Psychiatry, 17,* 35–56.

Ryan, N. D., Puig-Antich, J., Ambrosini, P., Rabinovich, H., Robinson, D., Nelson, B., et al. (1987). The clinical picture of major depression in children and adolescents. *Archives of General Psychiatry, 44,* 854–861.

Sandler, I. N., Miller, P., Short, J. & Wolchik, S. A. (1989). Social support as a protective factor for children in stress. In D. Belle (Ed.), *Children's social networks and social supports* (pp. 207–307). New York: Wiley.

Sanford, M., Szatmarc, P., Spinner, M., Munroe-Blum, H., Jamieson, E., Walsh, C., & Jones, D. (1995) Predicting the one-year course of adolescent major depression. *Journal of the American Academy of Child and Adolescent Psychiatry, 34*, 1618–1628.

Schilling, R., Koh, N., Abramovitz, R., & Gilbert, L. (1992). Bereavement groups for inner-city children. *Research on Social Work Practice, 2*, 405–419.

Schocket, I. & Dadds, M. (1997) Adolescent depression and the family: A paradox. *Clinical Child Psychology and Psychiatry, 2*, 307–312.

Schoeman, L. H., & Kreitzman, R. (1997). Death of a parent: Group intervention with bereaved children and their caregivers. *Psychoanalysis and Psychotherapy, 14*(2), 221–245.

Shaffer, D. (1988). The epidemiology of teen suicide: An examination of risk factors. *Journal of Clinical Psychiatry, 49*(Suppl. 9), 36–41.

Shaffer, D., & Finkelson, J. (Eds.). (2002). *Columbia treatment guidelines. Depressive disorders (version 2)*. New York: Columbia University, Department of Child and Adolescent Psychiatry.

Shaffer, D., Fisher, P., Dulcan, M. K., & Davies, M. (1996a). The NIMH Diagnostic Interview Schedule for Children version 2. 3 (DISC–2. 3): Description, acceptability, prevalence rates, and performance in the MECA study. Methods for the epidemiology of child and adolescent mental disorders study. *Journal of the American Academy of Child and Adolescent Psychiatry, 35*(7), 865–877.

Shaffer, D., Gould, M. S., Fisher, P., Trautman, P., Moreau, D., Kleinman, M., et al. (1996b). Psychiatric diagnosis in child and adolescent suicide. *Archives of General Psychiatry, 53*, 339–348.

Shaffer, D., & Greenberg, T. (2002). Suicide and suicidal behavior in children and adolescents. In D. Shaffer & B. D. Waslick (Eds), The many faces of depression in children and adolescents. *Review of Psychiatry, 21*(2), 129–178.

Simeon, J. G., Dinicola, V. F., Ferguson, B. H., & Copping, W. (1990). Adolescent depression: A placebo-controlled fluoxetine study and follow-up. *Progress in Neuro-Psychopharmacology and Biological Psychiatry, 14*, 791–795.

Sklar, F. & Hartley, S. F. (1990). Close friends as survivors: Bereavement patterns in a "hidden" population. *Omega—Journal of Death and Dying, 21*(2), 103–112.

Slesnick, N., & Waldron, H. B. (1997) Interpersonal problem-solving interactions of depressed adolescents and their parents. *Journal of Family Psychology, 11*, 234–245.

Sloane, R. B., Stapes, F. R., & Schneider, L. S. (1985). Interpersonal therapy versus nortriptyline for depression in the elderly. In G. D. Burrow, T. R. Norman, & L. Dennerstein (Eds.), *Clinical and pharmacological studies in psychiatric disorders* (pp. 344–346). London: Libbey.

Southard, M. J., & Gross, B. H. (1982). Making clinical decisions after Tarasoff. *New Directions for Mental Health Services, 16*, 93–101.

Stader, S., & Hokason, J. (1998). Psychosocial antecedents of depressive symptoms: An evaluation using daily experiences methodology. *Journal of Abnormal Psychology, 107,* 17–26.

Sullivan, H. S. (1953). *The interpersonal theory of psychiatry.* New York: Norton.

Swift, W. J., Andrews, D., & Barklage, N. E. (1986). The relationship between addiction disorder and eating disorder: A review of the literature. *American Journal of Psychiatry, 143*(3), 290–299.

Task Force on Promotion and Dissemination of Psychological Procedures. (1996). Training in and dissemination of empirically validated psychological treatments: Report and recommendations. *Clinical Psychologist, 8,* 3–24.

Velez, C., & Cohen, P. (1988). Suicidal behavior and ideation in a community sample of children: Maternal and youth reports. *Journal of the American Academy of Child and Adolescent Psychiatry, 27,* 349–356.

Vernberg, E. M. (1990). Psychological adjustment and experiences with peers during early adolescence: Reciprocal, incidental, or unidirectional relationships? *Journal of Abnormal Child Psychology, 18,* 187–198.

Wagner, K. D., Ambrosini, P., Rynn, M., Wohlberg, C., Yang, R., Greenbaum, M. S., et al. (2003). Efficacy of sertraline in the treatment of children and adolescents with major depressive disorder: Two randomized controlled trials. *Journal of the American Medical Association, 290,* 1033–1041.

Walker, M., Moreau, D., & Weissman, M. M. (1989). Parents' awareness of children's suicide attempts. *American Journal of Psychiatry, 147*(190), 1364–1366.

Warner, V., Weissman, M. M., Fendrich, M., Wickramaratne, P., & Moreau, D. (1992). The course of major depression in the offspring of depressed parents: Incidence, recurrence and recovery. *Archives of General Psychiatry, 49,* 795–801.

Waslick, B. D., Kandel, R., & Kakouros, A. (2002). Depression in children and adolescents. In D. Shaffer & B. D. Waslick (Eds.), *The many faces of depression in children and adolescents* (pp. 1–36). Washington, DC: American Psychiatric Publishing.

Weissman, M. M., Bland, R., Joyce, P. R., Newman, S., Wells, J. E., & Wittchen, H. U. (1993). Sex differences in rates of depression: Cross-national perspectives. *Journal of Affective Disorders, 29,* 77–84.

Weissman, M. M., Gammon, D., John, K., Merikangas, K. R., Warner, V., Prusoff, B. A., et al. (1987a). Children of depressed parents: Increased psychopathology and early onset of major depression. *Archives General Psychiatry, 44,* 847–853.

Weissman, M. M., Klerman, G. L., Paykel, E. S., Prusoff, B., & Hanson, B. (1974). Treatment effects on the social adjustment of depressed patients. *Archives of General Psychiatry, 30*(6), 771–778.

Weissman, M. M., Leckman, J. F., Merikangas, K. R., Gammon, D., & Prusoff, B. A. (1984a). Depression and anxiety disorders in parents and children. *Archives of General Psychiatry, 41,* 845–851.

Weissman, M. M., Markowitz, J. C., & Klerman G. L. (2000). *A comprehensive guide to interpersonal psychotherapy.* Albany, NY: Basic Books.

Weissman, M. M., Prusoff, B. A., DiMascio, A., Neu, C., Goklaney, M., & Klerman, G. L. (1979). The efficacy of drugs and psychotherapy in the treatment of acute depressive episodes. *American Journal of Psychiatry, 136, 555–558.*

Weissman, M. M., Prusoff, B. A., Gammon, G. D., Merikangas, K. R., Leckman, J. F., Kidd, K. K., et al. (1984b). Psychopathology in the children (ages 6–18) of depressed and normal parents. *Journal of the American Academy of Child and Adolescent Psychiatry, 23,* 78–84.

Weissman, M. M., Rounsaville, B. J., & Chevron, E. S. (1982). Training psychotherapists to participate in psychotherapy outcome studies: Identifying and dealing with the research requirement. *American Journal of Psychiatry, 139,* 1442–1446.

Weissman, M. M., Warner, V., Wickramaratne P., Moreau, D., & Olfson, M. (1997). Offspring of depressed parents: Ten years later. *Archives of General Psychiatry, 54*(10), 932–940.

Weissman, M. M., Warner, V., Wickramaratne, P., & Prusoff, B. A. (1988). Early onset major depression in parents and their children. *Journal Affective of Disorders, 15*(3), 269–278.

Weissman, M. M., Wickramaratne, P., Warner, V., John, K., Prusoff, B. A., Merikangas, K. R., et al. (1987b). Assessing psychiatric disorders in children: Discrepancies between mothers' and children's reports. *Archives of General Psychiatry, 44,* 747–753.

Weissman, M. M., Wolk, S., Goldstein, R. B., Moreau, D., Adams, P., Greenwald, S., et al. (1999a). Depressed adolescents grown up. *Journal of the American Medical Association, 281,* 1707–1713.

Weissman, M. M., Wolk, S., Wickramaratne, P., Goldstein, R. B., Adams, P., Greenwald, S., et al (1999b). Children with prepubertal onset major depressive disorder and anxiety grown up. *Archives of General Psychiatry, 56,* 794–801.

Weller, R., & Weller, E. (1991). Depression in recently bereaved prepubertal children. *American Journal of Psychiatry, 148,* 1535–1540.

Wilfley, D. E., MacKenzie, K. R., Welch, R. R., Ayres, V. E., & Weissman, M. M. (2000). *Interpersonal psychotherapy for group.* New York: Basic Books.

Williamson, D. E., Birmaher, B., Frank, E., Anderson, B. P., Matty, M. K., & Kupfer, D. J. (1998). Nature of life events and difficulties in depressed adolescents. *Journal of the American Academy of Child and Adolescent Psychiatry, 37*(10), 1049–1057.

Wu, P., Hoven, C., Bird, H., Cohen, P., Alegria, M., Dulcan, M., et al. (1999). Depressive and disruptive disorders and mental health service utilization in children and adolescents. *Journal of the American Academy of Child and Adolescent Psychiatry, 38,* 1081–1092.

Zajecka, J., Tracy, K. A., & Mitchell, S. (1997). Discontinuation symptoms after treatment with serotonin reuptake inhibitors: A literature review. *Journal of Clinical Psychiatry, 58*(7), 291–297.

Index

identifying patterns in, 172
IPT-A and, 20–21, 25–26
as a risk factor, 8
setting the treatment contract and, 65–66
Relevance of material presented by patient, 78–79
Renegotiation stage of disputes. *See also* Role disputes
and decision making, 133–135
description, 129
goals of treatment and, 129–130
parental involvement in treatment and, 138
Research
description, 250
on the effectiveness of IPT-A, 246–247
on the efficacy of IPT-A, 243–246
on group psychotherapy, 247–249
on interpersonal psychotherapy, 21–22, 24, 25
on IPT-A, 28
on the training of therapists, 249–250
on treatment options, 12
Resistance to treatment
compared to helplessness and hopelessness, 213–214
description, 208
Retardation, assessment of, 44
Risk factors, 8–9
Role disputes
case example of, 138–142, 262–272
description, 126–128
diagnosis of, 128–129
interpersonal functioning and, 65–66
running away and, 229
schedule of IPT-A and, 287
Role of the patient in treatment
description, 68–72
disruptions to treatment and, 207–212
during the middle phase of IPT-A, 74–75
Role of the therapist, 75
Role playing. *See also* Techniques
case example of, 269–272
description, 101–104
interpersonal deficits and, 171, 173–174
role transitions and, 161
Role transitions
in adolescence, 144–146
case example of, 162–164

description, 143–144, 161–162
diagnosis of, 146–147
educating patients and parents about, 149–152
reviewing old and new roles, 152–156
schedule of IPT-A and, 287–288
social skills and, 156–160
social support and, 160–161
treatment of, 147–149, 148*t*
Running away, 229–230. *See also* Crises

S

Sadness, 4–5. *See also* Symptoms
School difficulties
description, 5
refusal to attend, 221–222
School system, involving with treatment, 52–53
Selective serotonin reuptake inhibitors. *See also* Antidepressants; Pharmacotherapy
comorbidity and, 240–242
in conjunction with IPT-A, 235
the decision to treat with, 235–236
description, 17, 238
side effects of, 239–240
Self-report instruments. *See also* Assessment
description, 34
pharmacotherapy and, 236–237
Separation issues, assessment of, 43
Sertraline, 17. *See also* Pharmacotherapy
Session 1. *See also* Initial phase of IPT-A
confirming suitability for treatment, 47
description, 53
explaining treatment options, 48
giving the adolescent a limited "sick role," 48–50
introducing the principles of IPT-A, 50
obtaining a treatment commitment, 50–51
parental involvement in, 51–53
review of symptoms, 41, 42*t*, 43, 44–47
Session 2, 54–55. *See also* Initial phase of IPT-A; Interpersonal inventory
Sexual abuse, 224–225
Sexual assault, 230
Sexual behavior, 225–226
Sexual symptoms, 46. *See also* Symptoms
"Sick role," 48–50